African Americans and HIV/AIDS

Donna Hubbard McCree
Kenneth Terrill Jones · Ann O'Leary
Editors

African Americans and HIV/AIDS

Understanding and Addressing the Epidemic

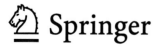 Springer

Editors

Donna Hubbard McCree, PhD, MPH, RPh
Division of HIV/AIDS Prevention
National Center for HIV
Viral Hepatitis, STD and TB Prevention
Centers for Disease Control and Prevention
1600 Clifton Road NE MS E-37
Atlanta, Georgia 30333
USA
zyr1@cdc.gov

Ann O'Leary, Ph.D.
Division of HIV/AIDS Prevention
Centers for Disease Control and Prevention
1600 Clifton Road, MS E-37
Atlanta, GA 30333
USA
aoleary@cdc.gov

Kenneth Terrill Jones, MSW
Division of HIV/AIDS Prevention
National Center for HIV
Viral Hepatitis, STD and TB Prevention
Centers for Disease Control and Prevention
1600 Clifton Road NE MS E-37
Atlanta, Georgia 30333
USA
kennethjones76@aol.com

ISBN 978-0-387-78320-8   e-ISBN 978-0-387-78321-5
DOI 10.1007/978-0-387-78321-5
Springer New York Dordrecht Heidelberg London

Library of Congress Control Number: 2010935484

Printed on acid-free paper

Springer is part of Springer Science+Business Media (www.springer.com)

Preface

Among U.S. racial and ethnic minority populations, African American communities are the most disproportionately impacted and affected by HIV/AIDS (CDC, 2009; CDC, 2008). The chapters in this volume seek to explore factors that contribute to this disparity as well as methods for intervening and positively impacting the epidemic in the U.S. The book is divided into two sections. The first section includes chapters that explore specific contextual and structural factors related to HIV/AIDS transmission and prevention in African Americans. The second section is composed of chapters that address the latest in intervention strategies, including best-evidence and promising-evidence based behavioral interventions, program evaluation, cost effectiveness analyses and HIV testing and counseling. As background for the book, the Introduction provides a summary of the context and importance of other infectious disease rates, (i.e., sexually transmitted diseases [STDs] and tuberculosis), to HIV/AIDS prevention and treatment in African Americans and a brief introductory discussion on the major contextual factors related to the acquisition and transmission of STDs/HIV.

Contextual Chapters

Johnson & Dean author the first chapter in this section, which discusses the history and epidemiology of HIV/AIDS among African Americans. Specifically, this chapter provides a definition for and description of the US surveillance systems used to track HIV/AIDS and presents data on HIV or AIDS cases diagnosed between 2002 and 2006 and reported to CDC as of June 30, 2007. The chapter also includes a discussion of the epidemiology of HIV/AIDS and describes how these data reflect different populations. The chapters that follow address HIV/AIDS among African Americans in the context of poverty and racism, organized religion, disparities in incarceration rates, trauma, substance use, mental health issues, violence, and a history of childhood sexual abuse.

Williams and Prather describe how experiences with racism and poverty and the interactions between racism and poverty affect sexual behavior and consequently HIV/AIDS transmission and acquisition among African Americans. They offer recommendations for measures of racism and poverty and methods for including these constructs in behavioral interventions. Eke, Willis and Gaither follow with a discussion of the "black church" and the influential role that this institution has on African American communities. They provide a summary of the church's historical activities in health promotion and disease prevention efforts associated with chronic diseases (e.g., diabetes, hypertension), and barriers to a role for the church in HIV/AIDS prevention activities.

Spikes, Willis and Koenig explored the available literature to identify potential links between exposure to traumatic events and HIV risk, mental health disorders and HIV risk, and utilization of mental health services for the general population and African Americans. Their chapter provides a discussion of these links and the implications of this research to HIV/AIDS prevention efforts among African Americans. El-Bassel, Gilbert, Witte, Wu and Vinocur describe the interpersonal contexts that link experiencing intimate partner violence and engaging in HIV/STI transmission risks among African American, drug-involved women and provide evidence supporting the need for strategies preventing HIV and sexually transmitted infections (STIs) for African American women that address individual, interpersonal, community, macro and structural risk factors. Finally, in the concluding chapter for this section, Sumner, Wyatt, Glover, Carmona, Loeb, Henderson, et al., focus on aspects of childhood sexual abuse that influence high-risk behaviors and discuss the importance and challenges of implementing community interventions that integrate HIV-risk reduction and child sexual abuse.

Intervention Chapters

The chapters in this section discuss evidence-based interventions developed for subgroups within the African American community. Marshall, O'Leary and Crepaz conducted a systematic review of evidence-based interventions (EBIs) for African American youth at risk for HIV; 11 EBIs were identified. Their chapter describes the process for identifying and evaluating the interventions, and discusses what was addressed in the EBIs, what research gaps exist, and research recommendations derived from the review. Henny, Williams and Patterson follow with a critical review of HIV behavioral prevention interventions for heterosexually active African American men (EBIs and other interventions) and the extent to which these interventions include elements of cultural competency. Further, the chapter includes a discussion of definitions and measures of cultural competency and identifies gaps and future directions regarding the use of cultural competency in HIV behavioral prevention intervention activities with these men. Wingood follows with a discussion of HIV prevention for heterosexually active African American women that describes correlates of HIV risk, how the Theory of Gender and Power may be used to understand women's HIV risk, and concludes with a critical review of the available literature on prevention interventions for this population. Jones, Wilton, Millett, and Johnson then provide a complimentary chapter on MSM that describes currently available interventions and describes a model to explain how racial social-ization and other culturally appropriate strategies might reduce the HIV risk of black MSM.

The next three chapters examine structural interventions, behavioral interven-tions for injection drug users (IDU), and interventions in correctional settings. Purcell, Mizuno and Lyles discuss the contribution of injection drug use to the HIV epidemic among African Americans and the interventions designed to reduce HIV transmission among IDUs, and specifically African American IDUs. Sanders and Ellen examine structural factors that may facilitate transmission of HIV and discuss the available literature on structural interventions that have been associated with decreasing HIV transmission risk. Finally, Seal, MacGowan, Eldridge, Charania, and Margolis provide a summary of the available literature on HIV prevention interventions for correctional populations in the United States and discuss gaps in the literature and needs for future intervention in this populations. This volume concludes with a final closing chapter by the co-editors that provides recommenda-tions for future HIV/AIDS prevention strategies among African Americans.

It is our intent that this book contribute to a greater understanding of HIV among African Americans and other emerging risk populations in the US and globally. As such, one goal of *African Americans and HIV/AIDS* is to provide practitioners, health workers, researchers, academics, students, and activists with an additional prevention tool to combat HIV. As evidenced by the book as a whole and individual chapters, much work has already occurred in halting the devastating spread of HIV in African American communities. However, also demonstrated in these chapters is the work that is yet to be completed. Only through collaborative efforts between community members, families, practitioners, activists, health officials, and research-ers will we have a positive impact on the HIV/AIDS epidemic among African Americans.

References

CDC. (2009) Fighting HIV Among African Americans. Atlanta, GA: US Department of Health and Human Services. http://www.cdc.gov/.
CDC. (2008) HIV/AIDS Surveillance Report, 2007, volume 19. Atlanta, GA: CDC.

About the Editors

Donna Hubbard McCree, PhD, MPH, RPh is Team Leader/Behavioral Scientist, Intervention Research Team, Prevention Research Branch, Division of HIV/AIDS Prevention, National Center for HIV, Viral Hepatitis, STD and TB Prevention (NCHSTP), Centers for Disease Control and Prevention (CDC) in Atlanta, Georgia. Dr. McCree has over 27 years of experience in Public Health and Pharmacy. She completed the Doctor of Philosophy *with Honors* (1997) and Master of Public Health (1987) degrees at The Johns Hopkins University School of Public Health, Baltimore, Maryland in Health Policy and Management with a specialty in Social and Behavioral Sciences. She also completed a postdoctoral fellowship through the former Association of Teachers of Preventive Medicine (ATPM) with a specialty in Sexually Transmitted Disease (STD) prevention. Additionally, she holds a Bachelor of Science degree, *summa cum laude*, in Pharmacy from Howard University (1982) and is a registered pharmacist in the states of Maryland and Connecticut, and the District of Columbia. She has held numerous positions in the fields of Public Health and Pharmacy including academia, bioavailability research, professional association management, and retail and hospital pharmacy practice. She was on the faculty of the former College of Pharmacy at Howard University for over 7 years where she served as Acting Chair of the Department of Pharmacy Administration. Her training and expertise are in developing and conducting STD/HIV behavioral interventions. Her work has resulted in over 80 peer-reviewed publications and presentations at both international and national scientific meetings. Additionally, she is the recipient of numerous awards and was recently awarded the 2009 Minority Health Mentor/ Champion of Excellence Award from the Division of HIV/AIDS Prevention for outstanding commitment and achievement as a mentor for the ORISE Community of Color Postdoctoral Research Fellowship.

Kenneth Terrill Jones, MSW, is a behavioral scientist with the Centers for Disease Control and Prevention's (CDC) Division of HIV/AIDS Prevention (DHAP). He has served as the project coordinator of the Social Networks Demonstration Project and the technical lead for d-up: Defend Yourself! (d-up!) – a culturally adapted evidence- and network-based intervention for young men who have sex with men (MSM). Also, he has served as the project officer for a randomized controlled trial of a community-level intervention adapted for young Black MSM. Most recently, he lead an initiative to package intervention and training materials for d-up!, which is being disseminated nationwide to community-based organizations (CBOs) and health departments through the CDC's Diffusion of Evidence-Based Interventions (DEBI) initiative. He has served on several planning committees and workgroups at the CDC, including the Workgroup to address HIV/AIDS and STDs among African Americans and the DHAP Executive Committee on HIV/AIDS among MSMs. Prior to joining the CDC, Jones served as the Director of Research for the Policy Institute of the National Gay and Lesbian Task Force, where he also participated in two liaison panels with the Institute of Medicine. He also coauthored and edited several research and policy reports including Say It Loud: I'm Black and I'm Proud, one of the largest multicity studies of Black lesbian, gay, bisexual, and transgender (LGBT) men and women attending Black Gay Pride celebrations in the United States, and Leaving Our Children Behind: Welfare Reform and the Gay, Lesbian, Bisexual, and Transgender Community, which examines the impact of 1996 legislation on a segment of Americans largely excluded from the debate. He has served as a research and curriculum consultant with various AIDS service organizations including Gay Men of African Descent and People of Color in Crisis. He is a founding member of the Black Gay Research Group, a multidisciplinary team of Black gay researchers brought together to address the dearth of research on Black MSM, and the former board president of In the Life Atlanta, a nonprofit community-based organization whose mission is to increase positive visibility of LGBT individuals of African Descent. Jones received a Bachelor of Arts degree in Sociology from the University of Michigana and a Masters of Science in Social Work degree from Columbia University in the City of New York. He has recently returned back to Columbia University where he is receiving doctoral training in social work and serving as a Predoctoral Research Fellow at the Social Intervention Group, a multidisciplinary intervention development and prevention organization at the Columbia University School of Social Work. Jones's recent manuscripts have appeared in the American Journal of Public Health, AIDS & Behavior, and Sexually Transmitted Diseases.

Ann O'Leary, PhD is a Senior Behavioral Scientist in the Division of HIV/AIDS Prevention, Centers for Disease Control and Prevention. Her training included a *summa cum laude* undergraduate degree from the University of Pennsylvania; a Ph.D. in Psychology from Stanford University, supported by a National Science Foundation fellowship; and 1 year of postdoctoral training in Health Psychology at the University of California at San Francisco. She served on the faculty of the Psychology Department at Rutgers University from 1986 to 1999. She has conducted research on HIV prevention for the past 27 years, and has also published many articles on other aspects of Health Psychology. Dr. O'Leary has published more than 150 scientific articles and chapters, and has edited or coedited three books, *Women at Risk: Issues in the Prevention of AIDS, Women and AIDS: Coping and Care, Beyond Condoms: Alternative Approaches to HIV Prevention, and From Child Sexual Abuse to Adult Sexual Risk: Trauma, Revictimization and Intervention.* She is a Fellow of the American Psychological Association and won the inaugural "Distinguished Leader" award from the APA's Committee on Psychology and AIDS. She serves on the editorial boards of several scientific journals, and is a frequent consultant to NIH and other scientific organizations.

Contents

Contributors

Jennifer Vargas Carmona
Associate Research Psychologist, UCLA Psychiatry & Biobehavioral Sciences, 760 Westwood Plaza, C9-539 Semel Institute, UCLA BOX 951759, Los Angeles CA, 90095-1759, USA

Mahnaz R. Charania
Behavioral Scientist, Research Synthesis & Translation Team - PRS Project, Prevention Research Branch, Division of HIV/AIDS Prevention, National Center for HIV, Viral Hepatitis, STD and TB Prevention, Centers for Disease Control and Prevention, 1600 Clifton Road NE, Mailstop E-37 Atlanta GA, 30333, USA

Dorothy Chin
Associate Research Psychologist, UCLA, Department of Psychiatry & Biobehavioral Sciences, 760 Westwood Plaza, C8-668 Semel Institute, BOX 951759, Los Angeles CA, 90095-1759, USA

Nicole Crepaz
Senior Behavioral Scientist, Centers for Disease Control and Prevention, 1600 Clifton Road, MS E-27 Atlanta GA, 30333, USA

Hazel D. Dean
Deputy Director, National Center for HIV/AIDS, Viral Hepatitis, STD, and TB Prevention, Centers for Disease Control and Prevention, 1600 Clifton Road Mailstop E-07 Atlanta GA, 30333, USA

Agatha N. Eke
Behavioral Scientist, Prevention Research Branch, Division of HIV Prevention National Centre for HIV/STD/TB Prevention, Centres for Disease Control and Prevention, 1600 Clifton Road NE Atlanta, GA 30333, USA

Nabila El-Bassel
Professor, Columbia University School of Social Work;
Director, Social Intervention Group (SIG);
Director, Global Health Research Center of Central Asia (GHRCCA)
Columbia University, Columbia University School of Social Work,
1255 Amsterdam Ave, Office 814 New York NY, 10027, USA

Gloria D. Eldridge
Associate Professor, Department of Psychology and Center
for Behavioral Health Research and Services, University of Alaska Anchorage,
3211 Providence Drive Anchorage AK, 99508, USA

Jonathan M. Ellen
Professor and Vice Chair, Department of Pediatrics,
Johns Hopkins School of Medicine; Director, Department of Pediatrics,
Johns Hopkins Bayview Medical center, Mason F. Lord, Center Tower,
5200 Eastern Ave, Ste 4200 Baltimore MD, 21224, USA

Juarlyn L. Gaiter
Senior Behavioral Scientist, Division of HIV/AIDS Prevention,
Centers for Disease Control and Prevention, 1600 Clifton Road,
N.E. M.S. E-37 Atlanta GA, 30333, USA

Louisa Gilbert
Associate Research Scientist, School of Social Work,
1255 Amsterdam Avenue Room 818 Mail Code 4600, New York NY, 10027, USA

Dorie (Dorothy) A. Glover
Assistant Professor in Residence, Child Division, Department of Psychiatry,
Semel Institute of Neuroscience and Human Behavior UCLA,
1118 N. Beverly Glen Blvd Los Angeles CA, 90077, USA

Tina B. Henderson
Visiting Scholar, UCLA Institute of American Cultures,
Murphy Hall 4067 Abourne Road, Unit D Los Angeles CA, 90008, USA

Kirk D. Henny
Behavioral Scientist Division of HIV/AIDS Prevention,
National Center for HIV/AIDS, Viral Hepatitis, STD and TB Prevention,
Centers for Disease Control and Prevention, 1600 Clifton Road NE, MS E-37
Atlanta GA, 30333, USA

Matthew Hogben
Division of STD Prevention, National Center for HIV,
Viral Hepatitis, STD and TB Prevention, Centers for Disease Control
and Prevention, Mail Stop E-44 Atlanta GA, 30333, USA

Anna Satcher Johnson
Epidemiologist, HIV Incidence and Case Surveillance Branch, Division
of HIV/AIDS Prevention, National Center for HIV/AIDS, Viral Hepatitis,
STD, and TB Prevention, Centers for Disease Control and Prevention,
1600 Clifton Rd NE MS E-47 Atlanta GA, 30333, USA

Wayne D. Johnson
Health Scientist, Division of HIV/AIDS Prevention, CDC,
Mailstop E-37 1600 Clifton Road NE Atlanta GA, 30333, USA

Kenneth Terrill Jones
Behavioral Scientist, Prevention Research Branch,
Division of HIV/AIDS Prevention, National Center for HIV, Viral Hepatitis,
STD and TB Prevention, Centers for Disease Control and Prevention,
1600 Clifton Road NE MS E-37 Atlanta GA, 30333, USA

Linda J. Koenig
Senior Scientist, Prevention Research Branch, Division of HIV/AIDS Prevention,
Centers for Disease Control and Prevention, 1600 Clifton Road,
Mailstop E37 Atlanta GA, 30333, USA

Tamra Burns Loeb
Associate Research Psychologist, Department of Psychiatry and
Biobehavioral Sciences, UCLA Semel Institute,
4458 Nogales Drive Tarzana CA, 91356, USA

Cindy Lyles
Mathematical Statistician, Prevention Research Branch,
Division of HIV/AIDS Prevention, Center for HIV, STD, and
TB Prevention, Centers for Disease Control and Prevention,
1600 Clifton Road, MS E-37 Atlanta GA, 30333, USA

LCDR Robin MacGowan
Expert Research Officer, US Public Health Service;
Deputy Team Leader, Interventions Research Team,
Prevention Research Branch, Division of HIV/AIDS Prevention,
National Center for HIV, Viral Hepatitis, STD and TB Prevention,
Centers for Disease Control & Prevention, 1600 Clifton Rd.,
MS E-37 Atlanta GA, 30333, USA

LCDR Andrew Margolis
Senior Research Officer, US Public Health Service,
Interventions Research Team, Prevention Research Branch,
Division of HIV/AIDS Prevention, National Center for HIV,
Viral Hepatitis, STD and TB Prevention, Centers for Disease Control
& Prevention, 1600 Clifton Rd., MS E-37 Atlanta GA, 30333, USA

Khiya J. Marshall
Division of HIV/AIDS Prevention, Centers for Disease Control and Prevention,
Atlanta, GA 30333, USA

Donna Hubbard McCree
Team Leader, Interventions Research Team,
Prevention Research Branch, Division of HIV/AIDS Prevention,
National Center for HIV, Viral Hepatitis, STD and TB Prevention,
Centers for Disease Control and Prevention, 1600 Clifton Road NE MS E-37
Atlanta GA, 30333, USA

Yuko Mizuno
Behavioral Scientist, Centers for Disease Control and Prevention,
1600 Clifton Road NE, MS-E37 Atlanta GA, 30033, USA

Ann O'Leary
Senior Biomedical Research Service, Prevention Research Branch,
Division of HIV/AIDS Prevention, Centers for Disease Control and Prevention,
1600 Clifton Road, MS E-37 Atlanta GA, 30333, USA

Jocelyn D. Patterson
Division of HIV/AIDS Prevention, National Center for HIV, Viral Hepatitis,
STD and TB Prevention, Centers for Disease Control and Prevention,
1600 Clifton Rd, NE Mail stop E-37 Atlanta GA, 30333, USA

Cynthia Prather
Commander, USPHS CDC/NCHHSTP/DHAP-IRS/PRB,
1600 Clifton Road, MS E-37 Atlanta GA, 30333, USA

David W. Purcell
Chief, Prevention Research Branch,
CDC/NCHHSTP/DHAP, 1600 Clifton Road, MS E-37 Atlanta GA, 30333, USA

Rotrease S. Regan
Doctoral Candidate, Department of Community Health Sciences,
UCLA School of Public Health, 3767 Mentone Avenue Apt. #208
Los Angeles CA, 90034, USA

Renata Arrington Sanders
Assistant Professor,
Division of General Pediatrics & Adolescent Medicine
Johns Hopkins School of Medicine,
200 North Wolfe Street, Room 2063 Baltimore, Maryland, 21287, USA

David Wyatt Seal
Qualitative Methods Core Director,
Departments of Psychiatry & Behavioral Medicine//Population Health,
Center for AIDS Intervention Research, Medical College of Wisconsin,
2071 N. Summit Avenue Milwaukee WI, 53202, USA

Pilgrim S. Spikes
Behavioral Scientist, Centers for Disease Control - NCHHSTP,
1600 Clifton Road - MS E-37 Atlanta GA, 30333, USA

Lekeisha A. Sumner
Clinical Psychologist, Assistant Research Psychologist
Department of Psychiatry & Biobehavioral Sciences, Center for Culture,
Trauma and Mental Health Disparities, UCLA,
3750 Jasmine Ave. #204 Los Angeles CA, 90034, USA

Danielle Vinocur
Supervising Psychologist, Women's Health Project,
Long Island University, Brooklyn Campus New York NY, USA

Aisha L. Wilkes
Behavioral Scientist, Prevention Research Branch/
DHAP/NCHHSTP, Centers for Disease Control and Prevention,
1600 Clifton Road, NE Mailstop E-37 Atlanta GA, 30333, USA

Kim M. Williams
Behavioral Scientist, Prevention Research Branch,
Division of HIV/AIDS, Prevention National Center for HIV, STD,
and TB Prevention, Centers for Disease Control and Prevention,
1600 Clifton Road, NE MS E-37 Atlanta GA, 30333, USA

Leigh A. Willis
Behavioral Scientist, Epidemiology Branch,
Division of HIV/AIDS Prevention,
Minority HIV/AIDS Research Initiative (MARI),
1600 Clifton Rd MS E-45 Atlanta GA, 30329, USA

Leo Wilton
CCPA Human Development, PO Box 6000,
Binghamton NY, 13902-6000, USA

Gina M. Wingood
Professor, Rollins School of Public Health,
Agnes Moore Faculty in HIV/AIDS Research, Emory University,
4279 Roswell Rd., Suite 102-256 Atlanta GA, 30342, USA

Susan Witte
Associate Professor, 1255 Amsterdam Ave Room 813
Mail Code: 4600, New York NY, 10027, USA

Elwin Wu
1255 Amsterdam Ave Room 830 Mail Code: 4600,
New York NY, 10027, USA

Gail E. Wyatt
Professor, Department of Psychiatry & Biobehavioral Sciences;
Director, UCLA Sexual Health Program; Director, Center for Culture,
Trauma and Mental Health Disparities; Associate Director, UCLA AIDS Institute;
Director, UCLA HIV/AIDS Translational Training Program (HATT);
Clinical Psychologist, UCLA Semel Institute for Neuroscience and Human
Behavior, BOX 951759 760 Westwood Plaza, C8-871C Semel Institute
Los Angeles CA, 90095-1759, USA

Part I
Introduction

Chapter 1
The Contribution to and Context of Other Sexually Transmitted Diseases and Tuberculosis in the HIV/AIDS Epidemic Among African Americans*

Donna Hubbard McCree and Matthew Hogben

Significant health disparities in chronic diseases, (e.g., cancer, cardiovascular diseases, hypertension, and diabetes) (CDC, January, 2005; Farmer & Ferraro, 2005; Gehlert et al., 2008; Glover, Greenlund, Ayala CDC, Croft, 2005; LaVeist, Bowie, & Cooley-Quille, 2000; Sudano & Baker, 2006; Williams, 1997) and infectious diseases like Human Immunodeficiency Virus (HIV)/Acquired Immunodeficiency Syndrome (AIDS) (Aral, Adimora, & Fenton, 2008; CDC Sexually Transmitted Diseases Surveillance report, 2008, 2009; CDC, 2008 HIV/AIDS Surveillance report, 2007), exist among ethnic minorities in the United States (US). Among US racial and ethnic minority populations, African American communities are the most disproportionately impacted. Further, rates of sexually transmitted diseases (STDs) like Chlamydia, gonorrhea and HIV in African American communities are the highest in the nation (CDC, 2007). Causes for these disparities are interrelated and fundamentally due to contextual and structural factors like higher poverty rates, lack of access to adequate health care, higher incarceration rates, lower income and educational attainment, and racism (Adimora et al., 2006; Aral et al.; Chu & Selwyn, 2008; Gehlert et al.; LaVeist et al., 2007). Therefore, interventions to address health disparities that exist between African Americans and Caucasians should be integrated and address the contextual and structural environment in which African Americans exist.

As background for the book, this Introduction provides a summary of other important infectious disease rates, i.e., STDs and tuberculosis (TB), and their contribution and importance to HIV/AIDS prevention and treatment in African Americans and a brief introductory discussion on the major contextual factors related to the acquisition and transmission of STDs/HIV.

D.H. McCree(✉)
Division of HIV/AIDS Prevention, Centers for Disease Control and Prevention,
1600 Clifton Road NE, MS E-37, Atlanta, GA 30333, USA
e-mail: zyr1@cdc.gov

D.H. McCree et al. (eds.), *African Americans and HIV/AIDS*,   3
DOI 10.1007/978-0-387-78321-5_1,

Importance of Co-infections with Other STDs and TB to HIV Rates Among African Americans in the US

The Centers for Disease Control and Prevention (CDC) estimates that about 19 million new STDs occur annually in the United States with the greatest burden of diagnosis among 15–24 year olds (Weinstock, Berman, & Cates, 2004), women and African Americans (CDC, January, 2009). Rates of Chlamydia, gonorrhea, and syphilis are higher among African Americans than any racial/ethnic group. More than 1.1 million cases of Chlamydia, a bacterial infection and the most commonly reported STD in the United States, were diagnosed in 2007 (CDC, March, 2009a, 2009b). Of these cases approximately 48% were diagnosed in African Americans, translating into a rate eight times as high as the rate among Caucasians (CDC, January, 2009; CDC, March, 2009a, 2009b). Additionally, of the approximately 356,000 cases of gonorrhea reported in 2007, about 70% of the cases were in African Americans (CDC, January, 2009; CDC, March, 2009a, 2009b). This trans-lates into a gonorrhea rate among African Americans that is 19 times the rate in Caucasians. Further, between 2005–2006 (CDC, November, 2007) and 2006–2007 (CDC, January, 2009), the rate of gonorrhea in African Americans increased by 6.3 and 1.8% respectively, while rates among all other US racial and ethnic groups declined (CDC, January, 2009).

While the racial gap in syphilis rates has narrowed since 1999, significant racial disparities still exist for African Americans. Approximately 11,466 cases of syphilis were reported in 2007 (CDC, January, 2009). The syphilis rate among African Americans (2.0 per 100,000 population) was seven times that among Caucasians and rates of primary and secondary syphilis (P&S syphilis) – the most infectious form of the disease – in African Americans increased for the fourth consecutive year (CDC, January, 2009). This increase was 16.5% between 2005 and 2006 (CDC, November, 2007) and 25% between 2006 and 2007 (CDC, January, 2009). Additionally, significant gender differences in syphilis diagnosis exits within the community. The largest increase, 28.2%, among African Americans was found in males, and mainly among men who have sex with men (MSM); rates of P&S among females increased 14.3% (CDC, January, 2009).

The disparities in STD diagnoses for African Americans are important because there is evidence that the presence of STDs like Chlamydia, gonorrhea and syphi-lis can increase the risk of HIV acquisition (Cohen, 2004; Weinstock et al., 2004) and transmission (Gavin & Cohen, 2004; Reynolds, Risbud, Shepherd et al., 2003; CDC, 1998). The available literature suggests that co-transmission of HIV and other STDs may be a common occurrence (Cohen, 2004) and that biological mechanisms, (e.g., impaired integrity of the genital mucosa creating an environ-ment more conducive to transmission) (Cohen, 2004; Gavin, & Cohen, 2004) and immunologic mechanisms, (e.g., immune activation) (Reynolds, Risbue, Shepherd, Zenilman, Brookmeyer, Paranjape, et al, 2003) are possible explanations for the increased risk for HIV transmission in persons infected with STDs.

Also of importance to HIV/AIDS disparities among African Americans are other infections that interact with an HIV infection. There are data linking tuberculosis (TB) to increase susceptibility to and worsening prognosis of an HIV infection (Bentwich, 2003; Fleming & Wasserheit, 1999; Hotz, Molyneux, Stillwaggon, Bentwich, & Kumaresan, 2006). The CDC estimates that 9–14 million Americans are infected with the TB bacterium, and, in 2005, approximately 16% of the TB cases among persons 25–44 years old were in those infected with HIV (CDC, January, 2008). Further, 63% of the TB patients reported in 2005 were African Americans (CDC, 2007). Given these data, identifying and treating co-infections, i.e., STDs and TB, among African Americans may be important methods for prevention and reduction of health disparities.

The Context of Behavioral Risk

A meaningful discussion of STD or HIV acquisition risk among African Americans requires examination of behaviors and context. In some geographic areas and among some African Americans, prevalence is sufficiently high that behaviors that confer minimal risk for others confer substantial risk among African Americans. For example, a syphilis outbreak in Rockdale County, Georgia almost a decade ago revealed an extensive network of concurrent sexual partnerships among predominantly white suburban adolescents (Rothenberg et al., 1998). Until a case of syphilis was introduced into the network, the putatively high-risk sexual behaviors among this group conferred no known STD acquisition risk (syphilis certainly spread quickly once the initial case entered the network). Had this network existed in a setting with the prevalence of nearby Fulton County, the *same* behaviors would have produced much faster spread of any STD. Given the racial demographics – Fulton County has a higher proportion of African Americans than does Rockdale – the example illustrates the important role of the context in which behaviors occur.

That noted, behaviors do matter, as do the psychosocial antecedents to behavior. There are numerous data linking psychological constructs, social networks and other contextual variables with risky sexual behaviors, and even data showing correspondence between variables in each of these categories and STD rates. (e.g., Locke & Newcomb, 2008; Paz-Bailey et al., 2005) These general data are relevant to STD and HIV among African Americans as they are relevant to any other sociodemographic partition of the US population. However, some data are relevant in particular ways to African Americans because (a) racial disparities in STD prevalence show some behaviors connote greater risk for African Americans than for most other Americans (e.g., Hallfors, Iritani, Miller, & Bauer, 2007) and (b) the prevalence of some risk factors or markers may actually be greater among African American populations.

We have categorized risk factors and markers into three broad levels: psychosocial antecedents, proximate social factors (e.g., peer networks), and broader context (e.g., health care availability). The levels are not cleanly delineated, mostly because they often interact with one another to produce multiplicative or even exponential effects upon the individual. Finally, each of the levels matters. To illustrate, if community prevalence were 0, the number of partners is irrelevant to disease acquisition; if community prevalence were 100% (and for ease of calculation, transmission probability were also 100%), any number of partners greater than 1 is irrelevant. But at any other level of prevalence, the odds of acquisition vary with number of partners; therefore both prevalence and number of partners interact to produce the odds of acquisition. Hallfors et al. (2007) is instructive: the authors provided an approximate continuum of risk behaviors ranging from categories such as "few partners, low alcohol and other drug use" to "marijuana and other drug use," together with the prevalence of STD by white and black race. Blacks with few partners and low drug use had a STD prevalence of 20.3% (3.2% for whites with the same behaviors); blacks engaging in marijuana and other drug use had a prevalence of 28.8% (7.5% for whites). The markedly different prevalences for the same behaviors across race indicate the greater risk blacks encounter, compared to whites, for each level of risk and illustrate the role of context.

Psychosocial constructs. Hallfors et al. (2007) also demonstrate that behaviors matter: the increasing prevalences in the previous paragraph within race across behaviors represent the effect of behavior. As influences upon, and explanations of, behaviors, psychosocial constructs also matter. Conceptual clarity about causality is often difficult because many psychosocial variables are both outcomes and antecedents to risky sexual behavior (i.e., the behaviors and psychosocial variables have recursive relationships). For example, a positive STD diagnosis may reduce self-esteem, especially if the STD is viral, ergo incurable, or if the STD is particularly associated with stigmatized behavior. A longitudinal analysis conducted in a cohort of HIV-infected African American women revealed an association between experience of intimate partner violence at one time point and subsequent incident STI, with depression as a mediating factor (Hogben et al., 2001). This particular analysis is also an example of how the levels proposed in the preceding paragraph combine: an experiential factor (violence) and a psychosocial measurement (depression) are both present to predict STD incidence.

Self-esteem and depression are frequently linked to risky sexual behavior as antecedents, with the putative mediating mechanisms ranging from poor negotiation skills associated with both conditions to lack of a belief in one's worth (e.g., Locke & Newcomb, 2008). Reduced self-esteem and increased depression do not arise from a vacuum. Depression may well have a substantial genetic component, although none of this research points to differences in pre-disposing genetic complements as a function of racial status. Negative life experiences are more clearly associated with depression and self-esteem, and negative life experiences are examples of social context. Childhood sexual abuse has often been shown to predict sexual risk, both directly and through the advent of survival sex among those who are fleeing abuse (e.g., van Roode, Dickson, Herbison, & Paul, 2009). When negative life experiences contain large racial disparities, they can produce disparities in psychosocial constructs like depression and contribute to the behavioral outcomes. A much larger proportion of African Americans are or have been incarcerated than whites. When that experience reduces a sense of control over one's life or when one is deprived of exercising control, risky behavior may increase, preserving the disparity generated through incarceration.

Behavioral self-efficacy is frequently associated with risk behaviors, generally through the prism of avoiding potential disease, "I could refuse to have sex," or the prism of harm reduction, "I could insist my partner wears a condom before we have sex." The association is often not reliable as typically measured, because self-reported broad self-efficacy is often high enough to compress variance and create a ceiling effect. If self-efficacy is measured with qualifiers, "I could insist my partner wears a condom … if I had not been drinking alcohol," responses tend to vary more widely across the response scale. In one study (Hogben, Lawrence, Hennessy, & Eldridge, 2003), incarcerated women averaged 35.4 (SD = 6.2) on a 40-point composite scale for being able to tell their partners to use a condom. With the qualification "…if I was high" added, efficacy dropped significantly, $p < 0.001$.

Better news is that many of these variables are amenable to remediation; social cognitive interventions that have focused upon such remediation have even shown efficacy in STD reduction, including among African American samples (e.g., Jemmott, Jemmott, Braverman, & Fong, 2005; Kamb et al., 1998; Shain et al., 2004). Most recently, Jemmott, Jemmott, and O'Leary (2007) conducted a trial of brief, skills-building interventions (one-on-one versus small-group by skills-building versus information plus a control group): skills-building groups reported fewer STD at 12-month follow-up visits than did control (15% versus 27%, $p < 0.05$). In setting the tone of the interventions, the authors emphasized a culturally sensitive, communal modality – "Sister To Sister! Respect Yourself! Protect Yourself! Because You Are Worth It!" The emphatic tone, assertion of worth, and peer to peer approach remove the sense of being lectured to and build mutual support for skills building (which in turn improves self-efficacy). Wingood, DiClemente and colleagues have produced a "suite" of interventions relying upon social cognitive changes to affect behaviors and STD rates (Wingood & DiClemente, 2006). Although the interventions within this suite (SISTA: DiClemente & Wingood, 1995; SiHLE: DiClemente et al., 2004; WiLLOW: Wingood et al., 2004) are principally aimed at HIV risk reduction, participants in SiHLE and WiLLOW intervention groups both showed statistically significant reductions in STD infection. Of psychosocial mediators, the interventions resulted in greater sexual self-control and assertiveness and reduced partner barriers to condom use.

Another class of psychosocial factors and markers pertains to health care seeking. Patient attitudes about sexuality in health care settings are correlated with the likelihood of STD-relevant discussions, like sexual histories, occurring. In one sample of 313 adolescents (81% African American, ages 11–21 years, mostly 15 and older), the likelihood of discussion of sexual behavior and STD prevention were both correlated with how comfortable the patients felt talking to a doctor and by whether the patient believed the topic was appropriate for a doctor to discuss with them (Merzel et al., 2004). If discomfort and community prevalence are high enough, disparities are likely to be preserved (even if the discomfort alone exists in other, lower-prevalence communities).

Social factors. A supportive peer network can reduce the risk of STD acquisition or transmission, as shown in the series of interventions described by Wingood and Diclemente (2006, and see above). However, networks can also increase the risk of disease, for example, with violent partners. Experience of intimate partner violence (IPV) is correlated with sexual behavior, most obviously when IPV takes the form of rape or other coercive sexual behavior. As noted previously, Hogben et al. (2001) found an association between IPV and incident STD acquisition among a sample of predominantly African American, HIV-infected women. Also among HIV-infected women, a more recent paper found no relationship between gender-based violence and sexually transmitted disease acquisition, but did find that experience of gender-based violence was associated with inconsistent condom use and abuse resulting from efforts to negotiate use (Lang, Salazar, Wingood, Diclemente, & Mikhail, 2007). In both studies, IPV was restricted to relatively recent experience (6 months in Hogben et al., 6–7% prevalence; 3 months in Lang et al., 10% prevalence).

A disrupted sexual network can also lead to elevated sexual risk, and African American women may be at more risk of network disruption. Using National Survey of Family Growth data and controlling for age and race, Liddon, Leichliter, and Aral (2007) reported divorced women were more than twice as likely than never-married women to have had multiple partners in the past year. While the risk conditional upon divorce may or may not differ by race, African American women (20%) were slightly more likely to be divorced than white or Hispanic women (both 16%), $p < 0.001$, and were therefore at higher risk, all else being equal.

Hurricane Katrina brought population-level social and economic dislocation to a majority African American city in 2002. Demonstrating the confluence between levels again, Cieslak et al. (2009) found social support was associated with coping self-efficacy among HIV-infected Katrina victims. As social support was disrupted, efficacy diminished.

Contextual factors. An increasing body of work, including in this volume, identifies racism and segregation as principal contextual factors in STD/HIV risk, as well as other negative health outcomes (Hogben & Leichliter, 2008; Krieger, 1999, 2003). St. Louis, Farley, and Aral (1996) identified racism as a key underlying factor in STD rates in the South almost 15 years ago. Krieger (2008) describes an ecosocial model that includes context and behavior; interestingly, she proposed moving away from the concept of proximal and distal measures, that is, the frequent classification of social determinants and similar contextual factors as distal and "upstream" against "proximate" behaviors, by level as predictors of health outcomes. This precept that is somewhat reflected here in the interactions among the levels we outline.

Health care of appropriate quality to prevent disease and stem transmission of infection is a factor immediately related to STDs among African Americans. Reduced provision of and access to appropriate services are one source of disparities (Parrish & Kent, 2008). In Merzel et al. (2004), the authors reported only 19% of the sample had been tested for chlamydial infection or gonorrhea, in spite of the fact that, not only are these STDs more common among adolescents and young adults than any other age groups, the study site was selected on the basis of high rates of gonorrhea. If we construe the adolescent–parent relationship as part of the context of sexuality, sexual behavior and sexual health care for adolescents, a second point from these data becomes relevant. The odds of the patient and doctor discussing sexual behavior and STD prevention also depended on whether the patient's parent knew the visit was taking place. In particular, patients whose parents knew about the health care visit were less than half as likely to discuss sexual behavior or STD prevention than those whose parents did not know (54% versus 25% and 61% versus 25%, respectively, both $p < 0.01$).

Returning to the Katrina-based research noted in the previous section, the subsequent influx of construction workers with high reported levels of sexual risk behaviors (Kissinger et al., 2008) illustrated a change in the overall social context that could facilitate STD or HIV acquisition and transmission among New Orleans residents staying or returning to the city. Another study tracking women (mostly African American) displaced by Katrina found disruptions in general health care access, employment, and pregnancy prevention services (Kissinger, Schmidt, Sanders, & Liddon, 2007). The same women reported elevated rates of reproductive tract discomfort and more than one sex partner in the previous few months. This last point ties a negative contextual factor squarely to behavioral risk.

Because of the contributions of co-infections with other STDs and TB and specific contextual and structural factors (as introduced in this chapter) to the acquisition, transmission, and/or worsening prognosis of an HIV infection, identifying and addressing these issues may be the best method for preventing HIV/AIDS among African Americans.

Summary of Chapters in this Volume

This volume is divided into two sections that focus on the history and context of HIV/AIDS in African Americans and interventions targeting specific subpopulations. The first part of the volume is composed of the context chapters that focus on specific contextual and structural issues related to HIV/AIDS transmission and prevention in African Americans. Johnson and Dean provide a background for this exploration in the opening chapter for this section. Their chapter discusses the history and the statistics of HIV/AIDS among African Americans. The chapters that follow address the role of racial disparities in incarceration, Gaither and O'Leary; contribution of substance use and mental health Spikes, Willis and Koenig; violence and substance use, El-Bassel et al.; and childhood sexual abuse, Wyatt and Summers, to HIV acquisition and transmission. Further, other context chapters discuss how poverty and racism (Williams & Prather), and organized religion (Eke and Gaither), affect HIV/AIDS rates among African Americans.

The second section of this volume is composed of the intervention chapters. These chapters summarize the available published literature on prevention interventions for adolescents, Marshall, O'Leary, and Crepaz; heterosexually active men, Henny, and women, Wingood; MSM, Jones, Wilton, Johnson and Millett; and intravenous drugs users, Purcell, Mizuno, and Lyles. This section concludes with a chapter authored by Arrington Sanders and Ellen on structural interventions for HIV/AIDS prevention with an emphasis on poverty and racism. Finally, the volume concludes with a discussion of future directions for HIV/AIDS prevention authored by the co-editors, O'Leary, Jones and McCree.

References

Adimora, A. A., Schoenbach, V. J., Martinson, F. E., Martinson, F. E., Coyne-Beasley, T., Doherty, I., et al. (2006). Heterosexually transmitted HIV infection among African Americans in North Carolina. *Journal of Acquired Immune Deficiency Syndromes, 41*, 616–623.

Aral, S. O., Adimora, A. A., & Fenton, K. A. (2008). Understanding and responding to disparities in HIV and other sexually transmitted infections in African Americans. *Lancet, 372*, 337–340.

Bentwich, Z. (2003). Concurrent infections that rise the HIV viral load. *Journal of HIV Therapy, 8*(3), 72–75.

CDC. (2007). Extensively drug-resistant tuberculosis – United States 1993–2005. *Morbidity and Mortality Weekly Report. Recommendations and Reports, 56*, 250–253.

CDC. (2009). *Fighting HIV among African Americans*. Atlanta, GA: US Department of Health and Human Services. http://www.cdc.gov/.

CDC. (January 2005). Health disparities experienced by Black or African Americans – United States. *Morbidity and Mortality Weekly Report. Recommendations and Reports*, 54(1):1–3.

CDC. (1998). HIIV prevention through early detection and treatment of other sexually transmitted diseases – United States recommendations of the Advisory Committee for HIV and STD Prevention. *Morbidity and Mortality Weekly Report. Recommendations and Reports, 47*(RR-12), 1–24.

CDC. (2008). HIV/AIDS Surveillance report, 2007, Volume 19. Atlanta, GA: CDC.

CDC. (March 2009a). *Most widely reported, curable STDs remain significant health threat*. Atlanta, GA: US Department of Health and Human Services. http://www.cdc.gov/std/.

CDC. (2008). *Sexually transmitted disease surveillance, 2007*. Atlanta, GA: US Department of Health and Human Services. http://www.cdc.gov/std/.

CDC. (January 2008). *TB and HIV/AIDS*. Atlanta, GA: US Department of Health and Human Services. http://www.cdc.gov/tb/.

CDC. (January 2009). *Trends in reportable sexually transmitted diseases in the United States, 2007. National surveillance data for Chlamydia, gonorrhea, and syphilis*. Atlanta, GA: US Department of Health and Human Services. http://www.cdc.gov/std/.

CDC. (November 2007). *Trends in reportable sexually transmitted diseases in the United States, 2006. National surveillance data for Chlamydia, gonorrhea, and syphilis*. Atlanta, GA: US Department of Health and Human Services. http://www.cdc.gov/std/.

CDC. (March 2009b). *Trends in tuberculosis – United States, 2008*. Atlanta, GA: US Department of Health and Human Services. http://www.cdc.gov/tb/.

Chu, C., & Selwyn, P. A. (2008). Current health disparities in HIV/AIDS. *The AIDS Reader, 18*(3), 144–146. 152–158.

Cieslak, R., Benight, C., Schmidt, N., Luszczynska, A., Curtin, E., Clark, R. A., et al. (2009). Predicting posttraumatic growth among hurricane Katrina survivors living with HIV: the role of self-efficacy, social support, and PTSD symptoms. *Anxiety, Stress, and Coping, 22*(4), 449–463.

Cohen, M. (2004). Perspective HIV and sexually transmitted diseases: lethal synergy. *Topics in HIV Medicine, 12*(4), 104–107.

DiClemente, R., & Wingood, G. (1995). A randomized controlled trial of an HIV sexual risk-reduction intervention for young African-American women. *Journal of the American Medical Association, 274*, 1271–1276.

DiClemente, R. J., Wingood, G. M., Harrington, K. F., Lang, D. L., Davies, S. L., Hook, E. W., III, et al. (2004). Efficacy of an HIV prevention intervention for African American adolescent girls: a randomized controlled trial. *Journal of the American Medical Association, 292,* 171–179.

Farmer, M. M., & Ferraro, K. F. (2005). Are racial disparities in health conditional on socioeconomic status? *Social Science & Medicine, 60,* 191–204.

Fleming, D. T., & Wasserheit, J. N. (1999). From epidemiological synergy to public health policy and practice: the contribution of other sexually transmitted diseases to sexual transmission of HIV infection. *Sexually Transmitted Infections, 75,* 3–17.

Gavin, S. R., & Cohen, M. S. (2004). The role of sexually transmitted diseases in HIV transmission. *Nature Reviews. Microbiology, 2,* 33–34.

Gehlert, S., Sohmer, D., Sacks, T., Mininger, C., McClintock, M., & Olopade, O. (2008). Targeting health disparities: a model linking upstream determinants to downstream intervention. *Health Affairs, 27*(2), 339–349.

Glover, M., Greenlund, K. J., Ayala, C., CDC, Croft, J. B. (2005). Racial/ethnic disparities in prevalence, treatment, and control of hypertension – United States, 1999–2002. *Morbidity and Mortality Weekly Report. Recommendations and Reports, 54,* 7–9.

Hallfors, D. D., Iritani, B. J., Miller, W. C., & Bauer, D. J. (2007). Sexual and drug behavior patterns and HIV and STD racial disparities: the need for new directions. *American Journal of Public Health, 97,* 125–132.

Hogben, M., Gange, S. J., Watts, D. H., Robison, E., Young, M., Richardson, J., et al. (2001). The effect of sexual and physical violence on risky sexual behavior and STD among a cohort of HIV-seropositive women. *AIDS and Behavior, 5,* 353–361.

Hogben, M., St. Lawrence, J. S., Hennessy, M. H., & Eldridge, G. D. (2003). Using the theory of planned behavior to understand STD risk behaviors of incarcerated women. *Criminal Justice and Behavior, 30,* 187–209.

Hogben, M., & Leichliter, J. S. (2008). Social determinants and sexually transmitted disease disparities. *Sexually Transmitted Diseases, 35*(12 Suppl.), S13–S18.

Hotz, P., Molyneux, D., Stillwaggon, E., Bentwich, Z., & Kumaresan, J. (2006). Neglected tropical diseases and HIV/AIDS. *Lancet, 368*(9550), 1865–1866.

Jemmott, J. B., III, Jemmott, L. S., Braverman, P. K., & Fong, G. T. (2005). HIV/STD risk reduction interventions for African American and Latino adolescent girls at an adolescent medicine clinic: a randomized controlled trial. *Archives of Pediatrics & Adolescent Medicine, 159,* 440–449.

Jemmott, L. S., Jemmott, J. B., III, & O'Leary, A. (2007). Effects on sexual risk behavior and STD rate of brief HIV/STD prevention interventions for African American women in primary care settings. *American Journal of Public Health, 97,* 1034–1040.

Kamb, M. L., Fishbein, M., Douglas, J. M., Jr., Rhodes, F., Rogers, J., Bolan, G., et al. (1998). Efficacy of risk-reduction counseling to prevent human immunodeficiency virus and sexually transmitted diseases: a randomized controlled trial. Project RESPECT Study Group. *Journal of the American Medical Association, 280,* 1161–1167.

Kissinger, P., Liddon, N., Schmidt, N., Curtin, E., Salinas, O., & Narvaez, A. (2008). HIV/STI Risk behaviors among Latino migrant workers in New Orleans post-Hurricane Katrina disaster. *Sexually Transmitted Diseases, 35,* 924–929.

Kissinger, P., Schmidt, N., Sanders, C., & Liddon, N. (2007). The effect of the hurricane Katrina disaster on sexual behavior and access to reproductive care for young women in New Orleans. *Sexually Transmitted Diseases, 34,* 883–886.

Krieger, N. (1999). Embodying inequality: a review of concepts, measures, and methods for studying health consequences of discrimination. *International Journal of Health Services, 29,* 295–352.

Krieger, N. (2003). Does racism harm health? Did child abuse exist before 1962? On explicit questions, critical science, and current controversies: an ecosocial perspective. *American Journal of Public Health, 93,* 194–199.

Krieger, N. (2008). Proximal, distal, and the politics of causation: what's level got to do with it? *American Journal of Public Health, 98,* 221–230.

Lang, D. L., Salazar, L. F., Wingood, G. M., Diclemente, R. J., & Mikhail, I. (2007). Associations between recent gender-based violence and pregnancy, sexually transmitted infections, condom use practices, and negotiation of sexual practices among HIV-positive women. *Journal of Acquired Immune Deficiency Syndromes, 46*, 216–221.

LaVeist, T. A., Bowie, J. V., & Cooley-Quille, M. (2000). Minority health status in adulthood: the middle years of life. *Health Care Financing Review, 21*(4), 9–21.

LaVeist, T., Thorpe, R., Bowen-Reid, T., Jackson, J., Gary, T., Gaskin, D., et al. (2007). Exploring health disparities in integrated communities: overview of the EHDIC study. *Journal of Urban Health: Bulletin of the New York Academy of Medicine, 85*(1), 11–32.

Liddon, N., Leichliter, J. S., Aral, S. O. (2007). *Divorce and sexual risk among US women: Findings from the National Survey of Family Growth.* Presented at the 17th International Society for STD Research, Seattle, WA.

Locke, T. F., & Newcomb, M. D. (2008). Correlates and predictors of HIV risk among inner-city African American female teenagers. *Health Psychology, 27*, 337–348.

St. Louis, M. E., Farley, T. A., & Aral, S. O. (1996). Untangling the persistence of syphilis in the South. *Sexually Transmitted Diseases, 23*, 1–4.

Merzel, C. R., Vandevanter, N. L., Middlestadt, S., Bleakley, A., Ledsky, R., & Messeri, P. A. (2004). Attitudinal and contextual factors associated with discussion of sexual issues during adolescent health visits. *The Journal of Adolescent Health, 35*, 108–115.

Parrish, D. D., & Kent, C. K. (2008). Access to care issues for African American communities: implications for STD disparities. *Sexually Transmitted Diseases, 35*(12 Suppl.), S19–S22.

Paz-Bailey, G., Koumans, E. H., Sternberg, M., Pierce, A., Papp, J., Unger, E. R., et al. (2005). The effect of correct and consistent condom use on chlamydial and gonococcal infection among urban adolescents. *Archives of Pediatrics & Adolescent Medicine, 159*, 536–542.

Reynolds, S. J., Risbud, A. R., Shepherd, M., Zenilman, J. M., Brookmeyer, R. J., Paranjape, R. S., Divekar, A. D., Gangakhedkar, R. R., Ghate, M. V., Bollinger, R. C., Mehendale, S. M. (2003). Recent herpes simplex virus type 2 infection and the risk of human immunodeficiency virus type 1 acquisition in India. *The Journal of Infectious Diseases, 187*, 1513–1521.

Rothenberg, R. B., Sterk, C., Toomey, K. E., Potterat, J. J., Johnson, D., Schrader, M., et al. (1998). Using social network and ethnographic tools to evaluate syphilis transmission. *Sexually Transmitted Diseases, 25*, 154–160.

Shain, R. N., Piper, J. M., Holden, A. E., Champion, J. D., Perdue, S. T., Korte, J. E., et al. (2004). Prevention of gonorrhea and Chlamydia through behavioral intervention: results of a two-year controlled randomized trial in minority women. *Sexually Transmitted Diseases, 31*, 401–408.

Sudano, J. J., & Baker, D. W. (2006). Explaining US racial/ethnic disparities in health declines and mortality in late middle age: the roles of socioeconomic status, health behaviors, and health insurance. *Social Science & Medicine, 62*, 909–922.

van Roode, T., Dickson, N., Herbison, P., & Paul, C. (2009). Child sexual abuse and persistence of risky sexual behaviors and negative sexual outcomes over adulthood: findings from a birth cohort. *Child Abuse & Neglect, 33*(3), 161–172.

Weinstock, H., Berman, S., & Cates, W. (2004). Sexually transmitted diseases among American youth: incidence and prevalence estimates, 2000. *Perspectives on Sexual and Reproductive Health, 36*(1), 6–10.

Williams, D. R. (1997). Race and health: basic questions, emerging directions. *Annals of Epidemiology, 7*(5), 322–333.

Wingood, G. M., & DiClemente, R. J. (2006). Enhancing adoption of evidence-based HIV interventions: promotion of a suite of HIV prevention interventions for African American women. *AIDS Education and Prevention, 18*(4 Suppl. A), 161–170.

Wingood, G. M., DiClemente, R. J., Mikhail, I., Lang, D. L., McCree, D. H., Davies, S. L., et al. (2004). A randomized controlled trial to reduce HIV transmission risk behaviors and sexually transmitted diseases among women living with HIV: The WiLLOW Program. *Journal of Acquired Immune Deficiency Syndromes, 37*(Suppl. 2), S58–S67.

Part II
Context Chapters

Chapter 2
Epidemiology and Surveillance of HIV Infection and AIDS Among Non-Hispanic Blacks in the United States

Anna Satcher Johnson, Xiangming Wei, Xiaohong Hu, and Hazel D. Dean

Surveillance of HIV Infection and AIDS

In June 1981, the first five cases of AIDS were recognized in the United States, and the Centers for Disease Control and Prevention (CDC) began tracking reported cases (Centers for Disease Control and Prevention, 1981). By June 1982, more than 400 AIDS cases had been reported to CDC, with 19% of these cases occurring among non-Hispanic blacks (Centers for Disease Control and Prevention, 1982). By 1996 and continuing through today, more cases have been diagnosed among blacks each year than among any other racial or ethnic population (Centers for Disease Control and Prevention, 1996). In 2006, blacks accounted for 13% of the population of the United States, yet they accounted for 49% (17,960) of new AIDS diagnoses that year (Centers for Disease Control and Prevention, 2008a; U.S. Census Bureau, 2006).

HIV/AIDS is considered a health crisis for blacks. This chapter reviews the epidemiology and surveillance of HIV infection and AIDS among blacks in the United States and describes the current state of the epidemic.

Public health surveillance is defined as "the ongoing, systematic collection, analysis, interpretation, and dissemination of outcome-specific data for use in the planning, implementation, and evaluation of public health programs."(Thacker, 2001) By that definition, CDC provides the only national population-based monitoring of the HIV epidemic in the United States – the HIV/AIDS Reporting System (HARS). Laboratories, physicians, hospitals, and other health care providers are required to report cases of HIV infection and AIDS confidentially to designated local and state health departments. Confidential case reports may include diagnostic information, risk factors for HIV exposure, demographic information, and other variables relevant to monitor the scope of the epidemic.

A.S. Johnson (✉)

Division of HIV/AIDS Prevention, National Center for HIV/AIDS, Viral Hepatitis, STD, and TB Prevention, Office of Infectious Diseases, Centers for Disease Control and Prevention, Mail Stop E-47, 1600 Clifton Road, Atlanta, GA 30333, USA e-mails: ATS5@cdc.gov; ASatcherJohnson@cdc.gov

D.H. McCree et al. (eds.), *African Americans and HIV/AIDS*,
DOI 10.1007/978-0-387-78321-5_2, © Springer Science+Business Media, LLC 2010

Since 1985, all 50 states, the District of Columbia (D.C.), and five U.S. dependent areas (American Samoa, Guam, the Northern Mariana Islands, Puerto Rico, and the U.S. Virgin Islands) have required the reporting of AIDS cases to state or local health departments. Using HARS software, state and local health departments transmit case report data to CDC without patient names or other personally identifying information. CDC analyzes, interprets, and disseminates these data nationally to help public officials plan for and evaluate prevention and care programs. During the early years of AIDS surveillance, case data alone provided an adequate picture of HIV trends. Today, with the advent of highly active antiretroviral therapy (HAART), the overall progression of HIV infection to AIDS and from AIDS to death has slowed (Palella et al., 1998). Consequently, AIDS surveillance data no longer serve as a reliable surrogate for monitoring HIV infection, although they do provide important information about where care and treatment resources are most needed.

New HIV diagnoses are better indicators of current trends in HIV transmission because they bring us closer to the front end of the disease spectrum. Since HIV antibody tests became available in 1985 (Centers for Disease Control and Prevention, 1984; Gallo, Salahuddin, & Popovic, 1984), states have implemented HIV infection reporting at different times and with different types of reporting (e.g., code-based, name-to-code). However, by April 2008, confidential reporting of cases of HIV infection by name was legally mandated in all 50 states, the District of Columbia, and five U.S. dependent areas.

This chapter presents data on HIV or AIDS cases diagnosed during 2002–2006 and reported to CDC as of June 30, 2007. The epidemiology of HIV/AIDS will be provided apart from the epidemiology of AIDS because the data reflect different populations. The term "HIV/AIDS" refers collectively to three categories of diagnoses: (1) a diagnosis of HIV infection (not AIDS), (2) a diagnosis of HIV infection with subsequent AIDS diagnosis, and (3) concurrent diagnoses of HIV infection and AIDS.

To ensure consistent data, this chapter presents only HIV/AIDS data from the 33 states that have had confidential, name-based HIV infection surveillance since at least 2001. These 33 states are Alabama, Alaska, Arizona, Arkansas, Colorado, Florida, Idaho, Indiana, Iowa, Kansas, Louisiana, Michigan, Minnesota, Mississippi, Missouri, Nebraska, Nevada, New Jersey, New Mexico, New York, North Carolina, North Dakota, Ohio, Oklahoma, South Carolina, South Dakota, Tennessee, Texas, Utah, Virginia, West Virginia, Wisconsin, and Wyoming. This chapter will also present data on persons in whom AIDS was diagnosed, as well as deaths among persons with AIDS, which includes deaths unrelated to AIDS. Data for AIDS cases and deaths were reported from all 50 states and the District of Columbia.

The data used here are estimates derived from cases of HIV infection, AIDS, and deaths reported to CDC, with some statistical adjustments made for reporting delays and redistribution of cases with missing risk factor information (Centers for Disease Control and Prevention, 2008a; Green, 1998). Statistical adjustments were not made for "diagnosed, but unreported cases" or for "cases yet to be diagnosed." Cases were classified according to "transmission" category, which is the term used to identify the risk factor most likely to have resulted in transmission of HIV infection. The following is a list of definitions of transmission categories:

- Male-to-male sexual contact (i.e., among men who have sex with men (MSM)).
- Injection-drug use (IDU).
- Both MSM and IDU (MSM/IDU).
- High-risk heterosexual contact (i.e., with a person of the opposite sex known to be HIV infected or at high risk for HIV infection (e.g., MSM or injection-drug user)).
- "Other" (e.g., hemophilia, blood transfusion, unidentified risk factors).

In addition, estimated numbers of HIV/AIDS and AIDS diagnoses were calculated for each racial and ethnic population by transmission category and other selected characteristics for the years 2002–2006. Estimated diagnosis and prevalence (i.e., persons living with HIV/AIDS) rates per 100,000 population for persons diagnosed with HIV/AIDS and for persons diagnosed with AIDS also were calculated for each racial and ethnic population. Rate calculations do not include cases among persons whose race was not reported, or who are of multiple races. Persons identified as white, black or African American, Asian/Pacific Islander, American Indian/Alaska Native, or other/unknown race are not Hispanic or Latino. Persons of Hispanic/Latino origin may be of any race.

HIV/AIDS in Blacks

The HIV/AIDS epidemic has evolved from primarily affecting white people to primarily affecting black people. When compared with other races and ethnicities in the United States today, the latest surveillance data consistently demonstrate that blacks are disproportionately affected by HIV/AIDS at all stages – from infection with HIV to death with AIDS. Of the estimated 173,956 adults and adolescents age 13 years and older diagnosed with HIV/AIDS in the 33 states with name-based HIV reporting during 2002–2006, nearly half (49.9%) were black. In comparison, whites age 13 years and older accounted for 29.9% of all HIV/AIDS diagnoses among adults and adolescents made during those years, while Hispanics/Latinos accounted for 18.1%, Asians/Pacific Islanders for 1%, and American Indians/Alaska Natives accounted for less than 1%. The distribution of transmission categories among adults and adolescents, by race/ethnicity and sex, is shown in Table 2.1.

During 2002–2006, among all adults and adolescents, blacks accounted for the largest percentages of HIV/AIDS diagnoses in the high-risk heterosexual (67.6%) and IDU transmission categories (54.9%). Of HIV/AIDS diagnoses among blacks, most were attributed to high-risk heterosexual contact (45.7%) and male-to-male sexual contact (34.2%). Blacks also accounted for the largest percentage of HIV/AIDS diagnoses in all age groups. Most (60.3%) HIV/AIDS diagnoses were among adults aged 25–44 years regardless of race or ethnicity, with blacks accounting for 46.6%. Racial disparities in HIV diagnoses were particularly severe among young

Table 2.1 Estimated number and percentage of HIV/AIDS[a] diagnoses among adults and adolescents, by race/ethnicity and selected characteristics – 33 states with confidential name-based HIV infection reporting, 2002–2006[b]

Characteristics	White, not Hispanic No.	(%)	Black, not Hispanic No.	(%)	Hispanic/Latino No.	(%)	Asian/Pacific Islander No.	(%)	American Indian/Alaska Native No.	(%)	Unknown/multiple races No.	(%)	Total[c] No.	(%)
All	51,944	29.9	86,747	49.9	31,498	18.1	1,723	1.0	874	0.5	1,170	0.7	173,956	100
Male														
Age group at diagnosis (years)														
13–24	3,412	22.5	8,571	56.5	2,851	18.8	133	0.9	74	0.5	125	0.8	15,167	100
25–34	11,009	33.3	13,017	39.4	8,136	24.6	494	1.5	189	0.6	205	0.6	33,050	100
35–44	17,325	39.3	17,365	39.4	8,422	19.1	474	1.1	213	0.5	255	0.6	44,053	100
45–54	8,759	36.6	11,173	46.6	3,588	15.0	185	0.8	104	0.4	146	0.6	23,957	100
55–64	2,716	36.3	3,525	47.1	1,130	15.1	41	0.5	30	0.4	49	0.7	7,492	100
≥65	679	31.0	1,049	47.9	426	19.5	12	0.5	5	0.2	17	0.8	2,188	100
Transmission category														
Male-to-male sexual contact (MSM)	34,472	42.3	29,685	36.4	15,554	19.1	919	1.1	397	0.5	470	0.6	81,496	100
Injection drug use (IDU)	3,630	22.0	8,805	53.4	3,703	22.5	134	0.8	88	0.5	133	0.8	16,494	100
MSM with IDU	2,764	42.4	2,434	37.4	1,159	17.8	50	0.8	53	0.8	53	0.8	6,513	100
High-risk heterosexual contact[d]	2,831	13.6	13,509	64.9	4,028	19.4	227	1.1	77	0.4	136	0.7	20,808	100
Other[e]	204	34.2	267	44.9	110	18.4	8	1.4	2	0.3	4	0.7	595	100
Total	43,901	34.9	54,701	43.4	24,554	19.5	1,338	1.1	616	0.5	798	0.6	125,906	100

Female

Age group at diagnosis (years)

	No.	%	No.	%	No.	%	No.	%	No.	%	No.	%	Total	%
13–24	1,196	15.9	5,153	68.3	1,032	13.7	44	0.6	43	0.6	71	0.9	7,541	100
25–34	2,074	15.7	8,876	67.3	1,899	14.4	158	1.2	76	0.6	102	0.8	13,184	100
35–44	2,601	17.6	9,726	65.9	2,146	14.5	89	0.6	81	0.5	110	0.7	14,752	100
45–54	1,583	17.7	5,912	66.0	1,300	14.5	57	0.6	43	0.5	60	0.7	8,954	100
55–64	479	17.2	1,807	65.0	428	15.4	28	1.0	14	0.5	23	0.8	2,780	100
≥65	112	13.3	571	68.1	139	16.6	9	1.1	1	0.1	7	0.8	839	100

Transmission category

	No.	%	No.	%	No.	%	No.	%	No.	%	No.	%	Total	%
Injection drug use	2,396	25.1	5,493	57.5	1,451	15.2	62	0.6	72	0.8	76	0.8	9,551	100
High-risk heterosexual contact[d]	5,558	14.7	26,170	69.0	5,401	14.2	316	0.8	181	0.5	293	0.8	37,919	100
Other[e]	89	15.4	384	66.1	92	15.8	7	1.3	6	1.0	3	0.5	581	100
Total[c]	8,044	16.7	32,046	66.7	6,945	14.5	385	0.8	258	0.5	372	0.8	48,050	100

[a] Includes persons diagnosed with HIV infection with or without AIDS

[b] Data as of June 2007, adjusted for reporting delays and risk factor redistribution

[c] Because subpopulation values were calculated independently, the values may not sum to the row or column total

[d] Heterosexual contact with a person known to be HIV infected or at high risk for HIV infection

[e] Other risk factors (e.g., hemophilia, blood transfusion) and all risk factors not reported or not identified

people. Overall, blacks accounted for half (49.9%) of all HIV/AIDS diagnoses during 2002–2006; however, among youth aged 13–24 years, blacks accounted for 60.4% (Table 2.1).

For each year, the HIV/AIDS diagnosis rates for black adults and adolescents in this study were consistently higher than the rates for adults and adolescents of other racial and ethnic groups. For example, in 2006, the estimated HIV/AIDS diagnosis rate was 85.6 per 100,000 in the black population. This rate was nearly nine times as high as the rate for whites (9.6 per 100,000) and more than twice as high as the rate for Hispanics/Latinos (33.7 per 100,000).

During 2002–2006, the overall estimated prevalence of HIV/AIDS was higher among blacks than among adults and adolescents of other race or ethnic groups. At the end of 2006, an estimated 485,081 adults and adolescents were living with HIV/AIDS in the 33 states, and of those, 47.4% (229,957) were black. The prevalence rate for blacks living with HIV/AIDS was 1,140.0 per 100,000. This rate was more than seven times as high as the HIV/AIDS prevalence rate among whites (148.7 per 100,000) and more than twice as high as the prevalence rate among Hispanics/Latinos (438.9 per 100,000).

AIDS in Blacks

Although the annual number of AIDS diagnoses among blacks has decreased in the past few years, disparities among racial groups persist (Centers for Disease Control and Prevention, 2006). Of the estimated 187,456 adults and adolescents with diagnosed AIDS in the 50 states and D.C. during 2002–2006, 49.9% were black. Whites accounted for 29.2% of AIDS diagnoses, Hispanics/Latinos for 18.3%, Asians/Pacific Islanders for 1.2%, and American Indians/Alaska Natives for less than 1% (Table 2.2).

The distribution of transmission categories by race/ethnicity and sex among adults and adolescents with diagnosed AIDS is shown in Table 2.2. During 2002–2006, blacks accounted for the largest percentage of AIDS diagnoses attributed to high-risk heterosexual contact and IDU (Table 2.2). Among blacks, most AIDS diagnoses were attributed to high-risk heterosexual contact (41.2%) or male-to-male sexual contact (30.1%).

Blacks also accounted for the largest percentage of AIDS diagnoses regardless of age at diagnosis. The highest proportions of adults with diagnosed AIDS were in the following age groups: 35–44 and 45–54 years, regardless of race or ethnicity. In these age groups, blacks accounted for 47.2 and 51.6%, respectively, of AIDS diagnoses. Racial disparities in AIDS diagnoses were particularly severe among young people. Overall, blacks accounted for half of all AIDS diagnoses during 2002–2006; among youth aged 13–24 years, blacks accounted for 60.9% of diagnoses. By region, blacks accounted for the largest percentage of AIDS diagnoses in every region (South, 62.0%; Northeast, 48.1%; and Midwest, 50.2%) except the West (18.4%).

Table 2.2 Estimated number and percentage of AIDS diagnoses among adults and adolescents, by race/ethnicity and selected characteristics – 50 states and the District of Columbia, 2002–2006[a]

Characteristics	White, not Hispanic No.	(%)	Black, not Hispanic No.	(%)	Hispanic/Latino No.	(%)	Asian/Pacific Islander No.	(%)	American Indian/Alaska Native No.	(%)	Unknown/ multiple races No.	(%)	Total[b] No.	(%)
All	54,811	29.2	93,492	49.9	34,265	18.3	2,283	1.2	858	0.5	1,748	0.9	187,456	100
Male														
Age group at diagnosis (years)														
13–24	1,101	16.6	3,765	56.7	1,612	24.3	81	1.2	28	0.4	56	0.8	6,643	100
25–34	8,275	28.6	12,010	41.5	7,753	26.8	527	1.8	158	0.5	246	0.9	28,969	100
35–44	20,589	37.4	22,617	41.1	10,365	18.8	768	1.4	267	0.5	485	0.9	55,092	100
45–54	12,080	35.8	15,756	46.7	5,074	15.0	345	1.0	141	0.4	316	0.9	33,712	100
55–64	3,663	35.9	4,858	47.5	1,470	14.4	104	1.0	31	0.3	91	0.9	10,217	100
≥65	912	32.3	1,323	46.9	530	18.8	31	1.1	9	0.3	16	0.6	2,820	100
Transmission category														
Male-to-male sexual contact (MSM)	33,674	42.3	28,155	35.4	15,491	19.5	1,257	1.6	359	0.5	617	0.8	79,553	100
Injection drug use (IDU)	5,216	21.2	13,568	55.2	5,231	21.3	188	0.8	110	0.4	276	1.1	24,590	100
MSM with IDU	4,014	41.1	3,813	39.1	1,623	16.6	102	1.0	96	1.0	114	1.2	9,762	100
High-risk heterosexual contact[c]	3,351	15.0	14,259	63.7	4,229	18.9	284	1.3	65	0.3	201	0.9	22,389	100
Other[d]	366	31.5	533	45.9	229	19.7	24	2.1	4	0.3	5	0.4	1,160	100
Region														
Northeast	9,290	28.1	14,293	43.2	8,460	25.6	415	1.3	50	0.2	577	1.7	33,085	100
Midwest	6,751	41.6	7,319	45.1	1,785	11.0	160	1.0	78	0.5	126	0.8	16,220	100
South	17,731	28.9	34,485	56.1	8,420	13.7	290	0.5	161	0.3	367	0.6	61,455	100
West	12,849	48.1	4,232	15.9	8,137	30.5	991	3.7	344	1.3	141	0.5	26,694	100
Total	46,621	33.9	60,329	43.9	26,803	19.5	1,856	1.4	634	0.5	1,212	0.9	137,454	100

(continued)

Table 2.2 (continued)

Characteristics	White, not Hispanic No.	(%)	Black, not Hispanic No.	(%)	Hispanic/Latino No.	(%)	Asian/Pacific Islander No.	(%)	American Indian/Alaska Native No.	(%)	Unknown/ multiple races No.	(%)	Total[b] No.	(%)
Female														
Age group at diagnosis (years)														
13–24	409	12.0	2,352	69.2	544	16.0	28	0.8	17	0.5	50	1.5	3,399	100
25–34	1,827	14.8	8,379	67.9	1,810	14.7	131	1.1	55	0.4	137	1.1	12,339	100
35–44	3,198	17.3	12,111	65.5	2,782	15.0	124	0.7	81	0.4	207	1.1	18,503	100
45–54	2,058	18.0	7,542	65.8	1,602	14.0	93	0.8	55	0.5	107	0.9	11,456	100
55–64	568	17.1	2,123	63.8	546	16.4	43	1.3	15	0.4	32	1.0	3,327	100
≥65	130	13.3	656	67.0	178	18.3	9	0.9	2	0.2	3	0.3	978	100
Transmission category														
Injection drug use	2,985	22.1	8,207	60.7	2,007	14.9	68	0.5	92	0.7	154	1.1	13,514	100
High-risk heterosexual contact[c]	5,041	14.2	24,280	68.5	5,263	14.9	338	1.0	126	0.4	374	1.1	35,422	100
Other[d]	164	15.4	675	63.4	192	18.0	20	1.9	6	0.6	8	0.8	1,066	100
Region														
Northeast	2,263	14.5	9,119	58.6	3,745	24.1	106	0.7	24	0.2	307	2.0	15,563	100
Midwest	1,017	21.6	3,198	67.9	406	8.6	43	0.9	23	0.5	26	0.6	4,712	100
South	3,660	14.4	19,379	76.2	2,057	8.1	108	0.4	59	0.2	178	0.7	25,440	100
West	1,251	29.2	1,467	34.2	1,254	29.3	170	4.0	119	2.8	26	0.6	4,286	100
Total[b]	8,190	16.4	33,163	66.3	7,462	14.9	427	0.9	224	0.4	536	1.1	50,002	100

[a]Data as of June 2007, adjusted for reporting delays and risk factor redistribution
[b]Because subpopulation values were calculated independently, the values may not sum to the row or column total
[c]Heterosexual contact with a person known to be HIV infected or at high risk for HIV infection
[d]Other risk factors (e.g., hemophilia, blood transfusion) and all risk factors not reported or not identified

Each year, during 2002–2006, the annual AIDS diagnosis rates among black adults and adolescents in the 50 states and D.C. were consistently higher than the rates for other racial and ethnic groups. In 2006, blacks in the 50 states and D.C. received a diagnosis of AIDS at a rate of 60.3 per 100,000. This rate was more than nine times as high as the rate among whites (6.4 per 100,000), and nearly three times as high as the rate among Hispanics/Latinos (20.8 per 100,000).

At the end of 2006, an estimated 431,969 adults and adolescents were living with AIDS in the 50 states and D.C., and blacks accounted for 44.1% of these persons. Each year, during 2002–2006, black adults and adolescents had the highest annual AIDS prevalence rate. In 2006, the prevalence rate for blacks living with AIDS in the 50 states and D.C. was 641.6 per 100,000. This rate was seven times as high as the AIDS prevalence rate among whites (90.5 per 100,000) and more than twice as high as the prevalence rate among Hispanics/Latinos (243.3 per 100,000). In 2006, the areas of the United States with the highest prevalence rates for blacks living with AIDS were D.C. (3,070.7 per 100,000), New York (1,343.4 per 100,000), Florida (1,056.0 per 100,000), New Jersey (970.9 per 100,000), Connecticut (899.8 per 100,000), and Maryland (875.3 per 100,000). Because D.C. is not a state, caution should be exercised when comparing its prevalence rate with those of the states.

Among persons diagnosed with AIDS during 1998–2005, the proportion surviving for more than 1 year after an AIDS diagnosis was greater among Asians/Pacific Islanders, whites, and Hispanics/Latinos than among blacks (Centers for Disease Control and Prevention, 2008a).

HIV/AIDS in Black Men

Although it has been shown that black people are disproportionately at risk for HIV/AIDS, black men bear the greatest burden of that risk. During 2002–2006, black men in the 33 states accounted for nearly one-third (31.4%) of all HIV/AIDS diagnoses and 43.4% of cases of HIV/AIDS diagnosed among men – with 63.1% (54,701) of that group consisting of black men.

Among black men diagnosed with HIV/AIDS during 2002–2006, more than half of those HIV infections (29,685, or 54.3%) were attributed to male-to-male sexual contact, 16.1% to IDU, and 24.7% to high-risk heterosexual contact. Of the HIV/AIDS cases attributed to male-to-male sexual contact, 29.4% of men were aged 35–44 years, 27.6% were aged 25–34 years, and 22.6% were among youth aged 13–24 years.

HIV/AIDS diagnosis rates were consistently higher for black men than for men of other racial and ethnic groups in the 33 states with name-based HIV reporting in each year of this study. In 2006, the rate of HIV/AIDS diagnosis among black men was 119.1 per 100,000. This rate was seven times as high as the rate among white men (16.7 per 100,000) and more than twice as high as the rate among Hispanic/Latino men (50.9 per 100,000) and black women (56.2 per 100,000).

At the end of 2006, of the estimated 353,026 men living with HIV/AIDS in the 33 states with name-based HIV reporting, 41.1% were black. In 2006, the prevalence rate for black men living with HIV/AIDS in the 33 states was 1,536.5 per 100,000. This rate was six times as high as the HIV/AIDS prevalence rate among white men (258.6 per 100,000) and more than twice as high as the prevalence rate among Hispanic/Latino men (642.7 per 100,000). The HIV/AIDS prevalence rate for black men was twice that of black women (791.7 per 100,000).

AIDS in Black Men

Of the 93,492 black adults and adolescents with diagnosed AIDS in the 50 states and D.C. during 2002–2006, 64.5% were men. The distribution of transmission categories among black men is shown in Table 2.2. Nearly half (46.7%) of AIDS diagnoses among black men were attributed to male-to-male sexual contact. High-risk heterosexual contact accounted for the second largest percentage (23.6%) among black men – a much larger percentage than that for all men (16.3%).

During 2002–2006, blacks accounted for the largest percentage of AIDS diagnoses among men regardless of age at diagnosis. Most (63.6%) black men diagnosed with AIDS were aged 35–44 (37.5%) or 45–54 (26.1%) years. Racial disparities in AIDS diagnoses were particularly severe among young men. Among young men aged 13–24 years, blacks accounted for 56.7% of diagnoses (Table 2.2). By region, black men accounted for more AIDS diagnoses than men of any other race or ethnic group in the South (56.1%), Midwest (45.1%), and Northeast (43.2%). (See Table 2.2.)

AIDS diagnosis rates also were consistently higher for black men than for men of other races and ethnicities in the 50 states and D.C. In 2006, the annual rate of AIDS diagnosis among black men was 82.9 per 100,000 – more than seven times as high as the rate among white men (11.2 per 100,000) and more than twice as high as the rate among Hispanic/Latino men (31.3 per 100,000) and black women (40.4 per 100,000).

At the end of 2006, an estimated 331,994 men in the 50 states and D.C. were living with AIDS. Blacks accounted for more than one-third (38.6%) of these men. The prevalence rate for black men living with AIDS in the 50 states and D.C. was 920.6 per 100,000. This rate was more than five times as high as the AIDS prevalence rate among white men (162.4 per 100,000) and more than twice as high as the rate among Hispanic/Latino men (371.1 per 100,000). The AIDS prevalence rate for black men was more than twice that of black women (395.9 per 100,000).

Among all men diagnosed with AIDS during 2002–2005 in the 33 states with name-based HIV reporting, a larger percentage of blacks received a diagnosis of AIDS within 1 year of HIV diagnosis than men of other races and ethnicities. Of all black men with diagnosed HIV infection during that time, 36.8% were diagnosed with AIDS within 1 year of HIV diagnosis, compared with 34.2% of white men. Among black men diagnosed with AIDS, larger percentages of diagnoses were made within 1 year of HIV diagnosis for men aged 65 years and older (53.6%) and IDUs (42.3%).

HIV/AIDS in Black Women

Black women also are severely affected by HIV/AIDS. During 2002–2006, blacks accounted for an estimated 66.7% (32,046) of HIV/AIDS diagnoses among women in the 33 states with name-based HIV reporting (Table 2.1). During this period, the number of annual HIV/AIDS diagnoses among black women exceeded the number of diagnoses among women and men of all other races and ethnicities, except for black or white men. The distribution of transmission categories by race and ethnicity among women with diagnosed HIV/AIDS is shown in Table 2.1.

Among all black women with diagnosed HIV/AIDS during 2002–2006 in the 33 states with name-based HIV reporting, more than three-fourths (81.7%) of infections was attributed to high-risk heterosexual contact. Of remaining cases, 17.1% were attributed to IDU, and 1.2% was attributed to "other" or unidentified risk factors. Of HIV/AIDS diagnoses among black women attributed to high-risk heterosexual contact, 29.5% were among women aged 35–44 years, 28.8% among women aged 25–34 years, 17.2% among women aged 45–54 years and 17.3% among youth aged 13–24 years.

In each year of this study, HIV/AIDS diagnosis rates were consistently higher among black women than among women of other races and ethnicities in the 33 states with name-based HIV reporting. In 2006, the estimated annual HIV/AIDS diagnosis rate among black women was 56.2 per 100,000, higher than any annual rate for women and men of all other race or ethnic groups except for black men. In 2006, the rate of HIV/AIDS diagnosis among black women was 19 times as high as the rate among white women (2.9 per 100,000) and nearly four times as high as the rate among Hispanic/Latino women (15.1 per 100,000).

During 2002–2006, the estimated number of black women living with HIV/AIDS increased steadily in the 33 states with name-based HIV infection reporting. At the end of 2006, an estimated 85,030 black women – or 64.4% of all women estimated to be living with HIV/AIDS in those areas – were living with HIV/AIDS. In 2006, black women had the highest HIV/AIDS prevalence rate, with 791.7 per 100,000 living with HIV/AIDS in the 33 states. This rate was 18 times as high as the prevalence rate among white women (44.4 per 100,000) and more than three times as high as the prevalence rate among Hispanic/Latino women (220.2 per 100,000).

AIDS in Black Women

Of the estimated 50,002 women with diagnosed AIDS in the 50 states and D.C. during 2002–2006, 66.3% were black (Table 2.2). During 2002–2006, blacks accounted for the largest percentage of AIDS diagnoses among women regardless of age at diagnosis. Most (61.8%) black women with diagnosed AIDS were aged 25–34 (25.3%) and 35–44 (36.5%) years. Racial disparities in AIDS diagnoses were particularly severe among young women. Among young women aged 13–24 years, blacks accounted for 69.2% of diagnoses. By U.S. region, black women accounted for more AIDS diagnoses than women of any other race or ethnic group in every region (South, 76.2%; Midwest, 67.9%; Northeast, 58.6%; and West, 34.2%) (Table 2.2).

Each year, during 2002–2006, the annual AIDS diagnosis rates were consistently higher among black women than for women of other races and ethnicities in the 50 states and D.C. In 2006, the annual rate of AIDS diagnosis among black women was 40.4 per 100,000. This rate was 21 times as high as the rate among white women (1.9 per 100,000) and four times as high as the rate among Hispanic/Latino women (9.5 per 100,000). At the end of 2006, an estimated 99,975 women were living with AIDS in the 50 states and D.C., and blacks accounted for nearly two-thirds (62.6%) of these women. The rate for black women living with AIDS in the 50 states and D.C. was 395.9 per 100,000. This rate was 18 times as high as the AIDS prevalence rate among white women (22.2 per 100,000) and nearly four times as high as the rate among Hispanic/Latino women (105.1 per 100,000).

Among all women with diagnosed AIDS during 2002–2005 in the 33 states with name-based HIV reporting, a larger percentage of blacks received a diagnosis of AIDS within 1 year of HIV diagnosis. Thirty-one percent of black women with diagnosed HIV infection during that time were diagnosed with AIDS within 1 year of HIV diagnosis, compared with 28.8% of white women. Among black women with diagnosed AIDS, larger percentages of diagnoses were made within 1 year of HIV diagnosis for women aged 65 years and older (52.0%) and women with HIV infection attributed to IDU (35.4%).

AIDS in Black Children

The decrease in mother-to-child (perinatal) HIV transmission is a notable public health achievement in HIV prevention in the United States (Centers for Disease Control and Prevention, 1998). Although significant progress has been made to prevent HIV/AIDS in children, there is still cause for concern for black children because the racial/ethnic gap in pediatric AIDS cases has not been eliminated. The increasing proportion of black women of reproductive age living with HIV/AIDS has major implications for black children because HIV transmission can occur from mother to child during pregnancy, labor, delivery, or breast-feeding.

Black children in the 50 states and D.C. accounted for 67.8% (217) of the estimated 320 AIDS diagnoses among children younger than age 13 years during 2002–2006. Mother-to-child HIV transmission accounted for nearly all (98.8%) of these AIDS diagnoses. At the end of 2006, an estimated 1,115 children were living with AIDS in the 50 states and D.C.. More than two-thirds (68.5%) of these children were black, compared with 12.3% that were white and 17.0% that were Hispanic/Latino. The overwhelming disparity in AIDS diagnoses affecting black children demonstrates the critical need to address access to testing, treatment, and care services for black women of child-bearing age.

Deaths of Blacks with AIDS

Sharp declines have been reported in both the annual numbers of persons with diagnosed AIDS and the number of deaths of persons with AIDS (Centers for Disease Control and Prevention, 2002, 2008a). This is due to the development of HAART, which for many HIV-infected people has delayed progression to end-stage HIV disease and increased survival. During 2002–2006, an estimated 80,059 adults and adolescents with AIDS in the 50 states and D.C. died. The largest number of deaths was among blacks, who accounted for 42,229 (52.7%) of estimated deaths among adults and adolescents with AIDS. At the same time, black women accounted for 67.7% (14,121) of all women who died with AIDS. The distribution of deaths with AIDS among black women was 37.3% (5,271) for women aged 35–44 years, 31.8% (4,485) for those aged 45–54 years, and 15.4% (2,179) for those aged 25–34 years. During 2002–2006, black men accounted for 47.5% (28,108) of all men who died with AIDS. Distribution of deaths with AIDS among black men was 36.9% (10,360) for men aged 45–54 years, 32.6% (9,155) for men aged 35–44 years, and 14.5% (4,081) for men aged 55–64 years.

CDC's National Center for Health Statistics compiles death certificate data from the 50 states and D.C. on underlying causes of deaths. In 2004, the year for which the most recent data are available, HIV disease was the ninth leading cause of death for all black persons (Heron, 2007). During this same period, HIV disease was the third leading case of death for black adults aged 35–44 and 45–54 years, and the fourth leading cause for black adults aged 25–34 years (Heron). By sex, black women account for an ever-growing number of U.S. deaths attributed to HIV disease. In 2004, HIV disease was the leading cause of death for black women aged 25–34 years and the third leading cause of death for black women aged 35–44 years (Heron). During this same period, HIV disease was the seventh leading cause of death for all black men, the second leading cause of death for black men aged 35–44, and the fourth leading cause of death for black men aged 25–34 and 45–54 years (Heron).

Limitations of Data Presented

The surveillance data presented in this chapter are subject to several limitations. First, estimated HIV/AIDS diagnoses are inherently underestimates of the true HIV-infected population because they only include people who have been tested for HIV and were reported to the state or local health departments that collected confidential name-based HIV infection case data during the period of analysis. In addition, trends in the HIV/AIDS epidemic are better reflected today by new HIV infections, which are more difficult to track.

The data in this chapter also describe when persons received a diagnosis of HIV infection, rather than when they became infected. This distinction is important because a person might have been infected with HIV for years before receiving a diagnosis.

The second limitation of the data presented here is that we must limit the temporal and geographic scope of our analyses until we have nationally representative data from mature surveillance systems (i.e., confidential, name-based reporting of HIV and AIDS cases for at least 4 years). Diagnoses of HIV/AIDS from areas with historically high AIDS morbidity that did not conduct confidential, name-based HIV surveillance as of 2006 (e.g., California, Illinois, and D.C.) were not included in this analysis. However, the racial/ethnic disparities described in this chapter are similar to disparities observed among persons with AIDS from all 50 states and D.C.

Finally, the data presented here may have been affected by statistical adjustments made to account for reporting delays and for cases reported with no identified risk factor. Such cases were reclassified on the basis of information obtained from follow-up investigations, and they were assumed to constitute a representative sample of all cases initially reported without a risk factor. However, this assumption might not prove valid, potentially affecting the accuracy of the estimated distribution of cases by transmission category. Since 1993, the proportion of HIV/AIDS cases reported to CDC without an identified risk factor for HIV infection has increased. In 2006, no risk factor was identified for 25% of HIV (not AIDS) cases among adults and adolescents reported to CDC (Green, 1998). This lack of data has resulted in an increasing proportion of cases that are assigned to transmission categories by statistical adjustment. Risk factor information often is missing because patients decline to disclose behaviors that place them at risk for HIV transmission, or they are simply unaware of their sex partners' high-risk behavior.

Future Directions

June 2006 marked the 25th anniversary of the first reported cases of AIDS in the United States. Although considerable progress has been made in reducing the impact of the HIV epidemic, HIV remains a persistent and pervasive threat to the health and well-being of many blacks. Disparities in HIV/AIDS diagnoses are most marked among black MSM, women, and children. Recent reports have found increases in annual diagnoses of HIV/AIDS among black MSM, and in particular, young MSM, which suggests a potential resurgence of HIV infection among this population (Centers for Disease Control and Prevention, 2008b). Prevention strategies must be strengthened, improved, and implemented more broadly to reduce HIV transmission, particularly among black MSM. The high rate of infection among blacks highlights the need to expand known, effective HIV-prevention interventions and to implement new, improved, and culturally appropriate HIV/AIDS strategies.

CDC is committed to continually reassessing, strengthening, and expanding its efforts to address the epidemic among African Americans. As a result, CDC joined with public health partners and community leaders in 2007 to spearhead the Heightened National Response to the HIV/AIDS Crisis among African Americans to reduce the toll of this disease (Centers for Disease Control and Prevention, 2007). That response focuses on the following areas:

- Expanding the reach of prevention services, including ensuring that federal prevention resources are expended where the need is greatest.
- Increasing opportunities for diagnosing and treating HIV, including encouraging more African Americans to know their HIV serostatus.
- Developing new effective prevention interventions, including behavioral, social, and structural interventions.
- Mobilizing broader action within communities to help change community perceptions about HIV/AIDS to motivate African Americans to seek early HIV diagnosis and treatment and to encourage healthy behaviors and community norms that prevent the spread of HIV.

CDC and its partners are committed to reducing the impact of HIV/AIDS among African Americans and helping to mobilize local, state, and national resources toward that goal. A comprehensive national program is required to address the substantial racial disparities in HIV/AIDS diagnoses among African Americans in the United States and its dependent areas. To reduce disparities, partnerships must be enhanced among a broad range of individuals and groups, including governmental agencies, community organizations, faith-based institutions, educational institutions, community opinion leaders, and the public.

References

Centers for Disease Control and Prevention. (1981). Pneumocystis carinii pneumonia – Los Angeles. *Morbidity and Mortality Weekly Report, 30*, 250–252.

Centers for Disease Control and Prevention. (1982). *Kaposi's sarcoma (KS), Pneumocystis carinii pneumonia (PCP) and other opportunistic infections (OI): Cases reported to CDC*. Atlanta: U.S. Department of Health and Human Services. Retrieved August 1, 2008, from http://www.cdc.gov/hiv/topics/surveillance/resources/reports/pdf/surveillance82.pdf.

Centers for Disease Control and Prevention. (1984). Antibodies to retrovirus etiologically associated with acquired immunodeficiency syndrome (AIDS) in populations with increased incidences of the syndrome. *Morbidity and Mortality Weekly Report, 33*, 377–379.

Centers for Disease Control and Prevention. (1996). *HIV/AIDS Surveillance Report*, 8, No. 2. Atlanta: U.S. Department of Health and Human Services.

Centers for Disease Control and Prevention. (1998). Success in implementing PHS guidelines to reduce perinatal transmission of HIV. *Morbidity and Mortality Weekly Report, 47*, 688–691 [Published errata appear in *Morbidity and Mortality Weekly Report, 47*, 718 (1998)].

Centers for Disease Control and Prevention. (2002). Deaths among persons with AIDS through December 2000. *HIV/AIDS Surveillance Supplemental Report*, 8, No. 1. Atlanta: U.S. Department of Health and Human Services.

Centers for Disease Control and Prevention. (2006). Cases of HIV infection and AIDS in the United States, by race/ethnicity, 2000–2004. *HIV/AIDS Surveillance Supplemental Report*, 12, No. 1. Retrieved August 1, 2008, from http://www.cdc.gov/hiv/topics/surveillance/resources/reports/index.htm.

Centers for Disease Control and Prevention. (2007). *A heightened national response to the HIV/AIDS crisis among African Americans*. Atlanta: U.S. Department of Health and Human Services. Retrieved August 1, 2008, from http://www.cdc.gov/hiv/topics/aa/resources/reports/heightendresponse.htm.

Centers for Disease Control and Prevention. (2008a). *HIV/AIDS Surveillance Report, 2006* (Vol. 18). Atlanta: U.S. Department of Health and Human Services.

Centers for Disease Control and Prevention. (2008b). Trends in HIV/AIDS diagnoses among men who have sex with men – 33 States, 2001–2006. *Morbidity and Mortality Weekly Report, 57,* 681–686.

Gallo, R. C., Salahuddin, S. Z., & Popovic, M. (1984). Frequent detection and isolation of cytopathic retroviruses (HTLV-III) from patients with AIDS and at risk for AIDS. *Science, 224,* 500–503.

Green, T. A. (1998). Using surveillance data to monitor trends in the AIDS epidemic. *Statistics in Medicine, 17,* 143–154.

Heron, M. P. (2007). *Deaths: Leading causes for 2004.* National Vital Statistics, Vol. 56, No. 5. Hyattsville, MD: National Center for Health Statistics.

Palella, F. J., Jr., Delaney, K. M., Moorman, A. C., Loveless, M. O., Fuhrer, J., Satten, G. A., et al. (1998). Declining morbidity and mortality among patients with advanced human immunodeficiency virus infection. *New England Journal of Medicine, 338,* 853–860.

Thacker, S. B. (2001). Historical development. In S. M. Teutsch & R. E. Churchill (Eds.), *Principles and practice of public health surveillance* (pp. 3–17). New York: Oxford University Press.

U.S. Census Bureau. (2006). Population estimates (specific files; entire data set no longer available). Retrieved March 17, 2008, from source http://www.census.gov/popest/archives/2000s/vintage_2006/.

Chapter 3
Racism, Poverty and HIV/AIDS Among African Americans*

Kim M. Williams and Cynthia M. Prather

Substantive evidence links racism and poverty to a host of chronic health conditions, adverse mental health outcomes and excess mortality, particularly among African Americans (Brondolo, ver Halen, Pencille, Beatty, & Contrada, 2009; Harrell, Hall, & Taliaferro, 2003; Jones, 2000, 2003; Krieger, 2000, 2005; Krieger, Rowley, Hermann, Avery, & Phillips, 1993; Kwate, Valdimarsdottir, Guevarra, & Vovbjerg, 2003; Mays, Cochran, & Barnes, 2007; Randall, 2006; Williams, 1999; Williams & Williams-Morris, 2000). The legacy of historic and contemporary forms of racism and discrimination towards African Americans (Latif & Latif, 1994; Washington, 2006), has also contributed to conditions of poverty and inequality (e.g., limited access to educational and employment opportunities and quality healthcare). According to the CDC (2009), African Americans are disproportionately affected by HIV/AIDS and continue to shoulder the burden of infections. However, prior prevention and control efforts have largely been limited in reducing such disparities. Critical inquiries into the range of social, economic and political forces impacting African Americans' health are urgently needed. Unfortunately, to date, there is but a dearth of research examining the complex interplay between these broader level contextual factors and HIV/AIDS-related outcomes. Although discussions about racism and poverty are mentioned in public health literature (Clark, 2001; Darity, 2003; Krueger, Wood, Diehr, & Maxwell, 1990; Utsey & Hook, 2007), few attempts have been made to extensively address their relationship to HIV in research or health promotion or prevention interventions. The authors assert that understanding the social and economic realities faced by African Americans is a necessary requisite to effectively address this epidemic. This chapter reviews definitions of racism

---

*The findings and conclusions in this report are those of the authors and do not necessarily represent the views of the Centers for Disease Control and Prevention.

K.M. Williams (✉)
Division of HIV/AIDS Prevention, Centers for Disease Control and Prevention,
1600 Clifton Road, MS E-37, Atlanta, GA 30333, USA
e-mail: KWilliams4@cdc.gov

D.H. McCree et al. (eds.), *African Americans and HIV/AIDS*,
DOI 10.1007/978-0-387-78321-5_3,

31

and poverty. The authors then discuss more generally disparate health outcomes associated with the effects of racism and poverty. The extent of these factors in the context of HIV among African Americans is elaborated. Lastly, recommendations are provided that address both theoretical and methodological implications for research and intervention development and implementation.

Definitions of Racism and Poverty

In his classic book entitled, *Prejudice and Racism* (1972), James Jones defined racism as the "use of power against a racial group identified as inferior by individuals and institutions with the intentional or unintentional support of the entire culture." Bulhan (1985) expounded on this definition as a "form of violence" whereby persons are violated on the basis of race. Further, Clark, Anderson, Clark, and Williams (2002) employed the definition as "attitudes and beliefs that demean individuals or groups as a result of physical attributes and/or ethnic group affiliation." Jones (2003) described racism as a "system that structures opportunity and value based on race, thereby undermining the full potential of the entire society because it unfairly disadvantages some communities while it unfairly advantages others." Overall, these definitions maintain that racism is used to justify inequity towards, supremacy over, and exclusion of particular individuals based on race, thereby infringing upon their physical, psychological and spiritual well-being of the community (Washington, 2006).

Poverty, a complex and multidimensional concept, has been defined in many different ways; however, more commonly it refers to "income deprivation." The World Bank defines poverty as "an income level below some minimum level necessary to meet basic needs." The greatest challenge however, lies in measuring poverty and determining a poverty line or a threshold at which an individual or a household is classified as poor (Coudouel, Hentschel, & Wodon, 2002). The official poverty measure used in the United States is an absolute one and is based on a formula developed in 1964 by the Social Security Administration (Dalaker, 2005). It is widely suggested that the current measure is outdated and no longer accurately portrays the amount needed for a decent living in the United States (Iceland, 2003). In contrast, more recently developed relative measures such as those created by the National Academy of Science (NAS) are believed to more accurately reflect those living in poverty (Iceland) by taking into account such factors as geographic location, family size, costs for food, housing, utilities, clothing, non cash benefits, and in some cases medical expenses and work related expenses (Dalaker). Depending on the definition used, poverty estimates can range substantially. However, according to the official poverty measure, 39.8 million people in the United States, in 2008, lived in poverty and one out of four blacks were poor (DeNavas-Walt, Proctor, & Smith, 2009).

Racism, Poverty and the Overall Health
of African Americans

Inequities in mortality and infirmity have remained consistent for African Americans from the inception of the government tracking these statistics (DHHS, 2001). In the United States, a history of deeply rooted racist ideologies resulted in widespread, institutionally-supported, discriminatory practices used to exclude African Americans from full participation in society (Bulhan, 1985; Randall, 2006; Washington, 2006; Williams, 1987). Some suggest that the resulting health conse-quences have been most profound among African Americans as evidenced by their suffering the brunt of health disparities (Clark et al., 2002; LaVeist, 2002; Mays et al., 2007; Paradies, 2006; Randall). For example, the effects of racism have been linked to disparities in chronic conditions such as cardiovascular health (Harrell et al., 2003; Krieger, 2000; Wyatt et al., 2000), mental health (Jackson et al., 1996; Kwate et al., 2003; Williams & Williams-Morris, 2000), emotional health (Lewis-Trotter & Jones, 2004; Morris-Prather et al., 1996), and HIV/AIDS (Bharat, 2003; Lemelle, 2003). The most commonly reported outcomes of studies on race-based discrimination are negative mental health outcomes (Klonoff & Landrine, 1999a, 1999b; Williams, Neighbors et al.). Depression, stress, anxiety and pessimism have been shown to be associated with experiences of racial oppression (Bowen-Reid & Harrell, 2002; Moore, 2000; Williams, Neighbors, & Jackson, 2008; Williams & Williams-Morris, 2000) and poverty (House & Williams, 2000; Williams, Yu, Jackson, & Anderson, 1997).

Although there are a number of causal pathways through which poverty affects health, it is critical to understand the cyclical nature of these relation-ships. Conditions of poverty (e.g., lack of access to quality healthcare) can result in poor health, and poor health can hinder one's ability to be economically self sufficient (e.g., not being able to maintain employment due to illness). Explanations for increasing levels of unemployment and income inequities among African Americans are vast and continue to be issues of growing concern and constant debate. In a recent analysis, Woolf, Johnson, and Geiger (2006) reported that poverty has increased most dramatically among the most marginal-ized, including African Americans. Although there have been increases in occu-pational mobility and wage parity over time, African Americans continue to experience stark disparities in employment rates and job earnings and are more likely to be chronically unemployed for a period of 6 months or more (Census, U.S. Census Bureau, 2007).

Racism also impacts the economic health and stability of the family. According to the 2008 Current Population Survey, African Americans were more likely to have never been married, and more likely to be divorced and separated when com-pared to other racial/ethnic groups (Census, 2009). Moreover, nearly one out of every three African American families with children under the age of 18 is main-tained by the mother only (Census, 2009). Early explanations about the origins of current trends in African American family structure (Johnson & Staples, 1993; Leary, 2005) pointed to the history of slavery as the root cause of the dismantling of the African American family. For example, reasons offered for the absence of African American men from their families today are deeply rooted in a history of slavery (Johnson & Staples), a time in which African American men were denied full and equal participation in humanity and stripped of the role of husband and father, and African American women were viewed as sexual objects that would be raped, beaten, whipped and sold at the will of their master. This was followed by decades of segregationist laws prohibiting African Americans from full and equitable participation in U.S. society. In current times, the absence of African American men in 'two-parent' households has been linked to an insecure economic environment, limited access to employment and training opportunities, stagnant wages, declining demand for lower skilled jobs/low wage work, discrimination in the workplace as well as damaging and non supportive cultural patterns and other adversative public and private policies (Holzer, 2007). Moreover, African American women are much more likely to experience economic deprivations as they are at increased risk for having incomes below the poverty threshold, have fewer financial resources, and receive less pay than men for the same work (Williams et al., 1997).

It is critical to note here the complex interplay between race, economic inequality and health. Tragically, the combination of these factors impedes the healthy development of individuals and communities. Racism not only has deleterious effects on the physical, psychological and emotional health of African Americans, but it also adversely impacts economic well-being. Race-based discriminatory practices have been a mechanism used for limiting educational and economic opportunities for African Americans and have resulted in higher rates of unemployment, inequities in wage earnings (Williams et al., 2008) and subsequently, limited access to health care (Darity, 2003; Randall, 2006; Williams, 1999). Williams (1999) asserts that "*socioeconomic status is part of the casual pathway by which race affects health.*" In other words, SES mediates the relationship between race and health. Thus, for example, one's racial/ethnic background can impact their employment status (if not hired due to race or not being paid equitable wages), and this subsequent lack of employment or underemployment may result in not having adequate health care coverage. Access to healthcare is largely a function of having jobs that offer health insurance. Many of the working poor do not have employers offering healthcare coverage and are unable to pay for care themselves. Although the poor are more likely to receive health care benefits through publicly funded programs (Copeland, 2005), nearly one out of every three persons living in poverty remains uninsured and one out of four reports no regular source of care (Woolf et al., 2006). Arguably any one or combination of the aforementioned consequences of racism and poverty can undermine African Americans' ability to care for their health, consistently provide financial support for their families, and maintain stable and healthy relationships.

The Interplay Between HIV/AIDS and the Dual Effects of Racism and Poverty

Prioritizing health, particularly as it relates to HIV/AIDS prevention, and accessing care in the presence of such formidable obstacles, such as racism and poverty, likely proves difficult, and for many African Americans impossible. The Tuskegee Syphilis Study had large-scale implications on the health and well being of African American men, women and children and also solidified a hearty distrust of the healthcare system among African Americans in general. In this study, the U.S. Public Health Service withheld treatment from African American men diagnosed with syphilis to study disease progression (Jones, 1993) over a period of 40 years. Unfortunately, this study was not the first nor the last experimental research project targeting African Americans (Washington, 2006).

Klonoff and Landrine (1999a, 1999b) explored beliefs that HIV was developed by the government to annihilate blacks in an investigation of 520 African American adults. Nearly half of the sample either believed in AIDS conspiracy theories or were undecided on whether or not they were true. Thomas and Quinn (1991) suggest that low levels of African American participation in HIV clinical trials is due in part to distrust in the healthcare system and beliefs that AIDS is an attempt to wideout African Americans. In a study by Boulware, Cooper, Ratner, LaVeist, and Poweand (2003) on the relationship between race and trust in the healthcare system, African Americans were more likely to report concerns related to harmful experimentation. More recently, Sullivan, McNaghten, Begley, Hutchinson, and Cargill (2007) reported that reluctance to participate in HIV clinical studies was associated with the perception of being "a guinea pig" and Moutsiakis and Chin (2007) found that mistrust and stigma were key reasons that African Americans were unwilling to participate in clinical trials. Thus, given the historical context, it is not surprising that conspiracy theories related to the emergence of HIV within the African American community surfaced in direct relation to experiences of racism (Klonoff & Landrine; Mays & Cochran, 1988; Thomas & Quinn).

Although evidence suggests that individual behaviors do not fully explain disparate rates of HIV/AIDS experienced by African Americans, prevention efforts have largely been limited in focus to reducing individual risk behaviors (Latkin & Knowlton, 2005; Sumartojo, 2000). With the exception of investigations examining access and use of healthcare services in general, studies of the relationship between racism, discrimination and HIV-related outcomes are limited. One such investigation of Latino gay men by Diaz, Ayala, and Bein (2004) found that men who reported experiences with racism, poverty and homophobia were more likely to report engaging in risky sexual situations, including having sex while on drugs or alcohol and with partners who do not want to use condoms. The authors posit that individual risk is a product of personal and contextual situations. In contrast however, others have found an inverse relationship between African American experiences with racism and engagement in risk behaviors (Jones et al., 2003;

LaVeist, Sellers, & Neighbors, 2001). The authors suggested that experiences with racism may have instilled a level of perseverance that buffers the negative effects of racism, thus fueling the individual's desire and efforts to protect against negative health outcomes.

Empirical evidence suggests that economic hardships plague many of those most at risk and affected by HIV/AIDS (Diaz et al., 1994; Ellerbrock et al., 2004; Fife & Mode, 1992; Forna et al. 2006; Krieger, Chen, Waterman, Rehkopf, & Subramanian, 2005; Krueger et al., 1990; Simon, Hu, Diaz, & Kerndt, 1995; Wohl et al., 1998; Zierler et al., 2000). Moreover, the geographic distribution of poverty often maps on to areas with high rates of morbidity and mortality as evidenced by States in the southern region of the U.S. that continue to experience the greatest burden of HIV/AIDS (CDC, 2009) and STDs (CDC, 2008). The South, now accounts for the highest estimated number of persons living with AIDS, and the highest estimated number of persons diagnosed and dying with AIDS for years 2003–2007 (CDC, 2009). This region, also having the greatest concentration of African Americans, continues to experience high rates of unemployment and healthcare uninsured, low levels of education attainment and the lowest median income when compared to other regions in the U.S. (Reif, Geonnotti, & Whetten, 2006; Southern AIDS Coalition, 2003). Furthermore, poverty largely remains centralized in metropolitan areas characterized by higher concentrations of low income housing and racially segregated neighborhoods. Zierler and Krieger (1997) suggest that racially segregated neighborhoods give rise to higher rates of HIV and STDs due to isolated pockets of sexual networks, limited access to educational and economic opportunities and quality health care in these areas.

In addition to high rates of unemployment and limited job availability, poor neighborhoods often reflect other interrelated characteristics impacting health, such as high rates of homelessness (Aidala, Cross, Stall, Harre, & Sumartojo, 2005), substandard housing and unsafe living conditions (Ross & Mirowsky, 2001). For example, being homeless or unstably housed has been linked to poverty and increases in substance use, sex exchange and unprotected sex among HIV-positive persons (Aidala et al.). In a recent examination of substance users, Latkin, Curry, Hua, and Davey (2007) reported significant associations between psychological distress, sexual risk behaviors, and several poverty-related neighborhood conditions, including vacant houses, loitering, and crime. Similarly, Cohen and colleagues (2000) constructed a "broken window index" which included items indicative of substandard living conditions, such as poor housing quality, deteriorating schools, abandoned cars and litter. They found that higher scores on the index were significantly associated with higher rates of gonorrhea.

In a review of literature examining the relationship between SES and sexual networks, Adimora and Schoenbach (2002) suggest that a combination of adversities, including poverty, unemployment, high incarceration rates and substance use decreases the pool of available and desirable male partners in African American communities, thus resulting in a lower sex ratio of men to women, and relationship instability. The authors assert that these conditions can lead to increased engagement in higher risk behaviors (i.e., sexual partner concurrency and lower risk individuals having sex with higher risk individuals) (Adimora & Schoenbach; Adimora, Schoenbach, & Doherty, 2006). Further, the dual challenges of disproportionate incarceration rates coupled with increasing numbers of African Americans with HIV has sounded an alarm in the public health arena. Harawa and Adimora (2008) state that incarceration disrupts stable relationships, resulting in increased HIV risk among the incarcerated as well as their partners. Post incarceration, some African Americans find themselves facing tough economic challenges as they attempt to re-enter society and are faced with financial insecurity due to limited employment opportunities.

Forna et al. (2006) reported data from a series of focus group discussions with African American women who reported that reliance on male partners for financial assistance to meet basic needs made it difficult to insist that their partners be monogamous, use condoms and be tested for HIV. Women in this study also reported that providing for basic needs took priority over their own health. According to Aral, O'Leary, and Baker (2006), depression and substance use, resulting from poverty, serve as the mechanisms for increased behavioral risk for HIV and STDs. They also suggest that sex exchange is a "poverty-related mechanism" linked to HIV because those with limited resources trade sex for needed or desired commodities including, money, shelter, food, drugs, companionship and comfort. Sex exchange can also lead to increased exposure to high-risk sexual contacts and multiple partnering to acquire items needed for subsistence (McNair & Prather, 2004).

Substance use and abuse have been linked to racism, poverty and risk for HIV as individuals may use illicit substances to "escape" adversative circumstances. Roberts, Wechsberg, Zule, and Burroughs (2003) concluded that individuals experiencing severe financial strain use drugs and alcohol to help cope with feelings of depression and despair and subsequently engage in risky sexual practices. Zierler and Krieger (1997) suggest that some engage in sexual relationships to seek comfort and as a way of temporarily escaping the harsh realities of racism.

Providing for HIV healthcare needs tends to lessen as a priority when individuals are faced with competing demands (Cunningham et al., 1999). Evidence suggests that the economically disadvantaged, particularly racial and ethnic minorities, often face a host of structural barriers, when interacting with the healthcare system (Smedley, Stith, & Nelson, 2003), including inadequate access to preventive care (e.g., health education, screenings, etc.) (Smedley et al.), access to only a limited number of providers and long wait times (Copeland, 2005). The dual effects of racism and poverty are demonstrated in unequal health care practices and the treatment provided to African Americans (Bach, Pham, Schrag, Tate, & Hargraves, 2004; Boulware et al., 2003). The Institute of Medicine reported that racial and ethnic minorities are less likely to receive patient education and more likely to receive incomplete information, experience discrimination and to indicate general distrust in the medical care system (Smedley et al.). Overall, the authors suggest that racial bias has led to substandard care from physicians towards African Americans (Smedley et al.). In an analysis of a nationally representative sample of HIV positive adults, Cunningham and colleagues found that more than a third postponed or went without care due to competing subsistence needs.

Racism and poverty are significant challenges that complicate HIV/AIDS prevention and care efforts for African Americans. Based on the available literature, these factors should be considered in prevention research and care efforts targeting African Americans.

Recommendations

Theoretical and methodological implications for assessing the relationship between poverty, racism and HIV-related outcomes will be explored in the recommendations that follow. The authors will also briefly discuss the importance of developing multidisciplinary partnerships to address the epidemic among African Americans. They suggest that these recommendations be considered because the current statistics indicate that HIV/AIDS continues to disproportionately impact African American communities; there has not been a significant decline in HIV within African American populations since the government reported it as a "state of emergency" in the 1990s; and no intervention studies, to our knowledge, have been designed for African Americans that specifically address the significance and complexity of experiences related to racism, poverty, and HIV.

Theoretical Considerations

As part of any scientific exploration of HIV among African Americans, it is necessary to identify and explain the multitude of factors potentially influencing risk. Selecting appropriate theoretical frameworks to guide scientific inquiry is necessary to more accurately conceptualize the relationships between varying constructs develop appropriate research designs; determine appropriate measures, interpret findings, and develop, implement and evaluate resulting intervention strategies and programs (Cochran & Mays, 1993; Kalichman, 1998). Understanding the burden of HIV among African Americans requires the use of culturally relevant theoretical frameworks that illuminate the relationships between a range of interrelated distal and proximal factors that may serve as plausible points of intervention. To date, the most common paradigms used in HIV prevention have been limited to viewing HIV as an individual level phenomenon, specifically seeking to change individual behavior, devoid of a greater social and economic context. Factors such as racism, discrimination and poverty, which are relevant to many African Americans at risk for and impacted by HIV, have largely been excluded from the most commonly used theoretical models in prevention research. As we come to understand and explore the range of factors influencing HIV-related outcomes, developing new theoretical frameworks and merging existing theories is likely warranted.

Ecological theory, a multilevel approach, is useful for conceptualizing the impact of a range of individual, social, economic and political factors on variations in health status (Smedley & Syme, 2000), and may be of utility for elucidating the causal pathways between racism, poverty and HIV-related outcomes among African Americans. This framework emphasizes that health behaviors are shaped by a host of interactive and interdependent physical and socio-environmental factors operating on multiple levels (Brofenbrenner, 1979; McLeroy, Bibeau, Steckler, & Glanz, 1988). Accordingly it is necessary to intervene at multiple levels (e.g., individual, interpersonal, organizational, societal) to address multiple levels of influence.

Embodied in an ecological perspective, community organization models are frequently used to identify and address "common problems" experienced by individuals and larger entities, including groups, organizations, institutions and communities (Minkler & Wallerstein, 1990, 2003; Rothman, Tropman, & Erlich, 2001). Community organization frameworks purport that through advocacy and mobilization, community members and organizations can more comprehensively promote change supportive of health promotion efforts. The basic premise supporting community organizing perspectives is that it is necessary to intervene at multiple levels to positively affect behavioral change and the "collective well-being" of communities (LaVeist, 2002).

Interpersonal behavioral theories, which have been more commonly utilized in HIV behavioral intervention research, also provide a useful framework for examining the influence of a myriad of factors influencing HIV/AIDS risk behaviors among African Americans. In particular, Social Cognitive Theory (SCT), emphasizes the reciprocal relationships between individual behaviors, interpersonal relationships and environmental factors and posits that past experiences influence behavior (Bandura, 1986). This paradigm lends support to addressing broader level contextual factors that have acute and pervasive influences on health, such as racism, poverty and other social determinants of health that may play a significant role in the diminishing health and well being of African Americans. However, Social Cognitive Theory has rarely been used in HIV prevention research to address the impact of broader level contextual influences.

Afrocentric and African American-centered behavioral change models are valuable for shaping the development and implementation of prevention interventions that acknowledge historical traditions endemic to their communities, such as interdependence, cooperation, collectivism, mutual responsibility, and egalitarianism (Beatty, Wheeler, & Gaiter, 2004; Cochran & Mays, 1993) and emphasize the shared cultural norms of communities (Gilbert & Goddard, 2007). Nobles (1985, 1986, 2006) suggests that Afrocentric theory can be used to explain behaviors of African Americans because this perspective is based on their history and experiences. Nobles, Goddard, and Gilbert (2009) employed the model as a framework for an HIV prevention intervention targeting African American women. The purpose of this study was to strengthen and enhance protective factors that promote traditional African and African American health and cultural values. Intervention participants engaged in activities including realigning women's thinking towards traditional African/African American cultural values (i.e., focus on community vs. individual) and restructuring thinking to embrace positive attitudes, values and perspectives of African American people to improve the development of protective factors. The study results suggested a significant increase in motivation, self worth and adoption of less risky sexual behaviors in the intervention group, and the researchers called for further investigation of culturally based interventions using more rigorous methods.

Methodological Considerations

It is beyond the scope of this chapter to provide an in-depth analysis of the range of methodological issues to be considered in examinations of the relationship between racism, poverty and HIV-related outcomes. However, the authors will highlight selected fundamental methodological issues that require attention. To empirically examine the relationship between racism, poverty and HIV, researchers must employ the appropriate research design methodologies. Selection of appropriate methods is critical for determining within a broad range of context, which aspects of an experience or an exposure regarding racism and poverty are relevant to specific HIV-related outcomes and why. At present, there is a dearth of research examining the various dimensions of racism and poverty and the complex interplay between these constructs and HIV. The authors acknowledge that it is not feasible for any one investigation to examine all the possible causal pathways in which racism and/or poverty impact a specific HIV-related outcome. For any analytic approach, major thought must be given to selecting the appropriate design and measures and assessing the amount of time and resources needed to conduct the investigation. To assess the relationship between racism, poverty and HIV-related outcomes, it is necessary to examine factors co-occurring on multiple levels (e.g., structural level factors – residential segregation vs. individual level factors – direct experiences with racism). Thus, the choice of method used to assess these relationships will vary as well.

Although use of experimental designs, particularly randomized controlled trials, provide increased rigor when assessing the influence of selected factors on a specified outcome, arguably it may not be the best method for assessing complex hypothetical pathways (as is the case in assessing the relationship between racism, poverty and HIV). Further, the authors suggest that because our understanding of the relationship between racism, poverty and HIV among African Americans is in its infancy, initial efforts should focus on conceptualizing, operationalizing and validating the various dimensions of these constructs with the target population.

Mixed method modalities (involving the use of qualitative and quantitative research methods) can also be used as part of formative research activities to inform development of testable hypotheses and HIV intervention programs. Ethnographic approaches and community-based participatory research (CBPR), in particular, are useful for obtaining in-depth information needed to more accurately understand the complex dimensions and effects of racism and poverty. Community-based participatory research is grounded in several principles, making this methodology potentially most useful in exploring the relationships between racism, poverty and HIV. This approach acknowledges the uniqueness and strengths of a community.

It underscores the importance of building partnerships of mutual regard and balanced power between researchers and community members to understand the complexities of adverse health outcomes from the perspective of the community and in developing sustainable interventions (Israel, Eng, Schulz, & Parker, 2005). Initially, qualitative methods, including focus groups, in-depth interviews, observations and quantitative surveys could be used to assess perceptions and experiences with racism and poverty and to explore plausible relationships to HIV-related outcomes. Use of these methods is critical for effectively designing and evaluating prevention interventions and ultimately decreasing disparate rates of infections experienced by African Americans.

Measures. Dependable, psychometrically sound measures of direct experiences of race-based discrimination (real or perceived) allow investigators to examine the impact of these factors on mental and physical well-being (Kressin, Raymond, & Manze, 2008; Krieger, 2005; Williams & Mohammed, 2009). Although currently there is not agreement regarding a standardized measure of racism, there are a growing number of measures available that assess multiple dimensions of racism and discrimination, including the different levels at which it occurs (e.g., individual, institutional), timing, frequency, duration, intensity and the context in which it occurs (e.g., work, school, healthcare setting, etc.) (Krieger, Pascoe & Sweet, 2009). Examples of such scales previously tested for reliability and validity with African American populations that may prove useful in HIV research include the following: Perceptions of Racism Scale (Murrell, 1996); Schedule of Racist Events (Landrine & Klonoff, 1996); Index of Race Related Stress (Utsey & Ponterotto, 1996); Perceived Racism Scale (McNeilly et al., 1996); Racism and Life Experience Scale (RaLES and RaLES-B) (Harrell, Merchant, & Young, 1997); the Experience of Discrimination Scale revised in Krieger and Sidney (1996); and the Everyday Discrimination Scale (Williams et al., 1997). These scales measure direct experiences with racism and discrimination at the individual level. Researchers can employ these measures to determine if there is an association with, for example, potential covariates, HIV-related risk behaviors and access to or utilization of healthcare services. At the population level, researchers can also examine co-factors such as residential segregation and concentrated poverty to assess if there are higher levels of HIV morbidity and mortality present and identify factors not readily apparent to individuals.

Public health has traditionally used income-based measures of poverty to examine its impact on available resources and health outcomes. While it is agreed that income and consumption are complex and interrelated constructs and are important to assess (Iceland & Bauman, 2007), several have argued that living conditions are determined by more than income and that income and consumption are not always positively correlated (Beverly, 2001; Mayer & Jencks, 1989; Rector, Johnson, & Youssef, 1999). As a result, researchers have increasingly sought measures that better capture a range of needs (i.e., material goods and resources) relative to expenses/consumption as an indicator of "hardship." For example, some measures assess selected material hardships including food insecurity (lack of availability and access to food); housing instability (homelessness, residing in overcrowded conditions); inadequate health insurance coverage and difficultly paying utilities (i.e., gas, water, electric, phone) (e.g., Beverly; Federman et al., 1996; Mayer & Jencks; Rector et al.). Using hardship measures in conjunction with traditional income measures may more accurately reflect African Americans' experiences with poverty. Braveman and colleagues (2005) mention important considerations when utilizing socioeconomic measures to assess impact on health. They state that the choice of a socioeconomic (SES) measure influences the outcome being studied. To address potential biases, they recommend that researchers assess as many SES indicators as possible, and critically examine as many explanatory pathways as possible that could potentially impact health, including institutional and personal experiences of racism and discrimination.

The authors suggest that researchers include measures of racism and discrimination, poverty and material hardship into investigations assessing, for example, African Americans risk for HIV and utilization of healthcare services to fully understand the complexities of these relationships. This can be done by incorporating such measures in small scale studies, large-scale surveys and longitudinal investigations.

Strengths perspectives. Prior research and HIV intervention programs have largely approached prevention for African Americans from a deficit model. Models that emphasize protective factors, such as "positive adaptive coping strategies" (Broman, 1996; Utsey, Ponterotto, Reynolds, & Cancelli, 2000; Wadsworth & DeCarlo Santiago, 2008), social support (Brown, 2008; Heckman, Kochman, & Sikkema, 2002) and spirituality (Prado et al., 2004) have been shown to buffer the effects of the deleterious effects of racism and poverty on health. These studies show that personal resilience and positive coping styles play an important role in mediating the relationship between distal risk factors such as poverty and racism and various health outcomes. Similar findings have been shown in the HIV literature. In a study of low income women living with HIV, Catz, Gore-Felton, and McClure (2002) reported that women who possessed fewer forms of social support and reported fewer active coping strategies experienced higher levels of anxiety and depression. Prado and colleagues found that among HIV-positive, low-income African American mothers, religious involvement was inversely associated with distress. The authors suggest that social support and coping mediated the relationship between religious involvement and distress. In a recent investigation, Konkle-Parker, Erlen, and Dubbert (2008) found that HIV medication adherence was facilitated by prayer and spirituality and the presence of social supports. Findings from these investigations have particular relevance for assessing the ways in which African Americans make healthy adaptations in the face of adverse conditions.

The authors recommend that HIV prevention interventions and care programs focus on the resiliency and perseverance of African Americans as this community has experienced some of the most brutal and oppressive treatment (i.e., slavery, segregationist laws and practices) in U.S. history. However, prior research and HIV intervention programs have largely failed to capitalize on these strengths. It is time that researchers and interventionists alike start placing greater emphasis on maximizing tools of empowerment that draw on individual, cultural and communal strengths existing within African American communities. These "assets" should serve as the basis for programs and efforts promoting health among African Americans.

Levels of interventions. Racism and poverty can and should be addressed in all levels of prevention interventions targeting African Americans. Structural, community, group, individual, as well as multilevel interventions pose unique opportunities to tackle these issues while at the same time promoting health. Although the following ideas for how various levels of interventions can be used to address racism, poverty and HIV among African Americans they have not been fully tested. The authors suggest that these recommendations merit testing in the future.

Structural interventions are most appropriate for altering conditions beyond the control of the individual (Sumartojo, 2000). Structural factors operate at multiple levels and can include key characteristics of the environment, such as resources, economic opportunities, laws, policies, and organizational and community structures (Gupta, Parkhurst, Ogden, Aggleton, & Mahal, 2008; Sumartojo). Because structural level interventions tend to be broad in scope, the authors suggest that they are well suited for addressing such complex phenomena as racism, poverty and HIV. Examples of structural level interventions that have been used to address poverty-related mechanisms associated with HIV risk include condom distribution programs (Cohen & Scribner, 2000; Cohen et al., 1999), free or affordable housing programs for HIV-positive persons (Aidala et al., 2005) and microenterprise programs that provide alternative sources of income for at risk women to increase economic dependence (Sherman, German, Cheng, Marks, & Bailey-Kloche, 2006). Stratford, Mizuno, Williams, Courtenay-Quirk, and O'Leary (2008) proposed using microenterprise as a strategy for HIV prevention among African American women. This approach has been widely used internationally to produce income as a means to improve health outcomes and has been shown to increase women's financial security while enhancing contraceptive use (Waters, Rodriguez-Garcia, & Macinko, 2001). More recently the implementation of a microenterprise program resulted in decreased engagement in sexual risk behaviors among young women in South Africa (Pronyk, Kim, Abramsky, Phetla, & Hargreaves, 2008).

Appropriate as well are community-level interventions which seek to affect change at the population level. Community-level interventions address community norms, allow members to share a common identity and consciousness, and support collective engagement in a broader network of systems and resources (Thompson & Kinne, 1990; Kalichman, 1998). Thus, empowering local communities is believed necessary to address co-mingling adversities influencing disparate rates of HIV in African American communities. Community level interventions addressing racism and poverty may, for example, use mass media campaigns to dispel prejudices against African Americans or mobilize communities to take action against unequal wage earnings, while at the same time promote health messages.

Group level interventions may be appropriate for addressing the complex pathways in which racism, discrimination and poverty impact health, as these types of interventions provide the opportunity to simultaneously intervene with several individuals. This strategy has several benefits (Kalichman, 1998). Among African Americans, experiences with racism and poverty are largely not viewed as unique or isolated phenomena but as shared experiences. Therefore, group-level interventions could allow members to reveal experiences among peers, gain confirmation, become more connected, strengthen supportive networks and increase ethnic pride, while at the same time increasing the ability and skills necessary to reduce HIV-related outcomes.

Individual-level interventions delivered one on one by a peer educator, counselor or other professional can address racism and poverty by, opening a session with the participants discussing experiences with racism, discrimination and poverty while providing them with a sensitive ear and acknowledging harsh realities, for example. This type of rapport building may allow the interventionist to set the stage for "meeting the participant where they are," thereby acknowledging and validating the participant within a broader social and economic context. Interventionists can integrate components that address the impact of history, tying in discussions about slavery and oppression, and informing the target population of the legacies of health-related consequences and their current relevance to the health status of African Americans.

Collaborative partnerships. Eradicating broader-level contextual factors such as racism and poverty should not be the charge of any one group, organization or establishment. What is required however is a broader quorum, a cadre of vested partners willing to work together to promote a relevant and tailored prevention agenda. (Sutton et al., 2009)). Thus, formulating effective partnerships is a necessary requisite and first step to addressing HIV/AIDS among African Americans. Multidisciplinary collaborations and approaches help to more clearly delineate the research agenda, and devise strategies to ensure that programs are appropriate and relevant for the affected population (Warnecke et al., 2008). As such, establishing effective partnerships with key stakeholders, including members of the target population, key community members and individuals representing public health, education, housing, labor, justice, transportation and religion, is necessary. Key policymakers and government agencies need to be at the table to create organizational and institutional changes to support fair and equitable practices, legislation and funding.

There is an African Proverb that states, "*Until lions have their own historians, tales of the hunt will always glorify the hunter.*" This proverb suggests that the development of HIV prevention intervention efforts seeking to reduce HIV/AIDS among African Americans may best be developed by researchers who share and understand similar experiences. Working in partnership with members of the affected population throughout the research process is particularly important, not only for gaining access to African American communities, but for ensuring that the methodological approaches taken are appropriate, relevant, and will result in the collection of valid and credible data. Engaging African Americans in setting a HIV prevention agenda that is relevant to their community and responsive to addressing needs will also help to ensure sustainability of efforts over time (Fitzpatrick, Sutton, & Greenberg, 2006).

Summary

Understanding and acknowledging the deleterious effects of complex social, economic and political realities are necessary to address HIV/AIDS infections impacting African Americans. Though many may view addressing racism and poverty as beyond the scope of HIV prevention, the authors assert that identifying and attacking root causes is a necessary requisite for eliminating disparities. However, we must first be willing to enter into open and honest, yet sometimes difficult, dialogue about these issues. Because racism and poverty are broader-level contextual factors, the most effective strategies will likely require using multiple methodologies at multiple levels. The recommendations herein offer an inclusive approach to investigate and begin to address racism and poverty in the U.S. and their implications for prevention and control of HIV among African Americans. As the root causes for HIV likely overlap with those of a multitude of adverse health outcomes, understanding the impact of the two constructs on health is integral to developing interventions that reduce HIV and other co-mingling health disparities among African Americans. Thus the field of HIV prevention could benefit from becoming part of an overarching agenda to eliminate overall health disparities and to promote health equity.

References

Adimora, A. A., & Schoenbach, V. J. (2002). Contextual factors and the black-white disparity in heterosexual HIV transmission. *Epidemiology (Cambridge, Mass.), 13*, 707–712.

Adimora, A. A., Schoenbach, V. J., & Doherty, I. A. (2006). HIV and African Americans in the southern United States: Sexual networks and social context. *Sexually Transmitted Diseases, 33*(Suppl. 7), S39–S45.

Aidala, A., Cross, J. E., Stall, R., Harre, D., & Sumartojo, E. (2005). Housing status and HIV risk behaviors: Implications for prevention and policy. *AIDS and Behavior, 9*, 251–264.

Aral, S. O., O'Leary, A., & Baker, C. (2006). Sexually transmitted infections and HIV in the southern United States: An overview. *Sexually Transmitted Diseases, 33*(Suppl. 7), S1–S5.

Bach, P. B., Pham, H. H., Schrag, D., Tate, R. C., & Hargraves, J. L. (2004). Primary care physicians who treat blacks and whites. *The New England Journal of Medicine, 351*, 575–584.

Bandura, A. (1986). *Social foundations of thought and action: A social cognitive theory.* Englewood Cliffs: Prentice Hall.

Beatty, L. A., Wheeler, D., & Gaiter, J. (2004). HIV prevention research for African Americans: Current and future directions. *The Journal of Black Psychology, 30*, 40–58.

Beverly, S. G. (2001). Measures of material hardship: Rationale and recommendations. *Journal of Poverty, 5*(1), 23–41.

Bharat, S. (2003). Racism and HIV/AIDS. *Dimensions of Racism, Proceedings of a workshop to commemorate the end of the United Nations third decade to combat Racism and Racial Discrimination* (HR/PUB/05/4). Paris, France: UN Office of the High Commissioner for Human Rights.

Boulware, L. E., Cooper, L. A., Ratner, L. E., LaVeist, T., & Powe, N. R. (2003). Race and trust in the health care system. *Public Health Reports, 118*, 358–365.

Bowen-Reid, T. L., & Harrell, J. P. (2002). Racist experiences and health outcomes: An examination of spirituality as a buffer. *The Journal of Black Psychology, 28*, 18–36.

Braveman, P. A., Cubbin, C., Egerter, S., Chideya, S., Marchi, K. S., Metzler, M., et al. (2005). Socioeconomic status in health research: One size does not fit all. *Journal of the American Medical Association, 294*, 2879–2888.

Brofenbrenner, U. (1979). *The ecology of human development: Experiments by nature and design.* Cambridge, MA: Harvard University Press.

Brondolo, E., Brady ver Halen, N., Pencille, M., Beatty, D., & Contrada, R. J. (2009). Coping with racism: A selective review of the literature and a theoretical and methodical critique. *Journal of Behavioral Medicine, 32*, 64–88.

Broman, C. I. (1996). Coping with personal problems. In H. W. Neighbors & J. S. Jackson (Eds.), *Mental health in Black America* (pp. 117–129). Thousand Oaks, CA: Sage.

Brown, D. (2008). African American resiliency: Examining racial socialization and social support as protective factors. *The Journal of Black Psychology, 34*, 32–48.

Bulhan, H. (1985). *Frantz Fanon and the psychology of oppression.* New York: Plenum.

Catz, S. L., Gore-Felton, C., & McClure, J. B. (2002). Psychological distress among minority and low-income women living with HIV. *Behavioral Medicine (Washington, D.C.), 28*, 53–60.

Centers for Disease Control and Prevention. (2008). *Sexually transmitted diseases surveillance, 2007.* Atlanta: US Department of Health and Human Services.

Centers for Disease Control and Prevention. (2009). *HIV/AIDS surveillance report, 2007.* Vol. 19. Atlanta: US Department of Health and Human Services.

Clark, V. (2001). The perilous effects of racism on blacks. *Ethnicity & Disease, 11*(4), 769–792.

Clark, R., Anderson, N. B., Clark, V. R., & Williams, D. R. (2002). Racism as a stressor for African Americans: A biosocial model. In T. A. LaViest (Ed.), *Race, ethnicity and health* (pp. 319–339). San Francisco, CA: Jossey-Bass.

Cochran, S. D., & Mays, V. M. (1993). Applying social psychological models to predicting HIV-related sexual risk behaviors among African Americans. *The Journal of Black Psychology, 19*(2), 142–154.

Cohen, D., Farley, T. A., Bedimo-Etame, J. R., Scribner, R., Ward, W., Kendall, C., et al. (1999). Implementation of condom social marketing in Louisiana, 1993 to 1996. *American Journal of Public Health, 89*, 204–208.

Cohen, D., & Scribner, R. (2000). An STD/HIV prevention intervention framework. *AIDS Patient Care and STDs, 14*, 37–45.

Cohen, D., Spear, S., Scribner, R., Kissinger, P., Mason, K., & Wildgen, J. (2000). "Broken windows" and the risk of gonorrhea. *American Journal of Public Health, 90*, 230–236.

Copeland, V. C. (2005). African Americans: Disparities in health care access and utilization. *Health & Social Work, 30*, 265–270.

Coudouel, A., Hentschel, J. S., & Wodon, Q. T. (2002). Poverty measurement and analysis. In J. Klugman (Ed.), *A sourcebook of poverty reduction strategies* (pp. 27–70). Washington, DC: World Bank.

Cunningham, W. E., Andersen, R. M., Katz, M. H., Stein, M. D., Turner, B. J., Crystal, S., et al. (1999). The impact of competing subsistence needs and barriers on access to medical care for persons with human immunodeficiency virus receiving care in the United States. *Medical Care, 37*, 1270–1281.

Dalaker, J. (2005). Alternative poverty estimates in the United States: 2003 (P60-227). *Current Population Reports:* Washington, DC: U.S. Census Bureau.

Darity, W. A. (2003). Employment discrimination, segregation and health. *American Journal of Public Health, 93*(2), 226–231.

DeNavas-Walt, C., Proctor, B. D., & Smith, J. (2009). Income, poverty, and health insurance coverage in the United States: 2008 (P60-236RV). *Current Population Reports: Consumer Income.* Washington, DC: U.S. Census Bureau.

Department of Health & Human Services. (2001). Closing the health gap: reducing health disparities affecting African-Americans. Retrieved from http://www.hhs.gov/news/press/2001pres/20011119a.html.

Diaz, R. M., Ayala, G., & Bein, E. (2004). Sexual risk as an outcome of social oppression: Data from a probability sample of Latino gay men in three U.S. cities. *Cultural Diversity & Ethnic Minority Psychology, 10*, 255–267.

Diaz, T., Chu, S. Y., Buehler, J. W., Boyd, D., Checko, P. J., Conti, L., et al. (1994). Socioeconomic differences among people with AIDS: Results from a multistate surveillance project. *American Journal of Preventive Medicine, 10*, 217–222.

Ellerbrock, T. V., Chamblee, S., Bush, T. J., Johnson, J. W., Marsh, B. J., Lowell, P., et al. (2004). Human immunodeficiency virus infection in a rural community in the United States. *American Journal of Epidemiology, 160*, 582–588.

Federman, M., Garner, T. I., Short, K., Cutter, W. B., Kiely, J., Levine, D., et al. (1996). What does it mean to be poor in America? *Monthly Labor Review, 119*, 3–17.

Fife, D., & Mode, C. (1992). AIDS incidence and income. *Journal of Acquired Immune Deficiency Syndromes, 5*, 1105–1110.

Fitzpatrick, L. K., Sutton, M., & Greenberg, A. E. (2006). Toward eliminating health disparities in HIV/AIDS: The importance of the minority investigator in addressing scientific gaps in black and Latino communities. *Journal of the National Medical Association, 98*, 1906–1911.

Forna, F. M., Fitzpatrick, L., Adimora, A. A., McLellan-Lemal, E., Leone, P., Brooks, J. T., et al. (2006). A case-control study of factors associated with HIV infection among black women. *Journal of the National Medical Association, 98*, 1798–1804.

Gilbert, D. J., & Goddard, L. (2007). HIV prevention targeting African American women: Theory, objectives and outcomes from an African-centered behavior change perspective. *Family & Community Health, 30*(Suppl. 1), S109–S111.

Gupta, G. R., Parkhurst, J. O., Ogden, J. A., Aggleton, P., & Mahal, A. (2008). Structural approaches to HIV prevention. *Lancet, 30*, 764–775.

Harawa, N., & Adimora, A. (2008). Incarceration, African Americans and HIV: Advancing a research agenda. *Journal of the National Medical Association, 100*, 57–62.

Harrell, J. P., Hall, S., & Taliaferro, J. (2003). Physiological responses to racism and discrimination: Assessment of the evidence. *American Journal of Public Health, 93*, 243–248.

Harrell, S. P., Merchant, M. A., & Young, S. A. (1997, August). *Psychometric properties of the racism and life experience scales (RALES)*. Paper presented at the annual convention of the American Psychological Association, Chicago.

Heckman, T. G., Kochman, A., & Sikkema, K. J. (2002). Depressive symptoms in older adults living with HIV disease: Application of the chronic illness quality of life model. *Journal of Mental Health and Aging, 8*, 267–279.

Holzer, H. (2007). Reconnecting Young Black Men: What policies would help? In S. J. Jones (Ed.), *The state of black America 2007: Portrait of the black male* (pp. 75–87). Silver Spring, MD: Beckhamm Publications Group.

House, J. S., & Williams, D. R. (2000). Understanding and reducing socioeconomic and racial/ethnic disparities in health. In B. D. Smedley & S. L. Syme (Eds.), *Promoting health: Intervention strategies from social and behavioral research* (pp. 81–124). Washington, DC: National Academy Press.

Iceland, J. (2003). *Poverty in America: A handbook*. Berkley, CA: University of California Press.

Iceland, J., & Bauman, K. J. (2007). Income poverty and material hardship: How strong is the association? *The Journal of Socio-Economics, 36*, 376–396.

Israel, B. A., Eng, E., Schulz, A. J., & Parker, E. A. (2005). Introduction to methods in community-based participatory research for health. In B. A. Israel, E. Eng, A. J. Schulz, & E. Parker (Eds.), *Methods in community-based participatory research* (pp. 3–26). San Francisco, CA: Jossey-Bass.

Jackson, J. S., Brown, T. N., Williams, D. R., Torres, M., Sellers, S. K. & Brown, K. (1996). Racism and the physical and mental health status of African Americans: a thirteen year national panel study. *Ethnicity & Disease, 6*, 132–47.

Johnson, L. B., & Staples, R. (1993). *Black families at the crossroads: Challenges and prospects*. San Francisco, CA: Jossey-Bass.

Jones, J. M. (1972). *Prejudice and racism*. New York: McGraw-Hill.

Jones, J. (1993). *Bad blood: The Tuskegee syphilis experiment*. New York and London: Free Press.

Jones, C. P. (2000). Levels of racism: A theoretic framework and a gardener's tale. *American Journal of Public Health, 90*(8), 1212–1215.

Jones, C. P. (2003). Confronting institutionalized racism. *Phylon, 50*, 7–22.

Kalichman, S. C. (1998). Preventing AIDS: A Sourcebook for Behavioral Interventions. Mahwah, NJ: Lawrence Erlbaum Associates.

Klonoff, E. A., & Landrine, H. (1999a). Do blacks believe that HIV/AIDS is a government conspiracy against them? *Preventive Medicine, 28*, 451–457.

Klonoff, E. A., & Landrine, H. (1999b). Racial discrimination and psychiatric symptoms among blacks. *Cultural Diversity & Ethnic Minority Psychology, 5*, 329–339.

Konkle-Parker, D. J., Erlen, J. A., & Dubbert, P. M. (2008). Barriers and facilitators to medication adherence in a southern minority population with HIV disease. *The Journal of the Association of Nurses in AIDS Care, 19*, 98–104.

Kressin, N. R., Raymond, K. L., & Manze, M. (2008). Perceptions of race/ethnicity-based discrimination: A review of measures and evaluation of their usefulness for the health care setting. *Journal of Health Care for the Poor and Underserved, 19*, 697–730.

Krieger, N. (1990). Racial and gender discrimination: Risk factors for high blood pressure? *Social Science & Medicine, 30*, 1273–1281.

Krieger, N. (2000). Discrimination and health. In L. Berkman & I. Kawachi (Eds.), *Social epidemiology* (pp. 36–75). Oxford, England: Oxford University Press.

Krieger, N. (2005). Embodying inequality: A review of concepts, measures, and methods for studying health consequences of discrimination. In N. Krieger (Ed.), *Embodying inequality: Epidemiologic perspectives* (pp. 101–158). New York: Baywood Publishing Company.

Krieger, N., Chen, J. T., Waterman, P. D., Rehkopf, D. H., & Subramanian, S. V. (2005). Painting a truer picture of US socioeconomic and racial/ethnic health inequalities: The public health disparities geocoding project. *American Journal of Public Health, 95*, 312–323.

Krieger, N., Rowley, D., Hermann, A. A., Avery, B., & Phillips, M. T. (1993). Racism, sexism and social class: Implications for studies of health, disease and well-being. *American Journal of Preventive Medicine, 9*, 82–122.

Krieger, N., & Sidney, S. (1996). Racial discrimination and blood pressure: The CARDIA study of young black and white adults. *American Journal of Public Health, 86*, 1370–1378.

Krueger, L. E., Wood, R. W., Diehr, P. H., & Maxwell, C. L. (1990). Poverty and HIV seropositivity: The poor are more likely to be infected. *AIDS (London, England), 4*, 811–814.

Kwate, N. O., Valdimarsdottir, H. B., Guevarra, J. S., & Vovbjerg, D. H. (2003). Experiences of racist events are associated with negative health consequences for African American women. *Journal of the National Medical Association, 95*, 450–460.

Landrine, H., & Klonoff, E. A. (1996). The schedule of racist events: A measure of racial discrimination and a study of its negative physical and mental health consequences. *The Journal of Black Psychology, 22*, 144–168.

Latif, S. A., & Latif, N. (1994). *Slavery: The African American psychic trauma.* Chicago: Latif Communications Group.

Latkin, C. A., Curry, A. D., Hua, W., & Davey, M. A. (2007). Direct and indirect associations of neighborhood disorder with drug use and high-risk sexual partners. *American Journal of Preventive Medicine, 32*(Suppl. 6), S234–S241.

Latkin, C. A., & Knowlton, A. R. (2005). Micro-social structural approaches to HIV prevention: A social ecological perspective. *AIDS Care, 17*(Suppl. 1), S102–S113.

LaVeist, T. A. (Ed.). (2002). *Race, ethnicity and health.* San Francisco, CA: Jossey-Bass.

LaVeist, T. A., Sellers, R. M., & Neighbors, H. W. (2001). Perceived racism and self and system blame attribution: Consequences for longevity. *Ethnicity & Disease, 11*, 711–721.

Lazarus, R., & Folkman, S. (1984). *Stress, appraisal and coping.* New York: Springer.

Leary, J. D. (2005). *Post-traumatic slave syndrome: America's legacy of enduring injury and healing.* Milwaukie, OR: Uptone Press.

Lemelle, A. J. (2003). Linking the structure of African American criminalization to the spread of HIV/AIDS. *Journal of Contemporary Criminal Justice, 19*, 270–292.

Lewis-Trotter, P. B., & Jones, J. (2004). Racism: Psychological perspectives. In R. Jones (Ed.), *Black psychology* (pp. 559–588). Oakland, CA: Cobb & Henry Publishers.

Mayer, S. E., & Jencks, C. (1989). Poverty and the distribution of material hardship. *The Journal of Human Resources, 24*, 88–113.

Mays, V. M., & Cochran, S. D. (1988). Issues in the perception of AIDS risk and risk reduction activities by Black and Hispanic/Latina women. *The American Psychologist, 43*, 949–957.

Mays, V. M., Cochran, S. D., & Barnes, N. W. (2007). Race, race-based discrimination and health outcomes among African Americans. *Annual Review of Psychology, 58*, 201–225.

McLeroy, K. R., Bibeau, D., Steckler, A., & Glanz, K. (1988). An ecological perspective on health promotion programs. *Health Education Quarterly, 15*(4), 351–377.

McNair, L. D., & Prather, C. M. (2004). African American women and AIDS: Factors influencing risk and reaction to HIV disease. *The Journal of Black Psychology, 30*, 106–123.

McNeilly, M., Anderson, N. B., Armstead, C. A., Clark, R., Corbett, M., Robinson, E. L., et al. (1996). The perceived racism scale: A multidimensional assessment of the experience of white racism among African Americans. *Ethnicity & Disease, 6*, 154–166.

Minkler, M., & Wallerstein, N. (1990). Improving health through community organization. In K. Glanz, F. M. Lewis, & B. K. Rimer (Eds.), *Health behavior and health education: Theory, research, and practice* (pp. 257–287). San Francisco, CA: Jossey-Bass.

Minkler, M., & Wallerstein, N. (Eds.). (2003). *Community based participatory research for health*. San Francisco, CA: Jossey-Bass.

Moore, L. (2000). Psychiatric contributions to understanding racism. *Transcultural Psychiatry, 37*, 147–183.

Morris-Prather, C. E., Harrell, J. P., Collins, R., Leonard, K. L., Boss, M., & Lee, J. W. (1996). Gender differences in mood and cardiovascular responses to socially stressful stimuli. *Ethnicity & Disease, 6*, 123–131.

Moutsiakis, D. L., & Chin, N. P. (2007). Why blacks do not take part in HIV vaccine trials. *Journal of the National Medical Association, 99*, 254–257.

Murrell, N. (1996). Stress, self-esteem, and racism: Relationships with low birth weight and preterm delivery in African American women. *Journal of National Black Nurses' Association, 8*(1), 45–53.

National Institute of Mental Health. (1983). *Research highlights: Extramural research*. Washington, DC: US Government Printing Office.

Nobles, W. W. (1985). *Africanity and the black family: The development of a theoretical model*. Oakland, CA: The Institute for the Advanced Study of Black Family Life and Culture, Inc.

Nobles, W. W. (1986). *African psychology: Towards its reclamation, reascension and revitalization*. Oakland, CA: Black Family Institute.

Nobles, W. W. (2006). *Seeking the sakhu: Foundational writings for an African psychology*. Chicago: Third World Press.

Nobles, W. W., Goddard, L. L., & Gilbert, D. J. (2009). Culturecology, women and African-centered HIV prevention. *The Journal of Black Psychology, 35*(2), 228–246.

Paradies, Y. (2006). A systematic review of empirical research on self-reported racism and health. *International Journal of Epidemiology, 35*, 888–901.

Pascoe, E. A., & Smart, R. L. (2009). Perceived discrimination and health: A meta-analytic review. *Psychological Bulletin, 135*(4), 531–554.

Prado, G., Feaster, D. J., Schwartz, S. J., Pratt, I. A., Smith, L., & Szapocznik, J. (2004). Religious involvement, coping, social support, and psychological distress in HIV-seropositive African American mothers. *AIDS and Behavior, 8*, 221–235.

Pronyk, P. M., Kim, J. C., Abramsky, T., Phetla, G., & Hargreaves, J. R. (2008). A combined microfinance and training intervention can reduce HIV risk behaviour in young female participants. *AIDS (London, England), 22*, 1659–1665.

Randall, V. (2006). *Dying while black: An in-depth look at a crisis in the American healthcare system*. Dayton, OH: Seven Principles Press.

Rector, R., Johnson, K., & Youssef, S. (1999). The extent of material hardship and poverty in the United States. *Review of Social Economy, 57*, 351–387.

Reif, S., Geonnotti, K. L., & Whetten, K. (2006). HIV infection and AIDS in the Deep South. *American Journal of Public Health, 96*, 970–973.

Roberts, A. C., Wechsberg, W. M., Zule, W., & Burroughs, A. R. (2003). Contextual factors and other correlates of sexual risk of HIV among African-American crack-abusing women. *Addictive Behaviors, 28*, 523–536.

Ross, C. E., & Mirowsky, J. (2001). Neighborhood disadvantage, disorder, and health. *Journal of Health and Social Behavior, 42*, 258–276.

Rothman, J., Tropman, J. E., & Erlich, J. L. (2001). Approaches to community intervention. In J. Rothman, J. E. Tropman, & J. L. Erlich (Eds.), *Strategies of community intervention* (pp. 27–64). Itasca, IL: F. E. Peacock Publishers.

Sherman, S. G., German, D., Cheng, Y., Marks, M., & Bailey-Kloche, M. (2006). The evaluation of the JEWEL project: An innovative economic enhancement and HIV prevention intervention study targeting drug using women involved in prostitution. *AIDS Care, 18*, 1–11.

Simon, P. A., Hu, D. J., Diaz, T., & Kerndt, P. R. (1995). Income and AIDS rates in Los Angeles County. *AIDS (London, England), 9*, 281–284.

Smedley, B. D., Stith, A. Y., & Nelson, A. R. (Eds.). (2003). *Unequal treatment: Confronting racial and ethnic disparities in health care.* Washington, DC: National Academy Press.

Smedley, B. D., & Syme, S. L. (Eds.). (2000). *Promoting health: Strategies from social and behavioral research.* Washington, DC: National Academy Press.

Southern AIDS Coalition. (2003). *Southern states manifesto-HIV/AIDS and STDs in the south: A call to action.* Retrieved March 2, 2003, from http://www.southernaidscoalition.org/policy/SouthernStatesManifesto_2003.pdf.

Stratford, D., Mizuno, Y., Williams, K., Courtenay-Quirk, C., & O'Leary, A. (2008). Addressing poverty as risk for disease: Recommendations from CDC's consultation on microenterprise as HIV prevention. *Public Health Reports, 123*, 9–20.

Sullivan, P. S., McNaghten, A. D., Begley, E., Hutchinson, A., & Cargill, V. A. (2007). Enrollment of racial/ethnic minorities and women with HIV in clinical research studies of HIV medicines. *Journal of the National Medical Association, 99*, 242–250.

Sumartojo, E. (2000). Structural factors in HIV prevention: Concepts, examples, and implications for research. *AIDS (London, England), 14*(Suppl. 1), S3–S10.

Sutton, M., Jones, R., Wolitski, R., Cleveland, J., Dean, H., & Fenton K. (2009). A review of the Centers for Disease Control and Prevention's response to the HIV/AIDS crisis among Blacks in the United States, 1981–2009. *American Journal of Public Health, 99*, S351–9.

Thomas, J. C., & Thomas, K. K. (1999). Things ain't what they ought to be: Social forces underlying racial disparities in rates of sexually transmitted diseases in a rural North Carolina county. *Social Science & Medicine, 49*, 1075–1084.

Thomas, S. B., & Quinn, S. C. (1991). The Tuskegee Syphilis Study, 1932 to 1972: Implications for HIV education and AIDS risk education programs in the black community. *American Journal of Public Health, 81*, 1498–1505.

Thompson, B. & Kinne, S. (1990). Social change theory: Applications to Community Health. In: Bracht N. (Ed.). *Health Promotion at the Community Level.* Newbury Park: Sage Publications.

U.S. Census Bureau. (2007). The American community – Blacks: 2004 (ACS-04). *American Community Survey Reports.* Washington, DC: U.S. Census Bureau.

U.S. Census Bureau. (2009). Current Population Survey, 2008: Annual social and economic supplement. Retrieved from http://www.census.gov/population/www/socdemo/hh-fam/cps2008.html.

Utsey, S. O., & Hook, J. N. (2007). Heart rate variability as a physiological moderator of the relationship between race-related stress and psychological stress. *Cultural Diversity & Ethnic Minority Psychology, 13*, 250–253.

Utsey, S. O., & Ponterotto, J. G. (1996). Development and validation of the index of race-related stress (IRRS). *Journal of Counseling Psychology, 43*, 1–12.

Utsey, S. O., Ponterotto, J. G., Reynolds, A. L., & Cancelli, A. A. (2000). Racial discrimination, coping, life satisfaction, and self-esteem among African Americans. *Journal of Counseling and Development, 78*, 72–80.

Wadsworth, M. E. & Decarlo Santiago, C. (2008). Risk and resiliency processes in ethnically diverse families in poverty. *Journal of Family Psychology, 22*(3), 399–410.

Warnecke, R. B., Oh, A., Breen, N., Gehlert, S., Paskett, E., Tucker, K. L., et al. (2008). Approaching health disparities from a population perspective: The National Institutes of Health Centers for Population Health and Health Disparities. *American Journal of Public Health, 98*, 1608–1615.

Washington, H. A. (2006). *Medical Apartheid: The Dark History of Medical Experimentation on Black Americans from Colonial Times to the Present*. New York: Doubleday Press.

Waters, W. F., Rodriguez-Garcia, R., & Macinko, J. A. (2001). *Microenterprise development for better health outcomes*. Westport, CT: Greenwood Press.

Williams, C. (1987). *Destruction of black civilization: Great issues of a race from 4500 BC to 200 AD*. Chicago: Third World Press.

Williams, D. R. (1999). Race, socioeconomic status, and health: The added effects of racism and discrimination. *Annals of the New York Academy of Sciences, 896*, 173–188.

Williams, D. R., & Mohammed, S. A. (2009). Discrimination and racial disparities in health: Evidence and needed research. *Journal of Behavioral Medicine, 32*, 20–47.

Williams, D. R., Neighbors, H. W., & Jackson, J. S. (2008). Racial/ethnic discrimination and health: Findings from community studies. *American Journal of Public Health, 98*, 29–37.

Williams, D. R., & Williams-Morris, R. (2000). Racism and mental health: The African American experience. *Ethnicity & Health, 5*, 243–268.

Williams, D. R., Yu, Y., Jackson, J. S., & Anderson, N. B. (1997). Racial differences in physical and mental health: Socioeconomic status, stress and discrimination. *Journal of Health Psychology, 2*, 335–351.

Wohl, A. R., Lu, S., Odem, S., Sorvillo, F., Pegues, C. & Kerndt, P. R. (1998). Sociodemographic and Behavioral Characteristics of African-American Women with HIV and AIDS in Los Angeles County, 1990–1997. Journal of Acquired Immune Deficiency Syndromes & Human Retrovirology, *1*, 413–420.

Woolf, S. H., Johnson, R. E., & Geiger, H. J. (2006). The rising prevalence of severe poverty in America: A growing threat to public health. *American Journal of Preventive Medicine, 31*, 332–341.

Wyatt, S. B., Williams, D. R., Calvin, R., Henderson, F. C., Walker, E. R., & Winters, K. (2000). Racism and cardiovascular disease in African Americans. *The American Journal of the Medical Sciences, 325*, 315–331.

Zierler, S., & Krieger, N. (1997). Reframing women's risk: Social inequalities and HIV infection. *Annual Review of Public Health, 18*, 401–436.

Zierler, S., Krieger, N., Tang, Y., Coady, W., Siegfried, E., DeMaria, A., et al. (2000). Economic deprivation and AIDS incidence in Massachusetts. *American Journal of Public Health, 90*, 1064–1073.

Chapter 4
Organized Religion and the Fight Against HIV/AIDS in the Black Community: The Role of the Black Church*

Agatha N. Eke, Aisha L. Wilkes, and Juarlyn Gaiter

Introduction

Religious faith and practices have long been an important consideration in health and well-being. Historically, religious institutions including the Black Church (i.e., any predominately African American religious congregation) have had important influences on public health and the practice of medicine (Chatters, Levin, & Ellison, 1998; Giger, Appel, Davidhizar, & Davis, 2008; Koenig, 2000). Over the last two decades there has been a resurgence of interest in the relationship between religion and health (Chatters, 2000; Ellison & Levin, 1998), because research has documented a correlation between religion and morbidity and mortality (Levin, 2003). There are over 1,200 published empirical studies of which 75–90% shows a positive association between aspects of religious faith and indicators of health status and emotional well-being at the population level (Koenig, McCullough, & Larson, 2001). Some of the most methodologically sophisticated, rigorously evaluated studies with the largest scope of health outcomes have been epidemiological studies of African Americans (Levin, Chatters, & Taylor, 2005). Levin et al. note that this body of work termed the "epidemiology of religion" contains findings showing associations between expressions of religiousness and mental health, psychological well-being, healthy lifestyles, health care utilization and health related outcomes. This is critical literature, given the growing disparities in HIV/AIDS particularly among disadvantaged (economically deprived/medically underserved individuals) African Americans and other racial/ethnic groups. Consequently, public health professionals are paying close attention to the unique and important role that religious and faith-based organizations such as the Black Church can play in addressing these disparities.

---

* "The findings and conclusions in this report are those of the authors and do not necessarily represent the views of the Centers for Disease Control and Prevention."

A.N. Eke (✉)
Division of HIV/AIDS Prevention, Centers for Disease Control and Prevention,
1600 Clifton Road, MS E-37, Atlanta, GA 30333, USA
e-mail: AEke@cdc.gov

African Americans have disproportionate morbidity and mortality associated with cancer, diabetes, infant mortality, obesity, high blood pressure, strokes, cardiovascular disease and especially HIV/AIDS (Centers for Disease Control and Prevention (CDC), 2005). Since the beginning of the HIV/AIDS epidemic in the United States, African Americans have been overrepresented among those living with and dying from AIDS. CDC statistics also show that African Americans are more likely to die from AIDS than people of any other race or ethnicity (CDC, HIV/AIDS surveillance report, 2008). These alarming statistics allude to the limitations of the public sector in preventing the spread of HIV/AIDS in African-American communities (Leong, 2003). African Americans, therefore, must rely more heavily on community resources for HIV/AIDS prevention and intervention, a system that is already reeling under the weight of responding to the excess morbidity and mortality from other conditions such as cardiovascular disease and diabetes (Fullilove, 2006).

Black Churches, which for decades have been responsive to the many health problems that plague African Americans (Logan & Freeman, 2000), have been slow to mobilize their communities to fight HIV/AIDS. This chapter will explore the role that organized religion has played in protecting public health and more closely examine how the Black Church can partner with public health professionals in preventing HIV/AIDS among African Americans.

The Role of Religion in Peoples' Lives

Religion has been defined as an organized system of beliefs, practices, rituals, and symbols that foster closeness to the sacred as in a higher power or God (Moreira-Almeida, Neto, & Koenig, 2006; Mystakidou, Tsilika, Parpa, Smyrnioti, & Vlahos, 2007). Religious practices, beliefs and values have played a vital role in shaping the lives and cultures of many people throughout the world. According to UNAIDS (2008), about 70% of the world's population identifies with a religious or faith community. Religious values and practices are often deeply rooted in the daily routines of individuals, and religious organizations such as churches, mosques, temples and other faith communities exert tremendous influence on a spectrum of human affairs including beliefs, and political, social and cultural viewpoints and practices (UNFPA, 2008). In a recent Gallup poll, 65% of Americans said that religion is an important part of their daily lives (Gallup, 2009).

The broad influence of religion is even more fundamental to the character and survival of African Americans as a community in the United States (Carver & Reinert, 2002; Newlin, Knafl, & Melkus, 2002). A nationally representative telephone survey by the Pew Forum on Religion and Public Life (2008) confirmed that African Americans are significantly more religious than the general U.S. population. This was evident from a variety of measures including level of religious affiliation, attendance at religious services, frequency of praying and the importance of religion in daily life decisions. Religious involvement, expressed either as personal spirituality or congregational participation, is a prominent component of African American culture, and permeates nearly every domain of life in the African American community (Newlin et al.).

Religious expression by African Americans is largely confined to the Black Church, which historically has served as a source of liberation, solace, hope, meaning and forgiveness, particularly in relationship to social, political and economic injustices (Dash, Jackson, & Rasor, 1997; Musgrave, Allen, & Allen, 2002; Newlin et al., 2002). Given the influence of religion and religious organizations, especially in the African American community, it is important to engage and persuade religious leaders to be partners with public health in addressing HIV/AIDS and other related health problems.

Organized Religion and Public Health

Faith based organizations, particularly those of the Christian tradition, were among the pioneers in the early practice of medicine (Amundsen, 1998). Inspired by the biblical injunction to "heal the sick" and "cleanse the lepers," Christian religious institutions built the first hospitals, and early physicians and nurses were often clerics, monks and other religious orders (Amundsen; Koenig et al., 2001). Religious institutions share a legacy of caring for the sick, the elderly and the needy with the public health community (Chatters et al., 1998; Foege, 1997). They have also been integral to the success of social reform movements throughout the world, having engaged in issues of social justice including health care, civil rights, apartheid, environmental justice, reproductive rights, poverty and hunger (Marsh, 2005; Pratt, 1997; Van Reken, 1999). They are, therefore, uniquely positioned to help bring health care to people that are in the most need of care, particularly poor and disenfranchised communities.

The growing disparities in HIV/AIDS and other health problems, particularly among African Americans and other poor racial/ethnic groups, coupled with dwindling financial resources requires even greater attention and help from religious and faith-based organizations. Fortunately, there is a track record of partnerships between public health and religious organizations (Cantor, 1996; Derose et al., 2000). Religious or faith-based organizations have long been essential supporters of public health (Foege, 1997). Congregations (including churches, synagogues, mosques, and temples) and social service organizations with religious roots (such as Catholic Charities, Lutheran Social Services and Salvation Army) provide food and shelter, child care, and other forms of emergency assistance, particularly for low-income people (Kramer, Finegold, De Vita, & Wherry, 2005). Furthermore, recent US federal administrations support the idea of faith-based organizations as ideal partners in providing health care and other services to the public (Francis & Liverpool, 2009). Thus, health professionals and agencies, including government agencies like the CDC, have developed policies that recognize the potential role of religious organizations in health care. Since 2000, CDC has directly funded faith-based organizations and particularly Black Churches as partners in efforts to address disparities in many health problems including HIV/AIDS (CDC, 2006).

The Historical Role of the Black Church

The Black Church is the oldest, uniquely African American institution (Brown & Gary, 1994) that has played a critical role in the development and survival of African American communities since the time of slavery (Blackwell, 1991, Franklin & Moss, 1994; Lincoln & Mamiya, 2001). The Black Church is not monolithic, but rather diverse and dynamic, and encompasses any predominately African American congregation, even if it is part of a white American religious denomination (Adksion-Bradley, Johnson, Sanders, Duncan, Holcomb-McCoy, 2005; Giger et al., 2008). Although more likely to be represented in Christian denominations including Methodist, Baptist and Pentecostal faith traditions as well as in African American Catholicism (Pinn & Pinn, 2002), the Black Church incorporates elements of African religion and Euro-Christianity as well as Islamic and Judaic sectarianism (Lincoln & Mamiya). Thus, the Black Church experience in its various forms may exhibit the unification of these disparate religious traditions (Sanders, 2002).

Beyond its central spiritual mission, the Black Church is a major factor in the social structure of many black communities. As such it functions almost as a community support center that promotes social cohesion, mutual support, and provision especially in times of oppression, tragedy, and illness (Franklin, 1997; Lincoln and Mamiya, 2001). Given the extreme difficulty of coping with dehumanizing forces beyond their control African Americans during slavery were protected by sacred space and a zone of freedom to worship God, to express emotions that helped them to transcend their circumstances (Eng, Hatch, & Callan, 1985; Franklin, 1997). Franklin noted that slaves threw themselves with fervor into the worship experience knowing that the crowd of loving, caring people was the safest place in the world. Since the time of reconstruction, the Black Church has been the cornerstone of civil right movements, and has offered strong support as an arbiter of social justice for African Americans (Taylor, 2006). As an institution it stands as a vital source of leadership, social capital and tangible assistance for its members, families, and communities (Harris, 1994). According to Levin (1984), the Black Church has also been the preserver and the perpetuator of the black ethos, that is, the base from which the community's values are defined. It has also served as an autonomous social institution that has provided order and meaning to the black experience in the United States (Lincoln and Mamiya). Scholars have noted (Richardson & June, 1997; Taylor, Ellison, Chatters, Levin, & Lincoln, 2000) that no other institution in the United States can claim the loyalty and attention of African Americans that the Black Church claims. Thus, the Black Church is seen as a potent partner in addressing the myriad of health problems facing the African American community, including HIV/AIDS.

The leaders of Black Churches have historically been involved in health promotion ministries and provided an effective arena for preventive services to black communities (Logan & Freeman, 2000). Black ministers in many instances have not only functioned as teachers, preachers, and politicians, but also as promoters of health and wellness (Levin, 1984). Health ministries in churches have traditionally taken the form of sermons from the pulpit, nurse guilds, health fairs, seminars, and prevention interventions. Many Black Churches either independently or collaboratively have hosted health promotion programs in areas such as health education, screening for and management of high blood pressure and diabetes, weight loss and smoking cessation, cancer prevention and awareness, nutritional guidance and mental health (DeHaven, Hunter, Wilder, Walton, & Berry, 2004). Similarly, many Black Churches have addressed the problem of drug use and abuse in the community by initiating or encouraging participation of members in prevention and treatment programs (Sutherland, Hale, & Harris, 1995; Sutherland & Harris, 1994). Public health scientists and other researchers have espoused strategies to effectively collaborate with faith-based organizations for health promotion (Ammerman et al., 2003; Campbell et al., 2007; Sutherland et al., 1995).

The Black Church's Response to HIV and AIDS

Given the urgency and persistence of the HIV/AIDS epidemic among African American communities, social scientists and public health researchers are exploring ways to involve the Black Church in raising awareness among African Americans about the urgent need to prevent the spread of HIV. The church's response to date has been slow, and only a few faith-based HIV prevention programs have been established (Francis & Liverpool, 2009). While some members of the Black Church have actively provided care (e.g., food, shelter, and other needs), for people in their communities who were infected and affected since the start of the HIV epidemic, many Black Church leaders have remained quiet about this growing epidemic. The CBS Evening News (2008) reported, "The Black Church, a loud, voice for social change, has been curiously silent on the crisis of AIDS in the African-American community, and some say, even negligent."

As the HIV/AIDS infection and death rates have escalated in the African American community, it has become more and more difficult for church leaders to stand back from the catastrophe unfolding around them (Niles, 1996). Many Black Church leaders across the country have recognized the great need for the church to become involved, and have begun initiatives aimed at breaking the silence and eliminating the stigma and prejudice associated with HIV/AIDS in the African American community (Swartz, 2002). A significant number of Black Churches are now actively engaged in ministries and programs that focus on promoting awareness for prevention and providing support for people living with AIDS (http://www.balmingilead.org/index.html, 2009; www.arkofrefuge.org, 2009).

The level of involvement in HIV/AIDS prevention outreach varies from one church to another. While some religious leaders openly discuss HIV/AIDS including issues such as condom use and homosexuality, others do not. Some churches have chosen to be involved in aspects of HIV/AIDS programs that do not contradict their doctrine or religious principle (Francis & Liverpool, 2009). For example, some Black Churches feel more comfortable providing assistance to people who are living with AIDS, consistent with the church's compassionate values, than engaging in prevention activities that would involve discussion of sensitive issues such as homosexuality and injection drug use. Other Black Churches involved in providing HIV/AIDS services choose not advertise their involvement (Swartz, 2002).

The following are examples of actions faith leaders have undertaken to address the HIV epidemic:

1. The Balm in Gilead Inc. in New York, works with Black Churches to stop the spread of HIV/AIDS in the African American community and to support those infected with and affected by the epidemic. This not-for-profit, non-governmental organization was created in 1989 by Pernessa Seele (Cohen, 1999; Niles, 1996) beginning with The Black Church National Week of Prayer for the Healing of AIDS. This annual national program mobilizes thousands of Black Church leaders to learn how to talk to their congregations about preventing the transmission of HIV. The Balm in Gilead provides comprehensive educational programs and offer compassionate support to encourage those who are HIV-infected to seek and maintain treatment (Niles). Another activity, the "Our Church Lights the Way" ministry, was launched in 1999 and encourages Black Churches to support and promote HIV Testing Month. In partnership with the CDC, this program engages the support of black ministers to empower and encourage African Americans to get tested for HIV and to know their status. The campaign supports faith institutions in offering their place of worship as community centers for AIDS education, and related services, making the program community owned and driven (http://www.balmingilead.org/index.html., 2009).

2. The ARK of Refuge is a faith-based HIV prevention program founded in 1988 by Bishop Yvette Flounder of the City of Refuge United Church of Christ in San Francisco. The Ark provides HIV/AIDS education and prevention services for African Americans (Public Media and the AIDS National Interfaith Network, 1997). The Ark recently opened a primary care facility, the Magic Johnson Clinic, in collaboration with AIDS Healthcare Foundation. The organization also provides substance abuse intervention programs, transitional housing for homeless youth, mentorship programs, and a computer lab, and audio/video training for community youth (The ARK of Refuge, 2009; http://www.arkofrefuge.org/flunder_bio_2004.shtml).

Leong (2003) describes the following two other examples of faith-based HIV/AIDS programs that reveal differences in approach and the levels of involvement by Black Churches in HIV/AIDS ministry which include:

The Universal Church, a predominantly African American church in an urban area of the West coast has an HIV/AIDS ministry whose mission is to reduce suffering and deaths due to HIV infection. This program increases the accessibility of HIV/AIDS-related health services and education and advocates for services for marginalized, overlooked, and underserved individuals, regardless of their demographics or sexual orientation. This contemporary church was founded in 1980 in response to the needs of gay individuals who were affected by HIV/AIDS. The pastors and congregation openly discuss HIV/AIDS and its impact during church services. The church's mission is inspired by the belief that "God is Love" and that love is the basis of all individuals, regardless of race, creed, color, religious affiliation, class or sexual orientation (Leong, 2003).

The Pacific African Methodist Episcopal Church (Pacific A.M.E.) is another metropolitan church and one of the first Black Churches in the western United States (Leong, 2003). This church approaches HIV prevention in a conservative manner that is congruent with the values of traditional African American churches (Pew Forum on Religion and Public Life, 2008). The church's main focus is to increase racial awareness by educating the public at large about racial disparities. Church leaders promote spiritual, economic, political and moral wellbeing among the members. There is not open discussion about issues of sexuality. This church is reluctant to engage in HIV/AIDS outreach to gays and bisexuals, however, it does provide an HIV/AIDS program to individuals the church considers to be "innocent" victims of HIV/AIDS. This group of innocent people includes mostly heterosexual women who contracted HIV from their male partners.

The stark differences in the approaches to HIV/AIDS issues by these two churches are attributed to their varying sociopolitical and ideological dispositions (Leong, 2003). Their perspectives are informed by their respective church origins (i.e., the founding philosophy of their churches), demographic characteristics of church members, and church leadership. These factors shape the churches' attitudes toward sexuality and HIV/AIDS. For example, the religious leaders and the members of the congregation at the Universal Church represent a range of minority groups (i.e., HIV-positive, racial/ethnic, low SES, and sexual minorities). Therefore, the leaders at Universal Church have re-defined the goals of religion and spirituality, and re-interpreted religion in ways that address their parishioners' unique needs, doing so in a manner that empowers all individuals (Leong, 2003). In contrast, the Pacific A.M.E. Church is comprised mostly of middle-class and working class African Americans. Their religious instructions and messages emphasize racial consciousness and a black theology that encourages self-help and personal responsibility (Leong, 2003).

Barriers to the Black Church's involvement in HIV/AIDS

It is important to note that religious leaders face multiple constraints that can restrict their participation in HIV/AIDS prevention efforts. Black Churches confront not only doctrinal limitations, but also significant political and sociocultural constraints that impede HIV/AIDS prevention efforts in church settings (Leong, 2003). Hammonds (1997) argued that African American religious leaders are wary about the larger society's tendency to perceive African Americans in pathological terms, i.e., not deserving of social protection. This assumption implies that African Americans are being held personally responsible for their disproportionate rates of

HIV/AIDS. Also, because of their high HIV prevalence rates, African Americans may be viewed as social contagions by the larger public (Hammonds). Consequently, Leong believes that the resistance by the Black Church leaders to confront HIV/AIDS as a serious health problem may have less to do with denial of HIV/AIDS in their community, but more to do with a rejection of racist assumptions and potential actions aimed at social control of African Americans. It is also possible that the role of public health in the legacy of the Tuskegee Experiment makes Black Churches very protective of African Americans (Thomas, 2000). Therefore, there may be varying levels of suspicion and resistance to collaborating with social scientists and public health researchers in the Black Church.

Furthermore, the Black Church faces contradictions in addressing the HIV/AID epidemic. On the one hand, church leaders have been vocal and in the front lines to help liberate African Americans from all forms of oppression (Leong, 2003). However, the church is perceived as the most conservative institution in the African American community. This perception constrains the willingness of the church to respond to HIV/AIDS. HIV/AIDS is perceived as a moral problem by many African American religious leaders (Leong). This attitude has led some pastors and ministers to either deny the existence of HIV/AIDS, or to be silent about the epidemic even though they may be personally involved in HIV/AIDS efforts. This conflict and reluctance on the part of some in the Black Church has helped to fuel discrimination against and stigmatization of people who are living with AIDS or perceived to be at risk for the disease (Brooks, Etzel, Hinojos, Henry, & Perez, 2005; Niles, 1996). The same barriers that impede HIV/AIDS prevention efforts in the Black Church are also present in the larger African American community (Niles). A discussion of specific barriers that confront the Black Church regarding HIV/AIDS prevention programming follows.

Stigma and Discrimination

HIV-related stigma has been a driving force behind the many failed efforts, be it church or secular, to respond to HIV (Brooks et al., 2005; Herek, Capitanio, & Widaman, 2003). Stigma has been particularly at the center of the silence and denial surrounding the existence of HIV/AIDS in the African American community (Doupe and World Council of Churches, 2005a, 2005b; Fullilove, 2006). Studies have shown that HIV-related stigma is often rooted in fear, ignorance, misconceptions and myths about AIDS and how the disease is transmitted (Kaiser Family Foundation, 2006). Misconceptions and myths about how HIV/AIDS is transmitted must be aggressively addressed, particularly among communities with high rates of poverty, low literacy and high unemployment (Melkote, Muppidi, & Goswam, 2000).

Stigma and discrimination can make living with HIV/AIDS and being part of the faith community exceedingly difficult for some African Americans. This is because HIV stigma may shut down open discussion about the risky behaviors that can lead to infection and ways to avoid infection. Additionally, HIV-related stigma can make individuals afraid to be tested and fearful of getting their test results and may cause infected people to avoid seeking treatment until they are ill (Herek et al., 2003; Public Media Center, 1997).

Homophobia

Same sex relationship is highly stigmatized in the African American community as it is in most communities (Ward, 2005). Homosexual behavior is regarded by most Christian religions as a "sin." Many church leaders justify their conviction that homosexuality is a sin by referencing scriptures in the Bible, many of which have been debated by theologians (Miller, 2007). Moreover, there are ministers in some Black Churches who preach from the pulpit to rebuke the sin of homosexuality and illustrate the belief that heterosexuality is natural or normal by saying in their sermons that, "God created Adam and Eve, not Adam and Steve" (Clarke, 2001).

In spite of the controversies, homosexuals or gay people are active members of many Black Churches and some hold key jobs such as choir directors or musicians (Fullilove & Fullilove, 1999). Yet, gay church members are expected not to say anything about their sexual orientation. Fullilove and Fullilove reported results from focus groups focusing on AIDS in the Black Church.

Findings indicated that the overwhelming avoidance of HIV/AIDS and condemnation of homosexuality or same sex loving lifestyles in Black Churches have caused some gay people to leave the church. For many homosexuals, the decision to leave their church can be bittersweet, because while it may be liberating to leave a place that continuously defames who they are; they are leaving a community that, for many, has been their home church since youth. Some gay people start their own churches, and others join churches that are less negative and condemning (Fullilove and Fullilove, 1999).

Lack of Resources

The reluctance of some Black Churches to respond to HIV/AIDS may be due to limited resources. A survey of 22 Black clergy in Rhode Island showed that most (83%) ministers felt that HIV/AIDS services were needed in their churches and communities. However, they felt unqualified or lacked financial and other resources to provide these services (Smith, Simmons, & Mayer, 2005). Faith based organizations like many community based organizations face significant operational challenges including lack of organizational infrastructure, few sources of stable and long term funding, reliance primarily on volunteer efforts, high personnel turnover, and limited networking and program coordination opportunities (Kelly et al., 2005). This is particularly true for many Black Churches whose congregations are socially and economically disadvantaged. These churches provide assistance to parishioners coping with other major health threats such as breast cancer, diabetes, cardiovascular disease, infant mortality, substance abuse and gang violence. HIV/AIDS is yet another challenge that threatens to stretch personnel and financial resources of both rural and urban churches.

Summary and Recommendations

Faith-based organizations have a long history and strong reputation for making a difference in people's lives by meeting spiritual needs and delivering crucial health and social services (Lincoln and Mamiya, 2001). In particular, the Black Church is a beacon in the African American community and an advocate for social justice and eradication of health disparities among African Americans (Adksion-Bradley et al., 2005). However, this unique and influential role of the Black Church has been slow to include the prevention of HIV/AIDS which is very crucial for African Americans. The HIV/AIDS epidemic has widened particularly among disadvantaged African Americans many of whom may be unaware of their infection and lack knowledge about how the disease is transmitted (CDC, 2009). The current era of denial, complacency, and fear must be confronted. African Americans must be warned of their potential risk for HIV and AIDS by trusted, authoritative communicators who will tell them the truth with love. Therefore, faith leaders are especially needed as partners with public health to not only issue a call to action and present information about how to prevent and reduce further spread of HIV/AIDS, but also provide vital leadership for a community that is under siege by HIV/AIDS. There is a much more urgent need now to not only acknowledge the size and scope of the epidemic among African Americans but also to make preventing HIV/AIDS a priority by Black Churches. Therefore, it is critical that public health officials and researchers identify mechanisms to educate and empower religious leaders to promote HIV prevention, HIV testing and high quality care for HIV infected individuals.

There are obvious advantages in partnerships between religious and faith-based organizations and public health. For one, religious organizations and public health practitioners share common principles and values such as serving and protecting those who are less fortunate and unable to protect themselves, sponsoring health promotion activities including primary, secondary, and tertiary prevention, and serving as educators and catalysts for health-related behavioral change (Chatters et al., 1998). In addition, religious organizations are stable and often the most trusted institutions in the community, and command the loyalty and attention of large numbers of people (Derose et al., 2000). Most Black Churches have well established communication networks that allow for easy dissemination of information to their members. For example, information can be shared through announcements during congregational worship, bulletin distributed at church services, phone networks and mailing to members' homes (Hale & Bennett, 2003).

Volunteerism is also a strong tradition in most faith-based organizations, a resource that can be tapped for delivery of health programs to the community (Hale & Bennett, 2003). Some large, urban Black Churches can increase access to care and prevention services for the underserved and invisible members of their communities such as the homeless, drug-addicted individuals, and men and women who have returned home from prison (Cantor, 1996; Derose et al., 2000). This is a critical opportunity for churches to build capacity for HIV/AIDS programming with the assistance of public health professionals.

Despite the many benefits that Black Churches offer public health, health professionals must be aware of potential challenges to launching HIV prevention efforts in church settings. Religious doctrine and cultural traditions may limit the participation of some Black Churches in HIV/AIDS. Conflicts between religion and science are well established and religious organizations are often resistant to scientific strategies employed by public health professionals (Chatters et al., 1998; Sternberg, Munschauer, Carrow, & Sternberg, 2007). For example, leaders in the Black Church may view HIV/AIDS from a moral perspective while public health researchers are focused on a scientific perspective (e.g., finding proven strategies for reducing HIV transmission including engaging in protective sexual behaviors and avoiding substance use). In addition, as in other research/community partnerships, religious leaders may sense a loss of autonomy, and resist a potential opportunity for collaboration.

Recommendations

The foregoing discussion implies that it is possible to engage Black Churches in public health effort to stem the spread of HIV/AIDS in African American communities. To do this successfully requires strategies that encourage mutual cooperation from both the church and public health professionals. Public health partnerships with Black Churches and other faith-based organizations in HIV/AIDS prevention should focus on aligning assets and leveraging each other's strengths, rather than imposing on each other strategies that contradict each partner's principles and goals.

McNeal and Perkins (2007) recommend that strategies include promoting communication between the Black Church and health professionals. Communication between the church and health professionals will result in sharing of information, and highlight the many ways in which HIV/AIDS presents challenges to the doctrine and practice of the Black Church. Such challenges may include: reconciling the perceived evil of HIV/AIDS with the goodness of God, having positive attitude about sexuality and the body, being a healing and inclusive community, eliminating stigma and discrimination associated with HIV/AIDS, dealing with poverty, and transforming unjust social structures (Doupe and World Council of Churches, 2005a, b). Understanding these challenges is critical to finding common grounds on best ways to involve the church in HIV prevention without compromising its basic tenets and principles.

Another strategy to effectively engage the Black Church in prevention efforts is to provide ongoing HIV/AIDS education and capacity building for black religious leaders and congregations (McNeal & Perkins, 2007). Ongoing HIV/AIDS training and workshops for Black Church leaders including information about how HIV is transmitted, the risk factors, prevention and treatment; and HIV testing, counseling and referral services will improve their understanding of HIV/AIDS. Church leaders and health professionals develop techniques and skills for incorporating HIV/AIDS into different church programs, (e.g., how to address stigma that links HIV/AIDS to drug use and homosexuality). They should also seek ways of leveraging resources within and outside the church. For example, public health professionals can guide church leaders on effective strategies for collaborating with other community organizations including other churches' ministries, as well as local scientists and researchers in HIV/AIDS. Furthermore, Church leaders need guidance on how to access funding including federal funding to support their HIV prevention efforts. This would not only enhance their knowledge and skills, but improve their ability to explore and discover innovative strategies of reaching and educating their congregations about the risk of HIV infection (McNeal & Perkins).

In conclusion, while public health professionals may bear responsibility for leading community health improvement efforts such as preventing the spread of HIV/AIDS, their success hinges on their ability to establish and maintain effective partnerships throughout the community. They need to identify and work with all entities that influence community health – from other government agencies to businesses to not-for-profit organizations including faith based institutions, to the general citizenry (U.S. Department of Health and Human Services, 2002). Partnerships with Black Churches and other faith-based organizations in HIV/AIDS prevention could elevate prevention efforts at levels that no other institution can achieve with African Americans, and could hasten a future where the spread of HIV/AIDS in this community is reversed.

References

Adksion-Bradley, C., Johnson, D., Sanders, J. L., Duncan, L., & Holcomb-McCoy, C. (2005). Forging a collaborative relationship between the Black Church and the Counseling Profession. *Counseling and Values, 49*(2), 147–154.

Ammerman, A., Corbie-Smith, G., St George, D. M., Washington, C., Weathers, B., & Jackson-Christian, B. (2003). Research expectations among African American church leaders in the PRAISE! Project: A randomized trial guided by Community-Based Participatory Research. *American Journal of Public Health, 93*(10), 1720–1727.

Amundsen, D. W. (1998). *Medicine, society, and faith in the ancient and medieval worlds.* London: Cambridge University Press.

Blackwell, J. E. (1991). *The black community: diversity and unity* (3rd ed.). Reading, MA: Addison Wesley Publishing Company.

Brooks, R. A., Etzel, M. A., Hinojos, E., Henry, C. L., & Perez, M. (2005). Preventing HIV among Latino and African American gay and bisexual men in a context of HIV-related stigma, discrimination, and homophobia: Perspectives of providers. *AIDS Patient Care and STDs, 19*(11), 737–744.

Brown, D. R., & Gary, L. E. (1994). Religious involvement and health status among African American males. *Journal of the National Medical Association, 86*(11), 825–831.

Campbell, M. K., Hudson, M. A., Resnicow, K., Blakeney, N., Paxton, A., & Baskin, M. (2007). Church-based health promotion interventions: evidence and lessons learned. *Annual Review of Public Health, 28*, 213–234.

Carver V. C., & Reinert, B. R. (2002). Faith-based organizations. encyclopedia of public health. http://www.encyclopedia.com/doc/1G2-3404000331.html. Accessed 17 June 2009

Cantor, C. (1996). Mobilizing faith into health care activities. *Advances: Robert Wood Johnson Foundation Quarterly Newsletter, 3,* 10.

CBS Evening News. (2008, August 17). Black churches confront HIV-AIDS crisis. http://www.cbsnews.com/stories/2008/08/17/eveningnews/main4356729.shtml. Accessed 22 June 2009.

Centers for Disease Control and Prevention (CDC) (2006). CDC consultation on faith and HIV prevention. http://www.cdc.gov/hiv/resources/other/PDF/faith.pdf. Accessed 13 July 2009.

CDC Fact Sheet (2009). HIV and AIDS among African Americans. http://www.cdc.gov/nchhstp/newsroom/docs/FastFacts-AA-FINAL508COMP.pdf Accessed 17 Sep 2009.

CDC (2008). HIV/AIDS Surveillance. http://www.cdc.gov/hiv/topics/aa/resources/factsheets/aa.htm. Accessed 29 June 2009.

CDC. (2006). Racial/ethnic disparities in diagnoses of HIV/AIDS – 33 states, 2001–2004. *Morbidity and Mortality Weekly Report, 55*(5), 121–125.

CDC. (2005). Health disparities experienced by Black or African Americans – United States. *Morbidity and Mortality Weekly Report, 54*(1), 1–3.

Chatters, L. M. (2000). Religion and health: Public health and practice. *Annual Review of Public Health, 21,* 335–367.

Chatters, L. M., Levin, J. S., & Ellison, C. G. (1998). Public health and health education in Faith Communities. *Health Education and Behavior, 25*(6), 689–699.

Clarke, V. (2001). What about the children? Arguments against lesbian and gay parenting. *Women's Studies International Forum, 24*(5), 555–570.

Cohen, C. J. (1999). *The boundaries of blackness: AIDS and the breakdown of Black politics.* Chicago, IL: University Of Chicago Press.

Dash, M. I., Jackson, J., & Rasor, S. C. (1997). *Hidden wholeness: An African American spirituality for individuals and communities.* Cleveland, OH: United Church Press.

DeHaven, M. J., Hunter, I. B., Wilder, L., Walton, J. W., & Berry, J. (2004). Health programs in faith-based organizations: Are they effective. *American Journal of Public Health, 94*(6), 1030–1036.

Derose, K. P., Hawes-Dawson, J., Fox, S. A., Maldonado, N., Tatum, A. A., & Kington, R. (2000). Dealing with diversity: recruiting churches and women for a randomized trial of mammography promotion. *Health Education & Behavior, 27*(5), 632–648.

Doupe, A. World Council of Churches (2005a). Partnerships between churches and people living with HIV/AIDS organizations. http://www.oikoumene.org/fileadmin/files/wcc-main/documents/p4/guidelines-e.pdf. Accessed 13 July 2009.

Doupe, A. World Council of Churches. (2005b). Working with people living with HIV/AIDS Organizations: Background document. http://www.oikoumene.org/fileadmin/files/wcc-main/documents/p4/background-e.pdf. Accessed 15 Sep 2009.

Ellison, C. G., & Levin, J. S. (1998). The religion-health connection: Evidence, theory, and future directions. *Health Education and Behavior, 25*(6), 700–720.

Eng, E., Hatch, J., & Callan, A. (1985). Institutionalizing social support through the church and into the community. *Health Education Quarterly, 12*(1), 81–92.

Foege, W. (1997). The Values of Religious Health Assets. In The carter center (Eds), *Strong Partners: Realigning Religious Health Assets for Community Health* (pp. 3–4). Atlanta, GA: The Carter Center.

Francis, S. A., & Liverpool, J. (2009). A review of faith-based HIV prevention programs. *Journal of Religion and Health, 48*(1), 6–15.

Franklin, J. H., & Moss, A. A. Jr. (1994). From slavery to freedom: A history of African Americans. (7th ed.). New York: McGraw-Hill College.

Franklin, R. M. (1997). *Another day's journey: Black churches confronting the American crisis.* Philadelphia, PA: Fortress Press.

Fullilove, M. T., & Fullilove, R. E. (1999). Stigma as an obstacle to AIDS action: The case of the African American community. *American Behavioral Scientist, 42*(7), 1117–1127.

Fullilove, R. E. (2006, November 17). African Americans, health disparities and HIV/AIDS, Recommendations for Confronting the Epidemic in Black America. http://nmac.org/index/grpp-publications. Accessed 17 Nov 2006.

Gallup (2009). State of the States: Importance of religion. http://www.gallup.com/poll/114022/state-states-importance-religion.aspx. Accessed 14 July 2009.

Giger, J. N., Appel, S. J., Davidhizar, D., & Davis, C. (2008). Church and spirituality in the lives of African American community. *Journal of Transcultural Nursing, 19*(4), 375–383.

Hale, W. D., Bennett, R. G. (2003). Addressing health needs of an ageing society through medical-religious partnerships: what do clergy and laity think? Gerontologist, *43*(6): 925–930.

Hammonds, E. M. (1997). Seeing AIDS: Race, gender, and representation. In N. Goldstein & J. L. Manlowe (Eds.), *The gender politics of HIV/AIDS in women: Perspectives on the pandemic in the United States* (pp. 113–126). New York, NY: New York University Press.

Harris, F. C. (1994). Something within: Religion as a mobilizer of African-American political activism. *The Journal of Politics, 56*(1), 42–68.

Herek, G. M., Capitanio, J. P., & Widaman, K. F. (2003). Stigma, social risk, and health policy: Public attitudes toward HIV surveillance policies and the social construction of illness. *Health Psychology, 22*, 533–540.

Kaiser Family Foundation (2006, February). African Americans and HIV/AIDS. http://www.kkf.org. Accessed 1 Oct 2006.

Kelly, J. A., Somlai, A. M., Benotsch, E. G., Amirkhanian, Y. A., Fernandez, M. I., Stevenson, L. Y., Sitzler, C. A., McAuliffe, T. L., Brown, K. D., & Opgenorth, K. M. (2006). Programmes, resources, and needs of HIV-prevention nongovernmental organizations (NGOs) in Africa, Central/Eastern Europe and Central Asia, Latin America and the Caribbean. *AIDS Care, 18*(1): 12–21.

Koenig, H. G. (2000). Religion, spirituality, and medicine: Application to clinical practice. *JAMA, 284*, 1708.

Koenig, H. G., McCullough, M. E., & Larson, D. B. (2001). *Handbook of religion and health.* New York, NY: Oxford University Press.

Kramer, F. D., Finegold, K., De Vita, C. J., & Wherry, L. (2005, July 28). Federal policy on the ground: faith-based organizations delivering local services. http://www.urban.org/UploadedPDF/311197_DP05-01.pdf. Accessed 20 June 2009.

Leong, P. (2003, August 16–19). *Sexuality, gender, HIV/AIDS, and the politics of the church: A comparison of two African-American churches.* Paper presented at the 2003 Annual Meeting of the American Sociological Association, Atlanta, GA. http://www.allacademic.com//meta/p_mla_apa_research_citation/1/0/8/2/1/pages108212/p108212-1.php. Accessed 22 June 2009.

Levin, J. S. (1984). The role of the Black church in community medicine. *Journal of the National Medical Association, 76*(5), 477–483.

Levin, J. (2003). Spiritual determinants of health and healing: an epidemiologic perspective on salutogenic mechanisms. *Alternative Therapies In Health And Medicine, 9*(6), 48–57.

Levin, J., Chatters, L. M., & Taylor, R. J. (2005). Religion, health, and medicine in African Americans: Implications for physicians. *Journal of the National Medical Association, 97*(2), 237–249.

Lincoln, C. E., & Mamiya, L. H. (2001). *The Black church in the African American experience.* Durham, NC: Duke University Press.

Logan, S. L., & Freeman, E. M. (2000). *Health care in the Black community: empowerment, knowledge, skills, and collectivism.* New York: Haworth Press.

Marsh, C. (2005). *The beloved community: How faith shapes social justice from the civil rights movement to today.* New York, NY: Basic Books.

McNeal, C., & Perkins, I. (2007). Potential roles of Black churches in HIV/AIDS prevention. *Health Care, Medical and Mental health Research, 15*(2), 219–232.

Melkote, S. R., Muppidi, S. R., & Goswam, D. (2000). Social and economic factors in an integrated behavioral and societal approach to communications in HIV/AIDS. *Journal of Health Communication, 5*, 17–22.

Miller, R. L. (2007). Legacy denied: African American gay men, AIDS, and the Black church. *National Association of Social Workers, 52*(1), 51–61.

Moreira-Almeida, A., Neto, F. L., & Koenig, H. G. (2006). Religiousness and mental health: A review. *Rev Bras Psiquiatr, 28*(3), 242–250.

Musgrave, C. F., Allen, C. E., & Allen, G. J. (2002). Spirituality and health for women of color. *American Journal of Public Health, 92*, 557–560.

Mystakidou, K., Tsilika, E., Parpa, E., Smyrnioti, M., & Vlahos, L. (2007). Assessing spirituality and religiousness in advanced cancer patients. *American Journal of Hospice & Palliative Medicine, 23*(6), 457–463.

Newlin, K., Knafl, K., & Melkus, G. D. (2002). African American spirituality: A concept analysis. *Advances in Nursing Science, 25*, 57–70.

Niles, W. S. T. (1996). The African-American Church & AIDS: Inevitable that they will succeed. *Health and Welfare Ministries, General Board of Global Ministries.* http://gbgm-umc.org/health/hivfocus/focus030.stm#2001. Accessed 13 July 2009.

Pew Forum on Religion and Public Life. (2008, February). U.S. religious landscape survey, religious affiliation: Diverse and dynamic. http://religions.pewforum.org/pdf/report-religious-landscape-study-full.pdf. Accessed 14 June 2009.

Pinn, A. H., & Pinn, A. B. (2002). *Black church history.* Minneapolis, MN: Fortress Press.

Pratt, R. (1997). *In good faith: Canadian churches against apartheid.* Canada: Wilfrid Laurier University Press.

Public Media Center. (1997). *The impact of homophobia and other social biases on AIDS.* San Francisco, CA: Public Media Center.

Public Media and the AIDS National Interfaith Network. (1997). *Faith and AIDS: American faith communities respond to the AIDS epidemic.* Francisco, CA: Public Media Center.

Richardson, B. L., & June, L. N. (1997). Utilizing and maximizing the resources of the African American church: Strategies and tools for counseling professionals. In L. C. Courtland (Ed.), *Multicultural issues in counseling: New approaches to diversity* (pp. 155–170). Alexandria, VA: American Counseling Association.

Sanders, R. G. (2002). The Black church: Bridge over troubled water. In J. Lipford Sanders & C. Bradley (Eds.), *Counseling African American families* (pp. 73–84). Alexandria, VA: American Counseling Association.

Sternberg, Z., Munschauer, F. E., Carrow, S. S., & Sternberg, E. (2007). Faith-placed cardiovascular health promotion: a framework for contextual and organizational factors underlying program success. *Health Education Research, 22*(5), 619–629.

Smith, J., Simmons, E., and Mayer, K. H. (2005). HIV/AIDS and the Black Church: What Are the Barriers to Prevention Services? Journal of the National Medical Association, *97*(12): 1682–1685.

Sutherland, M., Hale, C. D., & Harris, G. J. (1995). Community health promotion: The church as partner. *The Journal of Primary Prevention, 16*(2), 201–216.

Sutherland, M., & Harris, G. (1994). Church-based, youth drug prevention programs in African-American communities. *Wellness Perspectives, 10*(2), 3–23.

Swartz, A. (2002). Breaking the silence: The black church addresses HIV. In *HIV impact* (pp. 1–3). Office of minority health, Washington, DC: US Department of Health and Human Services, Public Health Services.

Taylor C. (2006). African American Religious Leadership and the Civil Rights Movement. History Now (online journal), Issue 8. http://www.historynow.org/06_2006/historian4.html. Accessed 29 September, 2009.

Taylor, R. J., Ellison, C. G., Chatters, L. M., Levin, J. S., & Lincoln, K. D. (2000). Mental health services in faith communities: The role of clergy in Black churches. *Social Work, 45*(1), 73–87.

The ARK of Refuge: ARK Programs. http://www.arkofrefuge.org/programs.html. Accessed 14 Sep 2009.

Thomas, S. B. (2000). The legacy of Tuskegee: AIDS and African-Americans. *The Body: The Complete HIV/AIDS Resource.* Retrieved September 29, 2009 from http://www.thebody.com/content/art30946.html#. Accessed 29 Sep 2009.

UNAIDS, Joint United Nations Programme on HIV/AIDS. (2008). Developing strategies to work with FBOs. http://www.aegis.org/news/UNAIDS/2008/UN080406.html. Accessed 13 July 2009.

UNFPA. (2008). Culturally sensitive approaches: Building bridges among faith-based organizations and secular development practitioners. http://www.unfpa.org/culture/fbo.html. Accessed 13 July 2009.

U.S. Department of Health and Human Services. (2002). Healthy people 2010 toolkit: Identifying and engaging community partners. September 17, 2009 from http://www.healthypeople.gov/state/toolkit/partners.htm. Accessed 17 Sep 2009.

Van Reken, C. P. (1999). The church's role in social justice. *Calvin Theological Journal, 34*, 198–202.

Ward, E. G. (2005). Homophobia, hypermasculinity and the US black church. *Culture, Health & Sexuality, 7*(5), 493–504.

Chapter 5
Disproportionate Drug Imprisonment Perpetuates the HIV/AIDS Epidemic in African American Communities

Juarlyn L. Gaiter and Ann O'Leary

Introduction

The U.S. inmate population increased by 700% between 1970 and 2005 (Austin, Naro, & Fabelo, 2007), mainly because correctional policies criminalize drug addiction. Almost one half of all prisoners are drug abusers (Karberg & James, 2002) despite evidence from molecular and imaging studies that addiction is a brain disorder with a strong genetic component (Chandler, Fletcher, & Volkow, 2009). The composition of prison admissions has shifted away from perpetrators of violent crimes towards less serious offenses such as parole violations and drug offenses (Clear, 2007). These offenses are largely responsible for the steep increases in the number of people who are incarcerated. Mauer (2006) notes that since there are no direct victims in drug selling and possession police rarely receive reports of these activities. Also, drug law enforcement is far more discretionary than for other offenses. The police decide when and where they will seek out people to arrest and most importantly what priority they will place on enforcing drug laws. Nearly six in ten persons in state prisons for a drug offense have no history of violence or significant selling activity. In 2005 four out of five drug arrests were for possession and only one out of five were for drug sales (Webb, 2007). States that have high numbers of drug arrests usually have higher incarceration rates (Mauer) and counties with burgeoning unemployment, persistent poverty and large percentages of African Americans have the highest incarceration rates for drug offenses (Beatty, Petteruti, & Ziedenberg, 2007).

African Americans are incarcerated for drug offenses at rates that are severely out of balance with their representation in the U.S. population. Most admissions for drug offenses are African American men, yet African American women are fast closing the gap in incarcerations for drug behaviors (Iguchi et al., 2002). Injection

J.L. Gaiter (✉)
Division of HIV/AIDS Prevention, Centers for Disease Control and Prevention,
1600 Clifton Road, N.E, MS E-37, Atlanta, GA 30333, USA
e-mail: JGaiter@cdc.gov

D.H. McCree et al. (eds.), *African Americans and HIV/AIDS*,
DOI 10.1007/978-0-387-78321-5_5,

drug users (IDU) who have used drugs such as heroin, cocaine and methamphetamine account for more than a third of new AIDS cases (Volkow, 2008). Repeated cycles of imprisonment for felony drug convictions, probation and parole not only disproportionately affect African Americans but increase the vulnerability of African American communities to crisis levels of HIV infection (Lane et al., 2004). This chapter describes the double burden of incarceration and HIV infection among African Americans and structural and contextual factors, such as correctional policies and concurrent partnerships that fuel these epidemics.

U.S. Incarceration Rates

The United States (U.S.) has less than 5% of the world's population but well over 23% of all incarcerated people (Hartney, 2006). Explosive growth in incarceration started in the 1970s when rates of inner city crime soared and the drug war intensified (King & Mauer, 2005a). Admissions for drug offenses severely inflated the prison population over the past three decades (Mauer & King, 2007). Consequently, by 2006 a quarter of a million drug offenders were among 1.4 million state prisoners and almost half of the 193,046 federal prisoners (Sabol, Couture, & Harrison, 2007).

The Epidemic of Incarceration Among African Americans

In 2006 African Americans, who were only 13% of the U.S. population were 42% of the total arrests for drug offenses (Sabol, Couture, et al., 2007). Beatty et al., 2007 noted that large pockets of disadvantaged people in poor areas within large counties were associated with vigilant policing, prosecuting and incarceration of individuals involved in drug behaviors. In fact, beginning in 1987 the rates of African Americans incarcerated for drug offenses quadrupled in only 3 years until in 2000 the rate was 26 times that of the early 1980s (Travis, 2005).

African Americans have been consistently more likely than European Americans to be convicted of drug felonies in state courts (Durose & Langan, 2001) and to be habitual offenders (Iguchi, Bell, Ramchand, Fain, 2005; Western, Kling, & Weiman, 2001). Half (50%) of African American inmates (496,900) were drug addicted or abusers compared to 59.1% of white (431,500), and 51% of Hispanic (222,700) inmates in 2004 (Mumola & Karberg, 2006). Yet, at the end of 2006 the incarceration rate for African American men was 3,042 per 1,000,000 residents, compared to 487 for white American men (Sabol et al., 2007). Also during 2006 1 in 21 African American adult men, 1 in 279 African American adult women and 1 in 41 African Americans of all ages were incarcerated (Warren, Gelb, Horowitz, & Riordan, 2008). African American men were hit the hardest as more than 19% of them between the ages of 25 and 29 years were in jail or prison in 2006 (Sabol et al., 2007).

These findings are noteworthy because European and African Americans report similar rates of illicit drug use and sales (Rouse, Sanderson, & Feldmann, 2006). Therefore, there is little evidence or reason to believe that African Americans have more substance abuse problems than European Americans (U.S. Department of Justice, 2003). Yet, it has been consistently shown that, in general, when a black man and a white man commit the same crime, the risk of incarceration is considerably greater for the black man than the white one (Zierler & Krieger, 1997).

In 2005 the Vera Institute reported that mandatory minimum sentences, were responsible for high incarceration rates of drug offenders in every state (Stemen, Rengifo, & Wilson, 2006). Not only were African Americans more likely than whites to be incarcerated for drug offenses; they also disproportionately received mandatory minimum sentences. Even more telling is that nationwide in every offense category – person, property, drug, and public disorder – African American youth are disproportionately incarcerated (Hartney & Silva, 2007).

African American Women

African American women are almost four times as likely than white women and three times as likely than Hispanic women to be incarcerated (Sabol, Minton, & Harrison, 2007). Prisons are the only places where HIV prevalence is higher for women (2.6%) than it is for men (1.8%). A report by the Center for Addiction and Substance Abuse (CASA, 1998) found that higher proportions of women inmates compared to men have histories of crack and injection drug use and relationships with multiple, risky sexual partners. For example data for state prisoners in 2004 showed that 60% of 82,800 incarcerated women and 53% of men (of 1.1 million) inmates were drug abusers or drug dependent (Mumola & Karberg, 2006). The more serious health problem for African American women is that they are two-thirds of all newly reported HIV cases among women as well as 34% of all female inmates (Harawa & Adimora, 2008). An especially alarming forecast is that the population of women inmates will grow more rapidly at 16% by 2011 compared to 12% for men (Austin et al., 2007). There is likely therefore to be commensurate increases in the proportion of HIV positive African American women behind bars.

Thomas and Torrone (2006) established a link between rates of incarceration among African Americans and high HIV and STI rates in African American communities. These researchers calculated correlations between rates of incarceration of the 76 prisons and 97 jails in the state of North Carolina and rates of STIs and teenage pregnancies for each of 100 counties between 1995 and 2002. They found that STI rates and teenage pregnancies adjusted for age, race and poverty distributions by county consistently increased with increases in incarceration. Thomas and Torrone concluded that high incarceration rates are strongly associated with health outcomes in the form of teenage pregnancies. They also noted that the incarceration variable most strongly related to health outcomes was number of prisoners per 100,000, the measure of the closest proxy for absence of individuals from a community.

Incarceration and Sexually Transmitted Infections

Sexually transmitted infections are secondary risk factors for HIV infection because individuals with untreated STIs are three to five times more likely to become HIV-infected (CDC, 1998). Dembo et al., (2009) examined the relationship between individual level-factors (gender, age, drug use) and community-level factors (concentrated disadvantage) and STI prevalence for Chlamydia and gonorrhea among adolescents (12–18 years of age) at intake during their first arrest. Demographic data and the adolescents home addresses were geocoded within a six county area.

The researchers conducted a two-level logistic regression analysis to determine the influence of individual-and community-level predictors on STI results from 1,368 urine assays (431 girls and 937 boys). They also created measures of residential stability, ethnic heterogeneity and an index of community disadvantage. The youth's positive STI results were predicted by individual level factors of gender (being female), age and race (being African American) and criminal history. Community level factors (concentrated disadvantage), defined as racially segregated housing combined with the proportion of the population that was: below the poverty line, identifying as black/African American; 16 years old and older; unemployed, and female-headed household with children predicted the youth's STI status. The individual-and community-level factors predicted sexually transmitted disease (STIs) among disadvantaged youth involved in the juvenile justice system. The researchers concluded that delinquents who lived in disadvantaged, stressful environments have a significantly elevated risk of STIs. They recommended that intense STI prevention efforts be mounted to improve the sexual health of disadvantaged youth to reduce their risk of contracting and spreading HIV infection.

Mechanisms for Disproportionate Incarceration worsening the epidemic

The effects of the disproportionate incarceration of African American adult men and their risk of HIV infection take both direct and indirect forms. Direct effects include the possibility of becoming infected while incarcerated and, for those already infected, health care in the institution and following release. Indirect effects are ones that influence sexual networks and partnerships.

HIV Risk Behavior in Prison

Nearly all HIV-infected prisoners entered prison with their infection. Not only are there more opportunities to engage in high-risk behavior such as injection drug use or risky sexual behavior in the community than while incarcerated (Wohl et al., 2000), but a number of studies show that incarcerated individuals report that they engage in more risky behaviors outside of prison than inside prison (Moseley & Tewksbury, 2006). Wohl et al.'s case-control study of incarcerated African American men at risk for HIV infection showed that men who reported sex with other men were also more likely to report this risky behavior before and after rather than during their incarceration.

Yet HIV transmission can occur while in prison or jail through unprotected sexual activity, needle sharing IDUs, tattooing with unsterilized sharp objects such as ball point pens and contact with HIV-infected blood or mucous membranes through violence (Krebs, 2006; Mahon, 1996). The majority of IDU will spend some time in prison and many IDU continue to use illicit drugs while they are incarcerated (Carvell & Hart, 1990). Needle sharing among injection drug users (IDUs) is highly associated with the transmission of HIV infection and is a major risk factor for incarcerated adults (Dufour et al., 1996). This association explains why a history of incarceration is an independent risk factor for HIV infection among IDUs (Clarke et al., 2001; Wood et al., 2005).

Much of the sexual contact between men in prison involves anal sex (Krebs & Simmons, 2002) which poses an especially high risk of HIV transmission. The actual incidence of anal and homosexual sex between men in jail and prison environments is unknown. Wardens typically refuse to allow inmates to be asked questions regarding sex between men. Most sexual contacts are unsafe because few correctional facilities give inmates free access to condoms and no U.S. jail or prison system permits the distribution of sterile needles (May & Williams, 2002).

Krebs and Simmons (2002) examined surveillance data for 5,265 men in prison over a 22-year period (Jan 1, 1978–Jan 1, 2000) to find out how many of them became HIV-positive while they were incarcerated. They found that a minimum of 33 men were HIV-infected in prison compared to 238 former inmates who became HIV-positive after they left prison. The investigators concluded that men having sex with each other was the main route of HIV infection transmission. Three studies with a total of 6,000 prisoners continuously incarcerated since 1977 or 1978 found only 52 HIV sero-conversions during incarceration periods of less than 15 years each. These data led Harawa and Adimora (2008) to conclude that most HIV transmission happens prior to rather than during incarceration.

The CDC studied HIV transmission in the Georgia state prison system (63% African American population) when 88 men who had tested HIV-negative at intake subsequently tested positive (CDC, 2006). Forty-five of the men had engaged in consensual sex with another man while in prison; 35 of the men said that they had not had sex with men during the 6 months prior to incarceration. Six men reported that they had been raped and forty men had been tattooed in prison. The CDC examined HIV sero-conversion in 68 of the 88 inmates known to have sero-converted between 1992 and 2005. The investigators found that men having sex with men, tattooing, a body mass index of less than 25.4 kg per square meter on prison entry and being African American were factors associated with HIV seroconversion (CDC). These known sero-converters were 9% of the HIV-infected prisoners in Georgia in 2005 (CDC).

In the context of an HIV prevention intervention for young men leaving state prison both quantitative (Seal et al., 2008) and qualitative (Seal et al., 2004) data were collected regarding their risk behavior while they were incarcerated. About half of sample of the 106 men the majority of whom were African American (54%) between the ages of 18 and 29 reported the most commonly used drugs in prison were alcohol and marijuana. Consensual sex was reported by 17% of the men; of these, 88% reported sex with a female partner and 21% with a man (Seal et al., 2008). The researchers noted that substance use and sexual behavior were correlated and that both were associated with being older, having spent more years in prison, having been sexually abused and involved with gangs and violence. Men with histories of sexual abuse, treatment for depression, anxiety or drug abuse, and who had been injured during a prison or jail fight were more likely to engage in risky behavior while incarcerated. Also, men were more likely to have had consensual sex inside prison if they had a male partner outside of prison. Only one man reported that he had been forced to have sex by another man. Seal et al. (2004) concluded that their data supported previous research findings that prisoners' substance use and consensual sexual behavior while in prison is indicative of similar, prior risky behavior in the community (Clarke et al., 2001; Kang et al., 2005).

Effects of Differential Incarceration on Sexual Networks

As discussed above, African Americans have vastly different experiences with the criminal justice system, and are far more likely to be incarcerated than members of other racial/ethnic groups. Beyond this, men are more likely than women to be incarcerated, and African American men are the highest-frequency incarcerated group of all. A closer look at sexually transmitted disease at a population, rather than an individual level, reveals that sexually concurrent partnerships stand out as important determinants of epidemics (Aral, 1999). Concurrent sexual relationships are simultaneous sexual relationships or relationships that overlap in time (Morris & Kretschmar, 1995). HIV transmission is made particularly more likely by concurrency, because HIV is highly contagious in the earliest phase of infection; newly infected people are much more likely to transmit to other partners than are chronically infected individuals (Morris & Kretschmar, 1997).

Because differential incarceration of men raises the ratio of women to men, it also promotes concurrent partnerships (for a review, see Adimora, Schoenbach, Martinson, Donaldson, Staneil, Fullilove, 2004). Some women would, even knowingly, share a man with another woman rather than have no man at all. A recent analysis of the population-based National Survey of Family Growth, showed that 11% of men reported concurrent sexual relationships during the preceding year, while the rate for African American women was more than twice as high (Adimora, Schoenbach, & Doherty, 2007).

Hammett and Drachman-Jones (2006) examined relationships between incarceration and increases in HIV and sexually transmitted diseases among poor African American women in the rural south. They learned that in small southern, rural towns with very low HIV prevalence sharp increases in HIV incidence were associated with sexual networks involving multiple partners, concurrent sexual relationships and co-occurrence of STIs. They hypothesized that large numbers of African American male inmates and recent increases in the incarceration of low income African American women as well as Latina women accounted for this finding. Large numbers of African American southern poor women with HIV/AIDS and STIs from rural areas were incarcerated. The researchers concluded that the HIV and STI epidemics among southern men and women are related to incarcerated populations more than in other parts of the U.S.

Comfort, Grinstead, McCartney, Bourgois, and Knight (2005) investigated the development and stability of intimacy between couples in a community where there were many men in prison away from their wives, girlfriends and families. They discovered that correctional control even extends to the bodies of women when they visit their sexual partners and are at home attempting to stay connected to their incarcerated men. For example, a review of qualitative interviews of 20 women who visited their men in prison and 13 correctional officers showed that prisons prohibit privacy and physical contact between women and their men. The researchers concluded that romantic scripts, the buildup of sexual tension during incarceration and restricted conditions of parole promote unprotected sexual contact and other HIV/STI risk behavior after men leave prison. Thus, this is a clear example of how the constant shortage of men as sexual partners and consequent increases in concurrent, high-risk sexual partnerships renders African American communities vulnerable to HIV infection.

HIV Care for Prisoners

The high prevalence of HIV infection among people who enter jails and prisons contributes to the alarming numbers of prisoners who are living with HIV. That number is about 10.8 times as high as that of the general population (Clarke et al., 2001; Sylla, 2008). State correctional systems are required by various Supreme Court decisions to provide reasonable care for offenders (Cropsey, Wexler, Melnick, Taxman, & Young, 2007). Despite the high prevalence of HIV in correctional institutions, the duration of treatment and the response to various highly active antiretroviral therapies (HAART) are largely unknown. Zaller, Thurmond, and Rich (2007) compared US correctional expenditures for antiretrovirals (ARVS) using Bureau of Justice Statistics data (Marusak, 2005) with an estimate of the medicine needed to effectively treat HIV-infected prisoners. They found that the total ARV sales in 2004 covered only 29% of the total necessary to treat all HAART-eligible inmates with known HIV infection. These data cast some doubt on how available HIV medications are to infected inmates who must rely on HAART to remain healthy while they are incarcerated.

Most US prisons do not provide inmates with the standard of care that is available to people in communities outside correctional institutions (WHO, 2006).

There are no mandatory guidelines for correctional medical care even though health care is a constitutional right of prisoners. Instead, there are voluntary guidelines for general correctional health and HIV treatment and no incentives for wardens of correctional facilities to comply with these voluntary standards. Over-crowded prison environments, exhausted medical staff with limited budgets who serve an ever-burgeoning population can be particularly dangerous for HIV-positive inmates (Sylla, 2008).

Recently, the CDC issued HIV testing Implementation Guidelines for Correctional Settings. Testing guidelines are critically important because early diagnosis and immediate antiretroviral treatment for positive inmates can suppress the virus (Springer, Friedland, Doros, Pesanti, & Altice, 2007). Altice, Mostashari, and Friedland et al. (2001) reported that 75% of HIV-infected inmates began their first antiretroviral treatment after they were incarcerated. The CDC HIV testing guidelines for correctional settings can be found at:

http://www.cdc.gov/Hiv/topics/testing/resources/guidelines/correctional-settings/index.htm (CDC webpage/to be published in AJPH/July 2009).

Baillargeon et al. (2009) conducted a retrospective cohort study of 2115 HIV-infected prison inmates who had received HAART before their release. Within 10 days of release only 115 (5.4%) of the inmates had filled their prescriptions and 634 (30%) had their medicines after 60 days. African American and Hispanic ex-offenders were less likely than white ex-offenders to fill their prescriptions within 10 and 30 days after they left prison. Those who typically got their medication in the community after 30 and 60 days were on parole. Others who had received help in completing an AIDS Drug Assistance Program application were more likely to fill their prescriptions for HAART within 10, 30 and 60 days.

Springer et al. (2007) evaluated the outcomes for 1,099 inmates on 6 months of continuous HAART and found that over half (59%) of the inmates had undetectable viral loads by the time they left prison. They concluded that their impressive results establish prison settings as critical for the initiation of effective antiretroviral therapy for HIV-infected inmates. Clements-Nolle et al. (2008) evaluated HAART therapy use and risk behaviors among 177 HIV-infected jail inmates over the course of 1 year. The investigators found that HIV transmission risk behaviors were widespread during the month before the inmates were reincarcerated. In addition, 59% of those who had started on HAART in prison had discontinued their medication. Initiating HAART and later discontinuing medication was associated with homelessness, marijuana use and not receiving medical care following release from jail. Ex-offenders who may relapse to drug use and discontinue their HAART during the first few weeks after they leave prison may increase their risk for adverse clinical outcomes, transmission of HIV infection to others and drug resistant HIV reservoirs in the community. This is a very serious public health problem because no one knows how many HIV-infected ex-offenders stop taking their medications or don't refill their prescriptions shortly after they are released from prison. Untreated HIV-positive individuals are more likely to transmit the virus to others (Quinn et al., 2000).

The Crisis of HIV/AIDS in Our Nation's Capital

The District of Columbia (DC; the District) is the only place in the country with a policy of annual HIV testing for every resident between the ages of 14 and 84. The District participates in the CDC funded National HIV Behavioral Surveillance System Study to determine the factors that place people at high risk for HIV infection in DC (DC Department of Health, 2007) The investigators interviewed 750 people (92% African American, 7.7% other) and the surveillance unit interviewed medical providers to find unreported HIV and AIDS cases.

Participants in this study had a median age of 36; had never been married and reported that they were heterosexual. Most had attained high school or higher education; yet 44% were unemployed, 60% had a yearly household income of less than $10,000 and 22% had a history of homelessness. Most notable is that 52% of the sample said that they had ever been to jail, prison or juvenile detention (DC Department of Health, 2007).

The epidemiology report noted that DC has every mode of HIV transmission. The HIV/AIDS epidemic affects every race, and gender across populations and neighborhoods in all but one of DC's eight wards. An astounding 5% of the study participants were HIV positive. In 2006 there were 12,428 people living with HIV and AIDS in the District of Columbia. African Americans account for 81% of new HIV infections although they are 57% of the DC population. The District of Columbia's prevalence rate of 5% is as high as the prevalence rate in sub-Saharan Africa (5%) which is the most seriously affected region in Africa (WHO, 2007). Furthermore, a general population prevalence rate over 1% is a threshold that defines a "generalized and severe" epidemic. Therefore, the 5% HIV prevalence rate in DC means that there is substantial heterosexual transmission and significant numbers of HIV infected children (Wilson, Wright, & Isbell, 2008).

A major finding was that half of the DC study sample ($N = 750$) reported that they believed that their partner was having sex outside of their relationship and half of the participants reported that they themselves had sex in the past year outside of their relationship. In addition, only half of the participants said that they knew their partner's HIV status. Almost half of the people who had connections to places with the highest AIDS prevalence and poverty rates in DC had concurrent sexual partners within the last year; and three in five were aware of their own HIV status. Yet only three in ten persons had used a condom during the last time that they had sex.

In the District, African American men have the heaviest disease burden with an infection rate of 7%. Three percent of African American women in the city have the virus and almost one in ten residents between the ages of 40 and 49, are HIV-infected. The majority of people in this study had never injected drugs, however nearly two-thirds of the sample had used drugs such as marijuana, crack cocaine and ecstasy within the past year. Most disturbing was that only one in eight people said that they any information or contact with an HIV prevention or outreach program.

Apparently, many impoverished District of Columbia residents incorrectly believe that they are not at risk for HIV infection. This can be inferred because study participants reported having sex outside of their main relationship, think that their main partner has sex with casual partners, do not know their partner's HIV status; and are not using condoms. This false assumption is alarming given that nearly half of the people who tested positive did not know their HIV status. Also, the fact that 52% of the sample had been incarcerated at some point in their lives makes it clear that many single, heterosexual African American residents of the District of Columbia area affected by disproportionate rates of incarceration and HIV infection.

Discussion

Drug-related incarcerations are not equally distributed. Impoverished African American men and women have a much higher chance than white men and women of serving a prison sentence for a felony drug conviction. The U.S. criminal justice system is a model of entrenched institutionalized racial disparity. Unprecedented numbers of African Americans are incarcerated for much longer sentences and those who leave prison return quicker than ever before (Clear, 2007). The failure of the "war on drugs" has shown that the criminal justice system cannot solve the complex societal problems of substance abuse and economic distress. Criminal justice statistics make it clear that there is no empirical evidence that incarcerating people for drug offenses reduces their illegal drug use. Unfortunately, for prisoners with drug abuse or addiction problems the most common service that they receive is drug education (Taxman, Perdoni, & Harrison, 2007).

Furthermore, failure to treat drug addiction as a medical condition, the lack of consistent access to treatment and inadequate social services make recidivism almost inevitable. The National Institute on Drug Abuse notes that drug addiction is a disease that causes changes in brain structure and function. Typically, the first time a person may choose to take drugs, but continued drug use over time alters the brain and impairs a person's self control and decision-making abilities, while sending intense impulses to take drugs (Volkow, 2008). Add this information to the fact that incarceration is independently associated with risky needle sharing by IDU makes clear that the rehabilitation of drug abusers requires a public health response.

Rhode Island's prison system has mandatory HIV testing for convicted felons, voluntary testing for individuals held prior to sentencing and may have one of the best counseling and testing, medical care and pre-release services in the nation. HIV specialists offer routine HIV testing, confidential care for HIV-infected inmate's, teach them how to avoid HIV transmission, overcome drug dependence and refer inmates at discharge to HIV care and methadone maintenance treatment in their communities (Okie, 2007). Between 1989 and 1999, the prison testing program identified 33% of all seropositive HIV tests in the state (Crosland, Poshkus, & Rich, 2002) easily getting voluntary testing compliance rates of greater than 90% (Spaete & Rich, 2005).

A felony drug conviction has an adverse ripple effect on the health and well-being of people who serve their sentence and leave prison. This is because most convicted felons have difficulty getting a job and associated health benefits; public housing, food stamps, certain employment licenses, permits and induction into military service, financial support for education and the right to vote in many states (Iguchi et al., 2005). Men especially have a hard time establishing relationships and a stable life when they are denied jobs.

Conclusion

Duncan Smith-Rohrberg and Basu (2007) argue that the two most critical actions that will control HIV infection are to avoid incarcerating drug users and mandating minimum sentences for drug possession (Courtwright, 2004). It must be understood that incarceration may be the root cause of the disproportionate rates of HIV infection among African Americans (Duncan Smith-Rohrberg & Basu).

The elimination of persistent racial disparities in the risk of HIV infection exacerbated by the crisis of widespread incarceration of African American drug offenders is an absolutely necessary and an achievable goal. Research has shown consistently that there are measureable, beneficial effects of drug treatment for drug abusers in the criminal justice system (Inciardi, Martin, Butzin, Hooper, & Harrison, 1997; Pearson & Lipton, 1999). Furthermore, alternatives to incarceration for drug abusers can help disrupt HIV infection transmission in African American communities.

The U.S. needs a comprehensive, national HIV/AIDS strategy for incarcerated African Americans because of the double crisis of incarceration and the generalized, severe HIV epidemic in disadvantaged urban communities. Until there are mandated standards of care for all inmates in prisons and jails African American communities will remain vulnerable to HIV and AIDS related infections and death.

High incarceration rates for African American men significantly lower the ratio of men to women and lower gender ratios not only affect rates of teenage pregnancy but syphilis and gonorrhea as well (Thomas & Gaffield, 2003). Sexual concurrency due to high levels of incarceration fuels the HIV epidemic, by disrupting social networks and partnerships among African Americans, and increasing the exposure of incarcerated men to high-risk sex and drug-using behaviors. Public awareness of this fact is low. This is a community-level effect on health that adds to others such as destabilization of communities and families, high rates of unemployment, and other health outcomes (Gaiter, Potter, & O'Leary, 2006). We must increase awareness of the dangers of concurrency among African American men and women.

The heterosexual transmission of HIV is following the epidemiologic pattern typical of sexually transmitted diseases such as syphilis and gonorrhea by disproportionately affecting African Americans. The racial disparity is not explained by traditional measures of socio-economic differences or individual-level determinants of sexual behavior but rather reflects deeper group-level social and environmental factors for which race is a marker (Farley, 2006). Therefore, a successful fight against the virus has to be waged against poverty, homelessness, unemployment, excessive incarceration, marginalization, homophobia and violence (Wilson et al., 2008).

These public health goals can and must be accomplished. The constant cycles that propel drug-involved men, women and adolescents into and out of prison must be halted. New infections must be prevented so that African American families can have a realistic chance of becoming and remaining healthy and productive far into and beyond the twenty-first century.

References

Adimora, A. A., Schoenbach, V. J., Martinson, F., Donaldson, K. H., Staneil, T. R, & Fullilove, R. E. (2004). Concurrent partnerships among African Americans in the Rural South. Annals of Epidemiology, 3, 155–160.

Adimora, A. A., Schoenbach, V. J., & Doherty, I. A. (2007). Concurrent sexual partnerships among men in the United States. American Journal of Public Health, 97, 2230–2237.

Altice, F. L., Mostashari, F., & Friedland, G. H. (2001). Trust and the acceptance of and adherence to antiretroviral therapy. Journal of Acquired Immune Deficiency Syndromes, 28, 47–58.

Aral, S. O. (1999). Sexual network patterns as determinants of STD rates: Paradigm shift in the behavioral epidemiology of STDs made visible. Sexually Transmitted Disease, 26, 262–264.

Austin, J. Naro, W., & Fabelo, T. (2007). Public safety, public spending: Forecasting America's Prison Population 2007–2011, A project of the Pew Charitable Trust, JFA Institute, 1-52. www.pewpublicsafety.org.

Baillargeon, J., Giordano, T. P., Rich, J. D., Wu, Z. H., Wells, K., Pollock, B. H., et al. (2009). Accessing antiretroviral therapy following release from prison. Journal of the American Medical Association, 301, 848–857.

Beatty, P., Petteruti, A., & Ziedenberg, J. (2007). The vortex: The concentrated racial impact of drug imprisonment and the characteristics of punitive counties (pp. 1–32). Washington, DC: Justice Policy Institute Report.

Carvell, A. L. M., & Hart, G. J. (1990). Risk behaviors for HIV infection among drug users in prison. British Medical Journal, 300, 1383–1384.

Center for Addiction and Substance Abuse (CASA). (1998). Crossing the bridge: An evaluation of the Drug Treatment Alternative to Prison (DTAP) Program, the National Center on Addiction and Substance Abuse at Columbia University, National Institute on Drug Abuse, 1–30.

Centers for Disease Control and Prevention. (1998). HIV Prevention through early detection and treatment of other sexually transmitted diseases: United States recommendations of the Advisory Committee for HIV and STD prevention. MMWR Recommendations and Reports, 47 (rr12), 1–24.

Centers for Disease Control and Prevention. (2006). HIV transmission among male inmates in a state prison system – Georgia, 1992–2005. Morbidity and Mortality Weekly Report, 55, 421–426.

Chandler, R. K., Fletcher, B. W., & Volkow, N. D. (2009). Treating drug abuse and addiction in the criminal justice system. Journal of the American Medical Association, 301, 183–190.

Clarke, J. G., Stein, M. D., Hanna, L., Sobota, M., & Rich, J. D. (2001). Active and former injection drug users report of HIV risk behaviors during periods of incarceration. Substance Abuse, 22, 209–216.

Clear, T. R. (2007). Imprisoning communities: How mass incarceration makes disadvantaged neighborhoods worse. New York: Oxford University Press.

Clements-Nolle, K., Marx, R., Pendo, M., Loughran, E., Estes, M., & Katz, M. (2008). Highly active antiretroviral therapy use and HIV transmission risk behaviors among individuals who are HIV infected and were recently released from jail. American Journal of Public Health, 98, 661–666.

Comfort, M., Grinstead, O., McCartney, K., Bourgois, P., & Knight, K. (2005). "You cannot do nothing in this damn place:" Sex and Intimacy among couples with an incarcerated male partner. *Journal of Sex Research, 42*, 3–12.

Courtwright, D. T. (2004). The Controlled Substances Act: How a "big tent" reform became a punitive drug law. *Drug & Alcohol Dependency, 76*, 9–15.

Cropsey, K. L., Wexler, H. K., Melnick, G., Taxman, F. S., & Young, D. W. (2007). Specialized prisons and services: Results from a national survey. *Prison Journal, 87*, 58–85.

Crosland, C., Poshkus, M., & Rich, J. (2002). Treating prisoners with HIV/AIDS: The importance of early identification, effective treatment and community follow-up. *AIDS Clinical Care, 14*, 67–76.

Dembo, R., Belenko, S., Childs, K., Wareham, J., & Schmeidler, J. (2009). Individual and community risk factors and sexually transmitted diseases among arrested youth: A two level analysis. *Journal of Behavioral Medicine, 32*(4), 303–316.

Dufour, A., Poulin, A. M., Allard, F. N., Trottier, G., Lepine, D., & Hankins, C. (1996). Prevalence and risk behaviors for HIV infection among inmates of a provincial prison in Quebec City. *AIDS, 10*, 1009–1015.

Duncan Smith-Rohrberg, M., & Basu, S. (2007). HIV control efforts should directly address incarceration, reflection and reaction. *The Lancet Infectious Disease, 7*, 568.

Durose, M. R., & Langan, P. A. (2001). Bureau of Justice Statistics, State Court Sentencing of Convicted Felons, 1998 Statistical Tables, U.S. Department of Justice.

Farley, T. A. (2006). Sexually transmitted diseases in the southeastern United States: Location, race and social context. *Sexually Transmitted Diseases, 33*(7 Suppl), S58–S64.

Gaiter, J., Potter, H., & O'Leary, A. (2006). Disproportionate rates of incarceration for people of color contribute to major health disparities in the U.S. [Letter]. *American Journal of Public Health, 96*, 1148–1149.

Hammett, T. M., & Drachman-Jones, A. (2006). HIV/AIDS, sexually transmitted diseases and incarceration among women: National and southern perspectives. *Sexually Transmitted Diseases, 33*(7 Suppl), S17–S22.

Harawa, N., & Adimora, A. (2008). Incarceration, African Americans and HIV: Advancing a research agenda. *Journal of the National Medical Association, 100*, 57–62.

Hartney, C. (2006). U.S. rates of incarceration: A global perspective, Fact Sheet, Research from the National Council on Crime and Delinquency, November, 1–8.

Hartney, C. & Silva, F. (2007). And justice for some: Differential treatment of youth of color in the justice system. *National Council on Crime and Delinquency*. www.nccd-crc.org.

Department of Health, Government of the District of Columbia HIV/AIDS Epidemiology Annual Report, Department of Health, HIV/AIDS Administration, Bureau of Surveillance and Epidemiology, November, 2007 Washington, DC. www.doh.dc.gov/hiv.

Iguchi, M. Y., Bell, J., Ramchand, R. N., & Fain, T. (2005). How criminal system racial disparities may translate into health disparities. *Journal of Health Care for the Poor and Underserved, 16*, 48–56.

Iguchi, M. Y., London, J. A., Forge, N. G., Hickman, L., Fain, T., & Reihman, K. (2002). Elements of well-being affected by criminalizing the drug user. *Public Health Reports, 117*(Suppl 1), 5146–5150.

Inciardi, J. A., Martin, S. S., Butzin, C. A., Hooper, R. M., & Harrison, L. D. (1997). An effective model of prison-based treatment for drug involved offenders. *Journal of Drug Issues, 27*, 261–278.

Kang, S. Y., Deren, S., Andia, J., Colon, H. M., Robles, R., & Oliver-Velez, D. (2005). HIV transmission behaviors in jail/prison among Puerto Rican drug injectors in New York and Puerto Rico. *AIDS and Behavior, 9*, 377–386.

Karberg, J. C., James, D. J., (2002). Substance dependence, abuse and treatment of jail inmates, Bureau of Justice Statistics, Office of Justice Programs, Washington, DC, July 2005, NCJ 209588.

King, R. S., & Mauer, M. (2005a).The War on Marijuana: The transformation of the war on drugs in the 1990s, Report of The Sentencing Project, Washington, DC, 1–33.

Krebs, C. P. (2006). Inmate factors associated with HIV transmission in prison. *Criminology and Public Policy, 5*, 113–136.

Krebs, C. P., & Simmons, M. (2002). Intra-prison HIV transmission: An assessment of whether it occurs, how it occurs and who is at risk. *AIDS Education and Prevention, 14*(Suppl. B), 53–64.

Lane, S. D., Rubinstein, R. A., Keefe, R. H., Webster, N., Cibula, D. A., Rosenthal, A., et al. (2004). Structural violence and racial disparity in HIV transmission. *Journal of Health Care for the Poor and Underserved, 15*, 319–335.

Mahon, N. (1996). New York inmate's HIV risk behaviors: The implications for prevention policy and programs. *American Journal of Public Health, 86*, 1211–1215.

Marusak, L. M. (2005). *HIV in prisons, 2003*. Washington, DC: Bureau of Justice Statistics. NCJ publication no. 210344.

Mauer, M. (2006). *Race to incarcerate*. New York, London: The New Press.

Mauer, M., & King, R. S. (2007). *Uneven justice: State rates of incarceration by race and ethnicity* (pp. 1–19). Washington, DC: The Sentencing Project Report.

May, J. P., & Williams, E. L. (2002). Acceptability of condom availability in a U.S. jail. *AIDS Education and Prevention, 14*(Suppl. B), 85–91.

Morris, M., & Kretschmar, M. (1995). Concurrent partnerships and transmission dynamics in networks. *Social Networks, 17*, 299–318.

Morris, M., & Kretschmar, M. (1997). Concurrent partnerships and the spread of HIV. *AIDS, 11*, 641–648.

Moseley, K., & Tewksbury, R. (2006). Prevalence and predictors of HIV risk behaviors among male prison inmates. *Journal of Correctional Health Care, 12*, 132–144.

Mumola, C. J., & Karberg, J. C. (2006). *Drug use and dependence, state and federal prisoners, 2004*. Washington, DC: U.S. Department of Justice, Office of Justice Programs, Bureau of Justice Statistics Special Report. NCJ 213530, 1-11.

Okie, S. (2007). Sex, drugs, prisons and HIV. *The New England Journal of Medicine, 356*, 105–108. Available at: http://www.nejm.org.

Pearson, F. S., & Lipton, D. S. (1999). A meta-analytic review of the effectiveness of corrections-based treatments for drug abuse. *Prison Journal, 79*, 384–410.

Quinn, T. C., Wawer, M. J., Sewankambo, N., Serwadda, D., Li, C., Wabwire-Mangen, F., et al. (2000). Viral load and heterosexual immunodeficiency virus type 1, Rakai Project Study Group. *The New England Journal of Medicine, 30*, 970–972.

Rouse, B., Sanderson, C., & Feldmann, J. (2006). *The 2005 National Survey on Drug Use and Health*. Washington, DC: Table J, Division of Population Surveys, Substance Abuse and Mental Health Services Administration (SAMHSA). Available at: http://www.samhsa.gov.

Sabol, W. J., Couture, H., & Harrison, P. M. (2007). *Prisoners in 2006*. Washington, DC: United Sates Department of Justice, Bureau of Justice Statistics Bulletin. NCJ 219416, 1-26.

Seal, D. W., Belcher, L., Morrow, K., Eldridge, G., Binson, D., Kacanek, D., et al. (2004). A qualitative study of substance use and sexual behavior among 18- to 29-year-old men while incarcerated in the United States. *Health Education and Behavior, 31*, 775–789.

Seal, D. W., Margolis, A. D., Morrow, K. M., Belcher, L., Sosman, J., Askew, J., et al. (2008). Substance use and sexual behavior during incarceration among 18-29-year old men: Prevalence and correlates. *AIDS and Behavior, 12*, 27–40.

Spaete, J. P., & Rich, J. D. (2005). HIV prevention and care in incarcerated populations. *Focus, 20*, 1–9.

Springer, S. A., Friedland, G. H., Doros, G., Pesanti, E., & Altice, F. L. (2007). Antiretroviral treatment regimen outcomes for HIV infected prisoners. *HIV Clinical Trials, 8*, 205–212.

Stemen, D., Rengifo, A., & Wilson, J. (2006). Of fragmentation and ferment: The impact of state sentencing policies on incarceration rates, 1975–2002, Final Report to the U.S. Department of Justice by the Vera Institute of Justice, 1–217.

Sylla, M. (2008). *HIV treatment in U.S. jails and prisons*. San Francisco AIDS Foundation, online newsletter retrieved from www.sfaf.org/beta/2008_win/jails_Prisons.

Taxman, F. S., Perdoni, M. L., & Harrison, L. D. (2007). Drug treatment services for adult offenders: The state of the state. *Journal of Substance Abuse and Treatment, 32*, 239–254.

Thomas, J. C., & Gaffield, M. E. (2003). Social structure race and gonorrhea rates in the south-eastern United States. *Ethnicity and Disease, 12*, 362–368.

Thomas, J. C., & Torrone, E. (2006). Incarceration as forced migration: Effects on selected community health outcomes. *American Journal of Public Health, 96*, 1762–1765.

Travis, J. (2005). *But they all come back: Facing the challenges of prisoner reentry*. Washington, DC: The Urban Institute Press.

U.S. Department of Justice. (2003). *The Federal Bureau of Investigation. Crime in the U.S. 2002* (pp. 252–259). Washington, DC: Government Printing Office.

Volkow, N. D. (2008). Drugs, brains and behavior: The science of addiction, National Institute on Drug Abuse, National Institutes of Health, U.S. Department of Health and Human Services, NIH Pub. No. 07-5605, 1–30. http://www.drugabuse.gov.

Warren, J., Gelb, A. Horowitz, J., & Riordan, J. (2008). One in 100: Behind bars in America 2008, The Pew Public Safety Performance Project, Pew Center on the States. www.pwertrusts.org.

Webb, J. (2007). U.S. Senator (VA). Mass incarceration in the United States: At what cost? Opening statement, Joint Economic Committee Hearing, October, 4. Washington, DC

Western, B., Kling, J. R., & Weiman, D. F. (2001). The labor market consequences of incarceration. *Crime and Delinquency, 47*, 410–427.

Wilson, P., Wright, K., & Isbell, M. T. (2008). *Left behind, Black America: A neglected priority in the global AIDS epidemic*. Los Angeles, CA: Black AIDS Institute. Available at: http://www.BlackAIDS.org.

Wohl, A. R., Johnson, D., Jordan, W., Lu, S., Beall, G., Currier, J., et al. (2000). High-risk behaviors during incarceration in African American men treated for HIV at three Los Angeles public medical centers. *Journal of Acquired Immune Deficiency Syndromes, 24*, 386–392.

Wood, E., Li, K., Small, W., Montaner, J. S., Schechter, M. T., & Kerr, T. (2005). Recent incarceration independently associated with syringe sharing by injection drug users. *Public Health Reports, 120*, 150–156.

World Health Organization, UNAIDS. (2007). AIDS epidemic update, Joint United Nations Programme on HIV/AIDS, 1–50, http://www.unaids.org.

World Health Organization/UNAIDS. (2006). *HIV/AIDS prevention, care, treatment and support in prison settings: A framework for an effective national response* (pp. 1–36). Vienna, NY: United Nations Office of Drugs and Crime, United Nations. Available at: http://www.unodc.org.

Zaller, N., Thurmond, P., & Rich, J. D. (2007). Limited spending: An analysis of correctional expenditures on anti-retrovirals for HIV infected prisoners. *Public Health Reports, 122*, 49–54.

Zierler, S., & Krieger, N. (1997). Reframing women's risk: Social inequalities and HIV infection. *Annual Review of Public Health, 18*, 401–436.

Chapter 6
Violence, Trauma, and Mental Health Disorders: Are They Related to Higher HIV Risk for African Americans?

Pilgrim S. Spikes, Leigh A. Willis, and Linda J. Koenig

Introduction

HIV disproportionately affects African Americans in the United States (Centers for Disease Control and Prevention (CDC), 2008a), and researchers have sought to understand the proximal and distal causes of this disparity. Although African Americans are knowledgeable about HIV risk factors and report fewer high-risk HIV-related behaviors than other high-risk racial or ethnic populations (Hallfors, Iritani, Miller, & Bauer, 2007; Kaiser Family Foundation, 1998; Millett, Peterson, Wolitski, & Stall, 2006), such knowledge may not translate into engaging in fewer risk behaviors or lower prevalence of HIV in African American communities. To date, most HIV prevention research has focused on determinants of infection at the individual level, such as sociodemographic characteristics and current sexual and drug risk behaviors, or increasing knowledge and improving decision making about behavior and risk. Few research studies focus on these more distal causes of HIV risk behavior, such as trauma and mental health issues. Research that addresses more distal causes of HIV risk behavior is less developed. However, over the past two decades, a growing body of literature suggests that experiences of violence and the psychological sequelae that follow, such as depression, stress syndromes, and substance use, may contribute to increased HIV risk behavior among African Americans.

Although a direct causal association between traumatic events, mental health, and HIV risk behavior has not been established, a number of studies have associated either traumatic events or mental health with behaviors related to increased risk for HIV. This suggests that mental health disorders could serve as mediators through which traumatic events impact HIV risk behaviors. In this chapter, we examine the extent to which traumatic events have been associated in African-American populations. We consider the possibility that increased exposure to certain traumatic events, such as exposure to violence or violence victimization,

P.S. Spikes (✉)
Prevention Research Branch, Division of HIV/AIDS Prevention, Centers for Disease Control and Prevention, 1600 Clifton Road, Mailstop E-37, Atlanta, GA 30333, USA
e-mail: PSpikes@cdc.gov

D.H. McCree et al. (eds.), *African Americans and HIV/AIDS*,
DOI 10.1007/978-0-387-78321-5_6, © Springer Science+Business Media, LLC 2010

particularly as they occur within the context of cultural norms that limit access to and use of mental health services, may serve as markers for increased risk for HIV among African Americans starting in young adulthood.

Goals of This Chapter

We reviewed three areas of literature to look for potential links between exposure to traumatic events and HIV risk, mental health disorders and HIV risk, and utilization of mental health services for the general population and African Americans. The review examines studies documenting the prevalence, predictors, outcomes, and associations of these three areas in the general population, including African Americans. In addition, we review some of the unique issues related to African Americans' use of mental health services. We also discuss considerations for future research that is needed to address these issues.

Exposure to Traumatic Events and Links with HIV

Traumatic events are unanticipated and uncontrollable events characterized by a sense of horror, helplessness, and threat of serious injury or death (CDC, 2003). The lingering effects of trauma vary and are largely a function of the type of trauma experienced, for example interpersonal or natural disaster; age and developmental level at the time of the traumatic event; perceived severity of the traumatic event; repetitiveness of the trauma; and relationship with the perpetrator of the traumatic event (Breslau, Chilcoat, Kessler & Davis, 1999; Briere & Elliott, 2003; Cusack, Frueh, & Brady, 2004; Felitti et al., 1998). Emotional and behavioral symptoms can be short-term (i.e., days or weeks) or long-term (i.e., months or years), and can first appear months or years after the original event occurred. Most people recover from traumatic events without intervention, but some, particularly those who have experienced previous traumatic events or face ongoing stress related to the event, require intervention (Gillespie et al., 2009; Wyatt, Guthrie, & Norgrass, 1992).

Prevalence rates of experiencing traumatic events vary widely, ranging from 20 to 89.6% (Alim et al., 2006; Breslau et al., 1998; Cusack et al., 2004). According to the National Comorbidity Study (NCS), the first nationally representative mental health survey of U.S. males and females aged 15–54 years, approximately 60.7% of males and 51.2% of females experienced at least one traumatic event in their lifetime (Kessler, Sonnega, Bromet, Hughes, & Nelson, 1995). The most commonly reported events were witnessing someone being injured or killed, being in a natural disaster, and being in a life-threatening accident. Males were significantly more likely to experience these traumatic events than females (19–36% vs. 14–15%), whereas females were more likely to report rape, sexual molestation, childhood parental neglect, and childhood physical abuse (3–12% vs. 1–3%). Race, sex, gender, age, income, personality traits (e.g., neuroticism, extroversion), early conduct problems, family history of psychiatric disorders, and previous assault history have been identified as risk factors of experiencing traumatic events (Acierno, Resnick, Kilpatrick, Saunders, & Best, 1999; Breslau, Davis, & Andreski, 1995; Zierler, Witbeck, & Mayer, 1996).

The immediate and long-term outcomes associated with trauma exposure include problems related to interpersonal and cognitive functioning; revictimization; mental health disorders, particularly posttraumatic stress disorder (PTSD) and other stress syndromes; major depression; and substance abuse and dependence. Engaging in HIV-related risk behaviors, such as early initiation of consensual intercourse, multiple sexual partners, unprotected sex, and sexual bartering as an adult, also are associated with trauma exposure (Briere & Elliott, 2003; Classen, Palesh, & Aggarwal, 2005; Felitti et al., 1998; Holmes & Sammel, 2005; MacMillan et al., 2001; Paxton, Myers, Hall, & Javanbakht, 2004; Roth, Newman, Pelcovitz, van der Kolk, & Mandel, 1997; Widom, 1999; Wyatt, Axelrod, Chin, Carmona, & Loeb, 2000).

African Americans and Traumatic Events

Exposure to Community Violence

Exposure to traumatic events may not be random; environment and location of residence can play a role (Breslau et al., 1995). Neighborhood characteristics and discrimination may contribute to increased exposure to and experiences of violence for residents living in impoverished communities. Compared with whites, African Americans appear to be at higher risk for certain types of traumatic events, related, in part, to the structurally and economically disadvantaged urban neighborhoods where they are more likely to reside (Alim et al., 2006; Breslau et al., 1998; Kisera & Black, 2005). Characteristics associated with such neighborhoods often include high unemployment rates, homelessness, crime, violence, and substance abuse (Wilson, 1987). Factors at the neighborhood level – such as poverty, residential instability, and ethnic heterogeneity – and discrimination may serve as underlying mechanisms through which structural inequalities operate. These mechanisms may impede the establishment of formal and informal institutions of neighborhood organization and social ties that are believed to maintain and foster strong and safe neighborhoods or communities (Browning & Cagney, 2002).

Data confirm that non-whites who live in urban settings are at increased risk for violence victimization. In a representative probability sample of 2,181 Detroit residents, Breslau (1998) estimated the lifetime prevalence of assaultive violence (rape, sexual assault, and being badly beaten-up) to be two times higher among non-whites than whites, persons who have not graduated from college versus college graduates, and persons living in low-income households versus persons living in high-income households. The probability of assaultive violence occurred less frequently among adults 21 and up. Furthermore, research on community violence in neighborhoods has documented a significant association between exposure to violence and engagement in high HIV risk behaviors among African Americans (Viosin, 2002, 2005). In a study examining assault and risky sexual behaviors among African American males ($n = 120$; mean age = 16), nearly 56% of participants had been robbed or mugged and almost a quarter (22.5%, $n = 27$) indicated that they had forced sexual contact before age 13 (Voisin, 2003). Nearly two-thirds engaged in one or more HIV risk behaviors or risk indicators in the last 12 months (e.g., sex without condoms, sex after drug use, sex with concurrent partners, testing positive for a sexually transmitted infection – STI). Multivariate analyses confirmed that males who were victims of community violence were significantly more likely than nonvictims to engage in HIV sexual risk behaviors.

Data show racial or ethnic disparities in exposure to and experience of violence begin before adulthood and are reported more commonly among African Americans than among any other ethnic or racial group (Purugganan, Stein, Silver, & Benenson, 2003; Rennison, 2002). Data from the United States Department of Justice (USDOJ) (2006) indicate that among young people aged 12–19, African Americans were more likely to experience violent crimes (robbery, aggravated assault, simple assault, and rape or sexual assault) than whites (59.5 vs. 39.9%, respectively). In 2005, African Americans accounted for 49% of all homicide victims (USDOJ, 2008), and 51% of homicide victims were aged 17–29 years, compared to about 37% of white victims. Given that the social networks of the victims are often persons of the same age and from the same neighborhoods, many African American youth are likely to be exposed to violence and its consequences, such as loss of friends or heightened risk of experiencing violence.

Youth of minority races and ethnicities might also experience increased exposure to violence because they have a higher likelihood of spending time in residential facilities, such as detention centers, jails, or prisons (Bykowicz, 2008; Cannon, 2004; Zweig, Naser, Blackmore, & Schaffer, 2006). Non-Hispanic African American teenage boys (1,279 per 100,000) had the highest rate of placement in juvenile detention centers relative to Hispanic (775), American Indian (600), and Non-Hispanic white (305) teen boys in 2003 (Sickmund, Sladky, & Kang, 2005). Non-Hispanic African American female adolescents exhibited higher rates of detention when compared with other racial and ethnic female teenagers as well. In 2005, among young adult men aged of 20–24, non-Hispanic African American men (10.5%) were more likely to be in prison than Hispanic (3.9%) and non-Hispanic white men (vs. 1.6%) (Harrison & Beck, 2006).

Intimate Partner Violence Exposure

Intimate partner violence (IPV) includes physical, sexual, economic, emotional, or psychological abuse by current or former partner, spouse, or lover. The goal of the abuse is to establish and maintain power and control over the other partner. Although IPV is mostly associated with violence against females, males in heterosexual relationships and same sex couples also report experiencing IPV. IPV is often underreported to law enforcement because of the personal and significant relationship between the victim and the perpetrator. Therefore, it is difficult to know the true prevalence of this type of abuse. Each year, approximately 1.5 million women and more than 800,000 men in the United States are raped or physically assaulted by an intimate partner (Tjaden & Thoennes, 2000). Lifetime prevalence levels of IPV of any form ranged from 25 to 55.1% for women and from 7.6 to 22.9% for men (Coker et al., 2002; Tjaden & Thoennes, Allison 1999). The rates of male to male IPV range between 11% and 44% (Herek & Simpson; Tjaden et al (1999). The variability in prevalence levels may be related to the different definitions of partner violence across studies.

According to a meta-analysis (Stith, Smith, Pee, Ward, & Tritt, 2004), risk factors associated with males who physically abused their female partners included emotional or verbal abuse, forced sex, illicit drug use, attitudes condoning violence, lower marital satisfaction, traditional sex-role ideology, anger or hostility, history of partner abuse, alcohol use, depression, younger age, lower educational attainment, and unemployment. For females, risk factors associated with victimization of male partners were low marital satisfaction, younger age, less education, violence by partner, fear, depression, and alcohol use. A prior history of violence victimization has also been identified as a risk factor for experiencing IPV (Wyatt et al., 2002).

Outcomes associated with IPV include increased engagement in high-risk sexual behaviors and negative health outcomes, such as inconsistent or no condom/contraceptive use, rough sex (resulting in vaginal lacerations), unwanted or unplanned pregnancy, multiple partners, STIs or HIV infection from partners of unknown status, PTSD, depression, anxiety, substance use or abuse, infidelity, and death (Coker et al., 2002; Heise & Garcia-Moreno, 2002; Plichta, 2004; Roberts, Auinger, & Klein, 2005; Roberts, Klein, & Fisher, 2003; Silverman, Raj, Mucci, & Hathaway, 2001; Wu, El-Bassel, Witte, Gilbert, & Chang, 2003).

Although IPV cuts across race and ethnicity, socioeconomic status, education levels, and income differences (Straus & Gelles, 1986), researchers have estimated that African American adults experience a disproportionate amount of IPV (rape, physical assault, and stalking) when compared with white American adults (Dearwater et al., 1998; Hampton & Gelles, 1994; Rennison & Welchans, 2000). However, depending on the sampling methodology and weighting characteristics (e.g., proportionality, differing probabilities of selection, and refusal rate), the statistical significance of this difference (the higher prevalence of IPV among African Americans compared with whites) disappears when sociodemographic and relationship variables are statistically controlled (Bauer, Rodriguez, & Perez-Stable, 2000; Rennison & Planty, 2003; Tjaden & Thoennes, 2000). These results suggest that IPV occurs less frequently among African Americans or at similar rates of the general population, partly because of sociodemographics and relationship characteristics.

Lifetime prevalence of IPV differs for African Americans and whites by type of violence. Whereas African American and white women are equally likely to report experiencing rape (7.4 vs. 7.7%), African American women are more likely to report physical assault than white women (26.3 vs. 21.3%). African American men are more likely report physical assault than white men as well (10.2 vs. 7.2%). Overall, African Americans are more likely to report higher lifetime victimization rates from IPV than whites (29.1 vs. 24.8% for women; 12.0 vs. 7.5% for men) (USDOJ, 2000).

Two studies (Caetano, Cunradi, Clark, & Schafer, 2000; Neff, Holamon, & Schluter, 1995) found that African American couples (23%) were more likely than Hispanic (17%) and non-Hispanic white (11.5%) couples to report an incident of male-to-female partner violence in the past 12 months. The rate of female-to-male partner violence between heterosexual couples was 30% among African Americans, 21% among Hispanics, and 15% among whites (Caetano, Nelson, & Cunradi, 2001). The researchers indicated that the higher prevalence of IPV among ethnic minorities compared with whites could not be explained by a single factor but seemed to be related to risk factors associated with the perpetrator, characteristics of the relationship, and neighborhood characteristics. Thirty to forty percent of men and 27–34% of the women who perpetrated violence against their partners were drinking at the time of the event.

Racial and ethnic disparities in IPV also occur among adolescents in grades 9–12. Dating violence, defined as being intentionally hit, slapped, or physically hurt by a boyfriend or girlfriend in the past 12 months, is highest among African Americans compared with other racial or ethnic groups. According to data from the Youth Risk Behavior Surveillance System (YRBSS), in 2007, African American youth attending high school were more likely to report experiencing dating violence than Hispanic and non-Hispanic white youth attending high school (14% vs. 11% and 8%, respectively) (CDC, 2008b).

Violence and HIV Risk

Physical or sexual abuse by an intimate partner can increase HIV risk. Maman, Campbell, Sweat, and Gielen (2000) identified three points of intersection between violence and a woman's risk for HIV infection (1) risk for infection through forced or coercive sexual intercourse with an infected partner; (2) limited ability to negotiate safer sexual behaviors, such as condom use, because of fear of or past experience with partner violence; and (3) increased likelihood of engaging in HIV risk-taking behaviors because of a past history of sexual assault. Studies suggest that although many women are fearful of making condom requests, only a small proportion actually experience violent reactions (Koenig & Moore, 2000). Nevertheless, some women in abusive relationships may not ask their partners to use condoms because they fear their partners' reaction. Finally, several studies have shown a relationship between IPV and greater risk of engaging in HIV high-risk behaviors. For example, in a study of 141 women attending urban health clinics, Morrill and Ickovics (1996) found that women who had been abused were more likely to have had partners who injected drugs, used coercion to have sex, and used coercion not to use a condom.

Similarly, in a pilot study of 143 women recruited from an inner-city emergency room, El-Bassel et al. (1998) found that abused women were four times as likely as women who had not been abused to report sex with a risky partner (e.g., has multiple partners, injects drugs).

Several large multisite cohort studies also have shown that prevalence of IPV is high among women with or at risk for HIV. In these cohort studies, prevalence of violence was equally high among seronegative and HIV-positive women (Burke, Thieman, Gielen, O'Campo, & McDonnel, 2005; Cohen et al., 2000; Koenig et al., 2002; Vlahov et al., 1998). The findings are explained by the matching of HIV-negative women to HIV-positive women on the basis of demographic and sexual and drug-use risk behaviors, suggesting that violence and HIV are likely linked through these sex and drug-risk behaviors (Koenig & Clark, 2004). In addition, although some women have experienced IPV as a direct response to disclosing their serostatus, this appears to be rare (Koenig & Moore, 2000).

Some HIV-positive men may be more likely than uninfected men to engage in IPV with their female partners. In a sample of 317 HIV-positive men who were injection drug users (IDUs), homelessness, psychological distress, and engaged in unprotected sex with main and non-main HIV-negative female partners were positively associated with IPV perpetration against main female partners (Frye et al., 2007). This finding suggest that IPV perpetration may be more prevalent among HIV-positive male IDUs and associated with sexual risk behaviors for HIV transmission than non-IDUs.

In addition, studies show that women with a history of childhood sexual assault are at greater risk of engaging in HIV risk behaviors and contracting HIV in adulthood compared with women without a history of childhood abuse (Koenig & Clark, 2004). Childhood abuse may continue to impact the behavior of adults with HIV. Among HIV-positive persons, childhood physical and sexual abuse were significant predictors of sexual risk behaviors such as multiple partners, injection drug use, and in some studies, unprotected sex in adulthood (Maker, Kemmelmeier, & Peterson, 2001; Paxton et al., 2004; Senn, Carey, & Vanable, 2006; Whetten et al., 2006; Wyatt et al., 2002) though not in others (Kalichman, 1999; Medrano, Desmond, Zule, & Hatch, 1999; Stein et al., 2005).

Mental Health Disorders and Links to HIV

Victimization experiences and other potentially traumatic events do not necessarily lead to mental health disorders or symptoms. It is not uncommon to experience certain stress symptoms following a traumatic event, but if responded to appropriately, these symptoms often dissipate over time. For some persons, however, such symptoms will develop into more serious problems. Although no one specific mental health disorder is associated with being a victim of or witness to violence, several mental health disorders, including PTSD, major depression, and substance abuse and dependence, are more commonly seen among trauma survivors.

Posttraumatic Stress Disorder (PTSD)

PTSD is an anxiety disorder that can develop after experiencing or witnessing an extreme, violent, overwhelming traumatic event during which the person experiences intense fear, helplessness, or horror. Symptoms associated with PTSD include emotional numbing (i.e., emotional non-responsiveness), hyperarousal (e.g., sleep difficulties, irritability, constant alert for danger), avoidance (e.g., avoiding places, thoughts, people, events associated with the traumatic event), and re-experiencing the trauma (e.g., flashbacks, intrusive emotions (APA,1994). These symptoms must be consistently present for at least 1 month to be considered for a PTSD diagnosis. Other mental health disorders, such as depression or drug abuse or dependence, can be present along with PTSD (Kessler et al., 1995). The psychological effects associated with experiencing a traumatic event can be immediate or delayed. Furthermore, an individual with PTSD may harbor feelings of mistrust, anger, shame, and rage, which can manifest through a variety of behaviors (Andrews, Brewin, Rose, & Kirk, 2000; Duncan et al., 1996; Najavits et al., 1998; Terr, 1991).

PTSD affects approximately 7.7 million adults in the United States, but can occur at any age, including childhood (Kessler, Berglund, Demler, Jin, & Walters, 2005). The lifetime prevalence of experiencing a traumatic event varies across studies, ranging from 40 to 60% (Breslau et al., 2006). Prevalence rates for PTSD are estimated to range from 8 to 12% in the general population (Kessler, Berglund, et al.). Lifetime prevalence rates of PTSD range from 9.2 to 10.4% for women and 5.0 to 6.2% for men in nationally representative samples (Breslau et al., 1998; Kessler, Berglund, et al.). According to one meta-analysis (Brewin, Andrews, & Valentine, 2000), the top three factors relating to events during and after the trauma – greater trauma severity, lack of social support, and more subsequent life stress – conveyed the strongest risk (effect size) for PTSD in addition to sociodemographic characteristics. Although Ozer, Best, and Lipsey (2003) found demographics to be important for predicting PTSD, she and colleagues found that peritraumatic psychological processes, intensely negative emotional responses or dissociative experiences during or immediately after the traumatic event, to be better predictors. The traumatic events most associated with the development of PTSD for males are rape, combat exposure, childhood neglect, and childhood physical abuse (Kessler, 1995). For females the most common events associated with PTSD include rape, sexual molestation, being physically attacked, being threatened with a weapon, and childhood physical abuse (Kessler, 1995). Sexual assault, nonsexual violence, and sudden unexpected death of a loved one are known to be high-impact traumatic events for both men and women that confer greater risk of developing PTSD than other traumatic events (Breslau et al., 1998).

African Americans and PTSD

Findings regarding African Americans' risk for PTSD are equivocal, with some indicating that African Americans are not at greater risk for PTSD than whites (Hutton, Treisman, Hunt, Fishman, Kendig, Swetz, et al., 2001) and others indicating that they are (Breslau et al., 1995; Butts, 2002). Two studies that examined trauma exposure and PTSD in predominantly African American convenience samples (100% African American for one study and 96% African American for the other) provide new information about prevalence of traumatic events among African Americans. Among 184 African Americans seeking long-term care at an outpatient center (Schwartz, Bradley, Sexton, Sherry, & Ressler, 2005), the estimated lifetime prevalence of PTSD, using the PTSD Symptom Scale, was 43%. Participants reported the following traumatic events: being attacked with a knife, gun, or other weapon (55%); being attacked by a perpetrator without a weapon with the intent to kill or injure (55%); being in a serious accident or experiencing a serious injury (48%); experiencing childhood sexual abuse before the age of 13 (39%); and forced sexual contact as an adult (33%). In another study of 617 African Americans seeking primary care (Alim et al., 2006), the most frequently reported traumatic events were transportation (car) accident (42%), sudden unexpected death of a loved one (39%), and physical assault (30%). Sixty-five percent had experienced a trauma that had a high impact on their wellbeing. The estimated PTSD lifetime prevalence rate for the sample was 33%. These estimates are higher than those found in the general population – 8 to 12% (Breslau et al., 1998; Kessler, Berglund, et al., 2005).

Prevalence of PTSD also may be underestimated among African Americans because researchers and health care providers may not categorize some traumatic events commonly experienced by African Americans as stressors. According to Butts (2002), the list of traumas associated with a diagnosis of PTSD in the *Diagnostic and Statistical Manual of Mental Disorders DSM* (DSM; American Psychiatric Association (APA), 1994) are too narrowly focused. He suggests that although experiences of discrimination and racism may not involve a threat to a person's life, they may lead to symptoms of PTSD. Butts suggests that persons who experience high levels of discrimination and racism exhibit the same outcomes as persons who experience stressors most commonly associated with a diagnosis of PTSD.

PTSD and HIV

PTSD may be related to HIV risk through its association with substance use. Individuals with PTSD are more likely to have problems with alcohol or drug use (Kessler, 1995), which can increase sexual HIV risk behaviors or lead to situations where risk behavior is likely to occur.

Studies indicate that the prevalence of PTSD and acute stress syndromes may be higher in HIV-positive populations. Estimates of PTSD prevalence rates among HIV-positive persons range from 35 to 46%, which is higher than the prevalence rate of PTSD among the general population (from 8 to 12%). To some extent, the higher rate may be related in part to the trauma of a diagnosis of and living with a life-threatening and stigmatized disease. After diagnosis, people with HIV must deal with the possibility of infecting others or dying of HIV, ongoing and unexpected illness, and experiencing stigma from family and friends. A few studies of persons with HIV have found that participants met the PTSD criteria specifically related to their HIV diagnosis (Kelly et al., 1998; Myers & Durvasula, 1999; Radcliffe et al., 2007). On the other hand, PTSD may dispose individuals to HIV. A number of studies have found that HIV-positive African American women often reported a history childhood abuse as well as adult abuse, rape, threats, assaults, and other traumatic life events (Brady, Gallagher, Berger, & Vega, 2002; Martinez, Israelski, Walker, & Koopman, 2002).

Depression

Depression can refer to a negative affective state; a collection of co-occurring affective, cognitive and physiological symptoms; or a disorder referred to as major depression. Major depressive disorder is characterized by changes in appetite and sleeping patterns; feelings of worthlessness, hopelessness, and inappropriate guilt; or loss of interest or pleasure in formerly important activities, leading to substantial role impairment (APA, 1994).

Episodes of depression may be triggered by traumatic or other stressful events. Sociodemographic characteristics that have been commonly associated with depression include being within the age range of 18–29, being female, living in a households with a family income of less than $20,000, being previously married, residing in an urban area, and being unemployed (Kessler et al., 2003; Williams et al., 2007). Outcomes that have been associated with depression include poor physical health, PTSD, substance abuse, engaging in unprotected sex, and suicide (Gilmer et al., 2005; Marks, Bingman, & Duval, 1998; United States Department of Health and Human Services (USDHHS), 1999a).

Prevalence of Depression in United States

Depression is one of the most prevalent mental health disorders in the United States and is often referred to as the common cold of psychopathology (Rosenhan & Seligman, 1995). Prevalence of experiencing an episode of major depressive disorder range from 5.4 to 47% (Blazer, Kessler, McGonagle, & Swartz, 1994; Kessler et al., 1994, 2003; Perdue et al., 2003; Riolo, Nguyen, Greden, & King, 2005; Williams et al., 2007). While studies conducted during the 1970s and 1980s suggested higher rates of major depressive disorder among African Americans compared with whites (Neighbors, Jackson, Bowman, & Gurin, 1983; Somervell, Leaf, Weissman, Blazer, & Bruce, 1989; Warheit, Holzer, & Arey, 1975), recent studies with more rigorous sampling and statistical techniques indicate otherwise. In almost every large, probability sample study conducted since the 1990s, prevalence for depression or experiencing depressive symptoms were higher for whites than non-whites (Blazer et al.; Kessler et al.; Riolo et al.; Williams et al.). However, Williams and colleagues point out that although the prevalence of depression is greater for whites, chronicity of depression is greater for African Americans than for whites, suggesting that the impact of depression for African Americans is more severe and debilitating.

Unique Stressors for African Americans

Racism

Racial or *ethnic discrimination* is defined as unfair, differential treatment on the basis of race or ethnicity. Within the United States, racial discrimination disproportionately affects African American adults (Kessler, Michelson, & Williams, 1999) relative to other ethnic or racial groups. Events associated with racial discrimination are stressful and can directly lead to psychological distress and physiological changes that affect mental health (Williams, Neighbors, & Jackson, 2003; Williams & Williams-Morris, 2000). A review of 138 studies on health and self-reported experiences of racism among oppressed racial groups found the strongest association with negative, mental health outcomes (such as psychological or emotional distress and depression or depressive symptoms) and health-related behaviors (Paradies, 2006).

Perceived racism has been found to be associated with depression among African American adults (Brown et al., 2000; Utsey & Payne, 2000). A few studies show the same association among younger African Americans. One study followed more than 700 African American children, starting when the children were aged 10–12 years, for 5 years, interviewing both them and their families about racism and other life experiences. The researchers found that children who reported more discrimination, such as name-calling or insults, were more likely to experience depression as they became teenagers (Brody et al., 2006). In a cross-sectional study of 5,135 fifth-graders, Coker et al. (2009) were more likely to find an association between perceived racial or ethnic discrimination and depressive symptoms for African American, Hispanic, and other minority youth than for white youth. Both studies showed that African American youth experienced racial discrimination at early ages, which has been linked to depressive symptoms and depression. Although depression occurs among all young people, its effect may be more debilitating for African American young adults than their white counterparts (Williams et al., 2007). Depression among younger African Americans has been linked to engaging in high-risk sexual behaviors (Brown et al., 2006; Diclemente et al., 2001; Seth, Raiji, Diclemente, Wingood, & Rose, 2009).

Homophobia

African Americans occupy multiple positions of minority statuses, particularly in terms of race and sexual orientation. They represent only 13% of the U.S. and report experiencing racism from white communities In addition, African American homosexual, bisexual, and transgender persons report discrimination from members of the African American community and the gay community. The dual influences of racism and discrimination can increase the risk for depression among racial and ethnic minorities.

Broadly defined, *homophobia* is the fear or irrational hatred of same-sex attraction or behavior on the basis of negative beliefs and attitudes. Homophobia and the verbal, emotional, physical, and social acts associated with it are systemic and perpetuated by religious or political beliefs. For victims of homophobia and homophobic acts, the effects are long lasting and may put some individuals at greater risk for isolation, physical violence, and mental health disorders.

Compared with heterosexual men, men who have sex with men (MSM) also report more frequent experiences with discrimination, a stressor, as both discrete events and everyday offenses (Cochran, 2001). In addition, MSM are three times as likely as heterosexual men to meet the criteria for major depression (Cochran, Sullivan, & Mays, 2003).

Kennamer, Honnold, Bradford, and Hendricks (2000) reported that homophobia appears to be "a major part of the African American culture, driven by both religious forces and political forces." Peer discrimination against African American men who do not conform to heterosexual identities begins during adolescence in some African American communities (Froyum, 2007). Research with African American homosexual and bisexual men suggests that internalized homophobia leads to lower self-esteem and to psychological distress (Stokes & Peterson, 1998). Higher depressive mood scores have been found among African American MSM (AAMSM) when compared with white and heterosexual African American men (Richardson, Myers, Bing, & Saltz, 1997). Racism and heterosexism are potential factors that may provide supporting evidence of AAMSM being at greater risk for depression than heterosexual men and women in general (Crawford, Allsion, Zamboni, & Soto, 2002).

Depression and HIV Risk

Studies that examine the relationship between depressive symptoms and high-risk sexual behaviors among various populations, such as HIV-positive gay men, IDUs, young gay men, female prisoners, serodiscordant couples, heterosexual men, and participants at an sexually transmitted disease (STD) clinic, have been mixed. Whereas some studies found an association between depressive symptoms and high-risk behaviors (Hutton, Lyketos, Zenilman, Thomposon, & Erbelding, 2004), others do not (Bradley, Remien, & Dolezal, 2008; Crepaz & Marks, 2002; Milam, Richardson, Espinoza, & Stoyanoff, 2006). In larger, multistudy reviews, factors such as risk and racial group were not compared, limiting the ability to determine whether one group was at greater risk for depression than others. The varying types of instruments used to measure depression in the studies (e.g., Center for Epidemiological Studies-Depression – CES-D, Symptom Checklist-90 Revised – SCL-90R, and Structured Clinical Interview for DSM Disorders – SCID interview) and altering the measures within the instruments may have contributed to the different results. In addition, the place where the population was recruited may have affected determinations of depression.

Depression and HIV Risk Among African Americans

Several studies have noted an association between depressive symptoms and HIV risk behaviors among samples of urban, African American adolescents (Brown et al., 2006; Diclemente et al., 2001; Seth et al., 2009). Seth et al. found that psychological distress was associated with inconsistent condom use, sex while under the influence of drugs or alcohol, high-risk sexual partners, and sexually transmitted infections. These studies indicate that depressive symptoms experienced by adolescents, particularly African American adolescents, can contribute to engaging in sexual practices that increase risk for HIV transmission.

Similar associations were found among African American adults. In a sample primarily composed of homosexual and bisexual African American men attending an outpatient clinic, Marks et al. (1998) found that negative affective states were significantly associated with participants' having unprotected sex with their most recent male-to-male sexual encounter. In another study of African American heterosexual, homosexual, and bisexual men, Myers, Javanbakht, Martinez, and Obediah (2003), using the SCL-90-R, found high psychological distress to be one of the best predictors for engaging in high-risk behaviors among HIV-positive and HIV-negative men.

Furthermore, gender may play a role in the types of risk behaviors in which depressed African Americans engage. In a sample primarily composed of African Americans (96%) seeking treatment at an STD clinic (Hutton et al., 2004), depressed women were more likely than women who were not depressed to have had sex for money or drugs, have had sex while "high" on alcohol, cocaine, or heroin, and have used cocaine or heroin in the preceding 30 days. Similarly, depressed men were more likely than men who were not depressed to have had sex while "high" on cocaine or heroine, abused alcohol or drugs in the past 30 days, and had a greater number of lifetime sexual partners. Both depressed men and women in the study were more likely to report histories of trading sex for drugs or money and having had a sex partner who used intravenous drugs than their nondepressed counterparts. However, depression was not related to unprotected sexual intercourse or an STI diagnosis for either sex. Although the differences are slight, we see that alcohol and drug use is associated with depression which may influence certain risk behaviors and not others. For example, substance use is associated with the selection of high-risk partners but not with engaging in unprotected sex. Similar results were found by Williams and Latkin (2005) using longitudinal data to examine the relationship between depressive symptoms and sexual risk behaviors in a community sample of 332 mostly African American urban drug users.

Substance Use Disorders

Substance use disorders are characterized as either disorders of dependence, a pattern of repeated self-administration of a substance that typically results in tolerance, withdrawal, and compulsive drug-taking, or disorders of abuse, characterized by a maladaptive pattern of use that involves adverse physical, legal, or social consequences (APA, 1994). Individuals may use alcohol or illicit drugs to relieve symptoms of an underlying emotional condition or disorder, such as fear, stress, or trauma. Research has demonstrated a strong relationship between experiencing traumatic events and substance use problems. For example, 25–75% of people who have survived abusive or violent traumatic experiences report problematic alcohol use. Adolescents who are sexually assaulted are nine times as likely as adolescents who have not been assaulted to experience hard drug dependence – such as cocaine, heroin, methamphetamine (International Society for Traumatic Stress Studies, 2009). Substance abuse also co-occurs with other mental health conditions, including depression and PTSD (Hasin, Stinson, Ogburn, & Grant, 2007). Continued use and abuse of these substances can further compound psychological and emotional problems.

Substance Use Disorders: Prevalence and Racial and Ethnic Differences

Alcohol Disorders

Hasin et al. (2007) used the 2001–2002 National Epidemiologic Survey on Alcohol and Related Conditions (NESARC) to calculate the current (12 month) and lifetime prevalence of alcohol abuse (4.7 and 17.8%) and alcohol dependence (3.8 and 12.5%) of adults ($n = 43,093$) in the United States. Current alcohol abuse was more prevalent among men, whites, young adults (18–29) and never-married individuals, while lifetime rates were highest among males, Native Americans, middle-aged Americans, and persons making more than $70,000. Reported prevalence rates of alcohol abuse at 12 month and lifetime for blacks were lower than whites, Native Americans, and Hispanics.

Injection Drug Use

The 1998 National Household Survey on Drug Abuse indicated that the lifetime prevalence for injection drug use was similar for whites, African Americans, and Latinos (1.5, 1.3, and 0.9%, respectively) (USDHHS, 1999b). However, health disparities associated with injection drug use is greater among African Americans than among whites (Cooper, Friedman, Tempalski, Friedman, & Keem, 2005). Injection drug use is directly associated with HIV transmission. Among IDUs, several demographic and behavioral characteristics are associated with a greater risk of acquiring HIV. These characteristics include low income, being African American, being male, and a diagnosis of antisocial personality disorder (Kalichman, 1999; Somlai, Kelly, McAuliffe, Ksobiech, & Lackl, 2003). Among adolescents and adults living with HIV, African Americans are more likely to report injection drug use as their mode of acquisition than whites. Approximately 22.2% of adult and adolescent African Americans living with HIV/AIDS and 12.5% of whites living with HIV/AIDS reported injection drug use as their primary mode of HIV acquisition (CDC, 2008a). Seven percent of cases of HIV/AIDS among African Americans and 8% of cases of HIV/AIDS among whites are related to both injection drug use and male same sex behavior, bringing the cumulative percentage of injection drug use related to HIV/ AIDS transmission to 26.4% for African Americans and 19.3% for whites (CDC).

Noninjection Drug Use

African Americans are less likely to report the use of most drugs except for crack (Ma & Shive, 2000), which is a derivative of cocaine. Crack is usually smoked and delivers large quantities of the drug to the lungs, producing an immediate and intense euphoric effect. It is abused because it produces an immediate high and is inexpensive to produce. The use of crack is most common among African Americans as well as males, adults aged 18–34 years, and adults who are unemployed (Ma & Shive; Sullivan, Nakashima, Purcell, Ward, & The Supplement to HIV/AIDS Surveillance Study Group, 1998).

Crack is highly addictive, and through its relationship with unprotected sex and multiple sex partners (Booth, Kwiatkowski, & Chitwood, 2000; Compton, Thomas, Stinson, & Grant, 2007), it fuels the epidemic of sexually transmitted HIV. Studies examining HIV and crack cocaine use identified the following as risk factors associated with its use: being African American, having a history of sexual abuse, having sexual partners of unknown or negative serostatus, having multiple sex partners, inconsistent condom use, younger age, having a difficult childhood, using alcohol daily, using marijuana frequently, trading sex for drugs or money, lack of permanent housing, being unemployed, having a lifetime history of syphilis, being female, and having a sex partner who injects drugs (El-Bassel et al., 2000; Hoffman, Klein, Eber, & Crosby, 2000; Iguchi & Bux, 1997; Klinkenberg & Sacks, 2004; Logan & Leukefeld, 2000; Logan, Leukefeld, & Farabee, 1998; Roberts, Wechsberg, Zule, & Burrough, 2003).

African American MSM are significantly more likely than MSM of other races or ethnicities to report using non-injected crack (Sullivan et al., 1998). African American females and males are more likely to report using non-injected crack than white males and females. In Timpson's study of African American crack users, participants reported an average of 17 sex partners in the previous 6 months, with men having an average of 19.8 partners and women having an average of 10.7 (Timpson, Williams, Bowen, & Keel, 2003). Crack use continues to fuel the transmission of HIV in African American communities.

Substance Use and HIV

Drug and alcohol use also increase the probability of a variety of HIV risk behaviors, including unprotected vaginal and anal intercourse, multiple sex partners, early sexual initiation, having a sex partner who injects or has ever injected drugs, and exchanging sex for drugs or money (Somlai et al., 2003; Stein et al., 2005; Windle, 1997). Moreover, substance use may interfere with a person's judgment or place them in high-risk situations, making them more vulnerable to participating in risky behaviors. Over time, the effects of alcohol or drugs on the brain can lead to significant impairment of cognitive functioning and judgment as well (MacDonald, MacDonald, Zanna, & Fong, 2000).

Utilization of Mental Health Services Among African Americans

Only a minority of persons with any mental health disorder in the general population receive treatment for it from health care services. Using data from the National Comorbidity Survey Replication Study ($n=4,319$) collected between 2001 and 2003, Kessler, Demler, et al. (2005) examined trends in the prevalence and rate of treatment of mental disorders among people 18–54 years of age using DSM-IV. The estimated prevalence of a 12-month mental disorder (e.g., anxiety, mood, substance abuse) was 30.5%, and approximately 20.1% received treatment. Predictors of use of mental health services were age greater than 24 years, female sex, non-Hispanic white race, and marital status (separated, widowed, divorced, or never married).

Only one of three African Americans who require mental health services receive them (USDHHS, 2001). African Americans' underutilization of mental health services has been associated with issues such as distrust and fear of the medical care system and the government, stigma associated with seeking mental health treatment, and lack of availability of or access to appropriate mental health services (Neighbors & Jackson, 1996; USDHHS). Underutilization of mental health services may play a role in African Americans' use of alcohol and drugs if these substances, rather than psychotropic drugs and therapy, are used to alleviate symptoms of distress. Self-medicating with drugs or alcohol can lead to engaging in HIV-related risk behaviors (Davis, Ressler, Schwartz, Stephens, & Bradley, 2008; Richman, Kohn -Wood, & Williams, 2007).

Distrust and Fear of Treatment

For some African Americans, distrust of health care providers and the government is a barrier to seeking care (USDHHS, 2001). Many studies have noted the provision of inadequate medical treatment for African Americans, their poor treatment and abuse since slavery, and their inhumane treatment in medical research (Gamble, 1993, 1997; Williams, 1986; Wynia & Gamble, 2006). The history of these injustices may have led to many African Americans to expect dishonesty from government institutions and health care providers today (Whaley, 2004).

The lack of cultural competency among institutions and service providers has also fueled perceptions of distrust (USDHHS, 2001). Services may not be responsive to the cultural concerns of African Americans and reflect a lack of awareness of their language, histories, traditions, beliefs, and values. Lack of cultural competency has been linked with the over-diagnosis of severe mental disorders and failure to prescribe medications for African American patients (Braithwaite & Taylor, 2001; Neighbors, Jackson, Campbell, & Williams, 1989). For example, if clinicians do not understand how racism, discrimination, or social environments influence the lives and mental health of African Americans, they may be more likely to diagnose a personality disorder (e.g., antisocial personality disorder) than an adjustment disorder for an African American who may deal with the effects of racism (Copland, 2006). Issues such as these may contribute to African Americans not returning for further treatment (USDHHS).

Stigma of Mental Disorder

Stigma associated with a mental disorder is one barrier to treatment for many African Americans (USDHHS, 2001). Some members in African American communities disapprove of seeking help for mental or emotional problems from nonreligious practitioners, an act viewed as "turning your back on God" (Cooper-Patrick et al., 1997). The stigma-related issues regarding mental illness that affect African Americans include viewing the seeking of treatment for mental illness as a sign of weakness or as embarrassing, the belief that African American people do not suffer from mental disorders, and the belief that mental illness can be cured through prayer and religious intervention (Early, 1992; Willis, Coombs, Cockerham, & Frison, 2002). African Americans who do seek mental health services must overcome the stigma associated with mental health problems. Outcomes associated with mental illness stigma include a delay in seeking treatment, use of primary care and emergency room services to receive treatment, and presenting with more severe symptoms at initiation of treatment (Gary, 2005; Snowden, 2001; USDHHS).

Availability of and Access to Mental Health Services

Availability of and access to health care influences the utilization of mental health services by African Americans in a number of ways. Proposed barriers to help seeking behaviors and mental health access among low-income African Americans were compiled by Hines-Martin, Malone, Kim, and Brown-Piper (2003). They included individual factors s (e.g., stigma, competing responsibilities, knowledge deficits), institutional factors (e.g., bureaucratic red tape), and cultural factors (e.g., family opposition). In other studies, issues associated with the availability and access to mental health services by African Americans included lack of transportation, negative therapy experiences of others, community disapproval, lack of awareness regarding the steps necessary to obtain services, inability to pay insurance copayments, understaffed facilities, and poor service quality (Davis et al., 2008; Livingston, 2004; USDHHS, 2001; Williams, 1998).

Conclusion

The link between of traumatic experiences, such as exposure to violence and abuse, and increased HIV risk has been well established. In this review, we found African Americans were at greater risk for exposure to violent victimization (community violence and IPV) than other racial or ethnic populations across their lifespan. The higher prevalence may be related to the areas in which they reside. We also found that African Americans were less likely to be diagnosed with depression, posttraumatic stress syndrome, or substance abuse disorders than the general population. Additional research is required to gain greater understanding why this is the case. Understanding how psychological trauma fosters HIV risk behaviors, particularly among African Americans, is important for the development of public policies and programs to reduce HIV transmission.

Based on the data currently available, we were unable to determine whether mental health problems mediate the relationship between exposure to violence and HIV risk behavior for African Americans. PTSD, depression, and substance abuse were all associated with HIV risk behavior for African Americans as they were for the general population, but African Americans were not at increased risk for HIV acquisition as a result of a mental health diagnosis. However, we see that drug use, injection and non-injection, specifically with Crack places African Americans at higher risk for HIV. Drug use (including alcohol) or exposure to it may-be associated with increased levels of IPV and community violence. Drugs may in part be fueling the HIV epidemic among African Americans, and thus could be the link between trauma experiences and HIV risk in this population.

In many of the large probability studies, whites, not African Americans, were at higher risk for PTSD, depression, and abuse of certain substances (Hasin et al., 2007; Kessler et al., 1994; Williams et al., 2007). Yet, most of these studies were conducted only with noninstitutionalized participants. This limitation may underestimate prevalence for some disorders among African Americans, since African Americans are overrepresented in some institutionalized populations, such as prisons and detention centers.

It is also possible that the impact of mental health problems that stem from traumatic events may be heightened for African Americans because these problems are less likely to be ameliorated through mental health treatment. Whether due to poor access to services and culturally competent providers, financial limitations, mistrust of the mental health community, or stigma of mental illness, African Americans are less likely to receive treatment for mental health problems than whites. Untreated, individuals experiencing the mental effects of trauma may begin using substances to self-medicate and relieve emotional distress, which could then develop into abuse and dependence, further increasing risk for both trauma and HIV.

A review of the literature found that factors associated with increased risk for violence or certain mental health problems are similar to factors recognized as increasing African Americans' risk for HIV transmission and acquisition. These factors include prior victimization, poverty, residing in an urban environment, low educational attainment, unemployment, and drug use. People of low socioeconomic status may be at higher risk of experiencing certain traumatic events because of the social and physical environments in which they reside. Socioeconomic status often determines place of residence (through racial segregation), partner selection, schools attended, and exposure to greater levels of violence and traumatic events. Exposure to violence and traumatic events may independently increase risk for both mental health disorders and for HIV risk behaviors, or mental health disorders may further increase risk for HIV-related behaviors. In addition to trauma and mental health issues co-occurring and contributing to HIV risk behaviors, other issues may be contributing to the engagement in unsafe behavior as well thereby making it difficult to establish causal or time-ordered relationships. Moreover, a cumulative effect of risk may be caused by experiencing a number of traumas across a lifetime, which, increases risk for both mental health problems and HIV risk behaviors.

Although the current literature shows connections between violence, HIV, and posttraumatic stress, depression, and substance abuse, relationships for affected subpopulations, particularly African Americans, have not been fully examined. The relationship between trauma, mental health, and HIV risk for African Americans is complex, and more targeted research is needed to clarify these relationships. The following are suggestions for future research:

- Expand mental health research to include homosexual, bisexual, and heterosexual African American men because much of the existing HIV-related research focuses on women.
- Examine ongoing traumatic events, such as racism and discrimination, as they relate to mental health disorders and influence sexual risk-taking behaviors among African Americans.
- Establish baseline frequencies of current and lifetime mental health disorders among African Americans at high risk for HIV infection as part of longitudinal assessments of mental health and trauma.
- Refine mental health-related scales and assessment practices to enhance cultural relevance for African Americans.
- Develop interventions that assist with helping to destigmatize seeking mental health services.
- Implement and evaluate the effects of structural interventions to address poverty and substance use among African Americans, particularly as the interventions relate to HIV risk.

Findings from such research will help in planning proper HIV prevention efforts for the African American community.

References

Acierno, R., Resnick, H., Kilpatrick, D. G., Saunders, N., & Best, C. L. (1999). Risk factors for rape, physical assault, and posttraumatic stress disorder in women: Examination of differential multivariate relationships. *Journal of Anxiety Disorders, 13*(6), 541–563.

Alim, T. N., Graves, E., Mellman, T. A., Aigbogun, N., Gray, E., Lawson, W., et al. (2006). Trauma exposure, posttraumatic stress disorder and depression in an African-American primary care population. *Journal of the National Medical Association, 98*(10), 1630–1636.

American Psychiatric Association (APA). (1994). *Diagnostic and statistical manual of mental disorders* (4th ed.). Washington, DC: American Psychiatric Association.

Andrews, B., Brewin, C. R., Rose, S., & Kirk, M. (2000). Predicting PTSD symptoms in victims of violent crime: The role of shame, anger, and childhood abuse. *Journal of Abnormal Psychology, 109*(1), 69–73.

Bauer, H. M., Rodriguez, M. A., & Perez-Stable, E. J. (2000). Prevalence and determinants of intimate partner abuse among public hospital primary care patients. *Journal of General Internal Medicine, 15*(11), 811–817.

Blazer, C., Kessler, R. C., McGonagle, K. A., & Swartz, M. S. (1994). The prevalence and distribution of major depression in a national community sample: The National Comorbidity Survey. *American Journal of Psychiatry, 151*, 979–986.

Booth, R. E., Kwiatkowski, C. F., & Chitwood, D. D. (2000). Sex related HIV risk behaviors: Differential risks among injection drug users, crack smokers, and injection drug users who smoke. *Drug and Alcohol Dependence, 58*, 219–226.

Bradley, M. V., Remien, R. H., & Dolezal, C. (2008). Depression symptoms and sexual HIV risk behavior among serodiscordant couples. *Psychosomatic Medicine, 70*, 186–191.

Brady, S., Gallagher, D., Berger, J., & Vega, M. (2002). Physical and sexual abuse in the lives of HIV-positive women enrolled in a primary medicine health maintenance organization. *AIDS Patient Care and STDs, 16*, 121–125.

Braithwaite, R. L., & Taylor, S. E. (2001). *Health issues in the Black community* (2nd ed.). San Francisco, CA: Jossey-Bass.

Breslau, J., Aguilar-Gaxiola, S., Kendler, K. S., Su, M., Williams, D., & Kessler, R. C. (2006). Specifying race-ethnic difference in risk for psychiatric disorder in a US national sample. *Psychological Medicine, 36*(1), 57–68.

Breslau, N., Chilcoat, H. D., Kessler, R. C., & Davis, G. C. (1999). Previous exposure to trauma and PTSD effects of subsequent trauma: Results of the Detroit area survey of trauma. *American Journal of Psychiatry, 156*(6), 902–907.

Breslau, N., Davis, G. C., & Andreski, P. (1995). Risk factors for PTSD-related traumatic events: A prospective analysis. *American Journal of Psychiatry, 152*, 529–535.

Breslau, N., Kessler, R. C., Chilcoat, H. D., Schultz, L. R., Davis, G. C., & Andreski, P. (1998). Trauma and posttraumatic stress disorder in the community. *Archives of General Psychiatry, 55*, 626–632.

Brewin, C. R., Andrews, B., & Valentine, J. K. (2000). Meta-analysis of risk factors for posttraumatic stress disorder in trauma-exposed adults. *Journal of Consulting and Clinical Psychology, 68*, 748–766.

Briere, J., & Elliott, D. M. (2003). Prevalence and psychological sequelae of self-reported childhood physical and sexual abuse in a general population sample of men and women. *Child Abuse & Neglect, 27*, 1205–1222.

Brody, G. H., Chen, Y., Murry, V. M., Ge, X., Simons, F. X., Gibbons, M. G., et al. (2006). Perceived discrimination and the adjustment of African American youths: A five-year longitudinal analysis with contextual moderation effects. *Child Development, 77*, 1170–1189.

Brown, L. K., Tolou-Shams, M., Lescano, C., Houck, C., Zeidman, J., Pugatch, D., et al. (2006). Depressive symptoms as a predictor of sexual risk among African American adolescents and young adults. *Journal of Adolescent Health, 39*(3), 444.e1–444.e8.

Brown, T. N., Williams, D. R., Jackson, J. S., Neighbors, H. W., Torres, M., & Sellers, S. L. (2000). Being black and feeling blue: The mental health consequences of racial discrimination. *Race and Society, 2*, 117–131.

Browning, C. R., & Cagney, K. A. (2002). Neighborhood structural disadvantage, collective efficacy, and self-reported physical health in an urban setting. *Journal of Health and Social Behavior, 43*, 383–399.

Burke, J. G., Thieman, L. K., Gielen, A. C., O'Campo, P., & McDonnel, K. A. (2005). Intimate partners violence, substance use, and HIV among low-income women: Taking a closer look. *Violence Against Women, 11*(9), 1140–1161.

Butts, H. F. (2002). The black mask of humanity: Racial/ethnic discrimination and posttraumatic stress disorder. *The Journal of the American Academy of Psychiatry and the Law, 30*, 336–339.

Bykowicz, J. (2008, March 28) Violence at juvenile center up again – Assaults at state facility increase nearly 40% in year. *Baltimore Sun Newspaper* (www.baltimoresun.com/news/maryland/bal-te.md.juveniles28mar28,0,6084825.story).

Caetano, R., Cunradi, C. B., Clark, C. L., & Schafer, J. (2000). Intimate partner violence and drinking patterns among White, Black, and Hispanic couples in the U.S. *Journal of Substance Abuse, 11*(2), 123–138.

Caetano, R., Nelson, S., & Cunradi, C. (2001). Intimate partner violence, dependence symptoms and social consequences from drinking among White, Black and Hispanic couples in the United States. *American Journal of Addictions, 10*(Suppl. 1), 60–69.

Cannon, A. (2004, August 1). *Juvenile injustice* – Overcrowding, violence, and abuse – state juvenile justice systems are in a shockingly chaotic state. Now, finally, the feds are stepping in. *US News and World Reports* – Politics Section, August 1, 2004.

Centers for Disease Control and Prevention (CDC) (2003). Coping with a traumatic event. http://www.bt.cdc.gov/masscasualties/copingpro.asp (accessed March 13, 2008).

Centers for Disease Control and Prevention (CDC). (2008a). *HIV/AIDS Surveillance Report, 2006* (Vol. 18). Atlanta, GA: U.S. Department of Health and Human Services, Centers for Disease Control and Prevention.

Centers for Disease Control and Prevention (CDC) (2008b). Percentage of students in grades 9–12 who report being victims of dating violence, by Race/Hispanic Origin, 2007. Surveillance summaries, June 6, 2008, MMWR:57(No. SS-4) (Table 11).

Classen, C. C., Palesh, O. G., & Aggarwal, R. (2005). Sexual revictimization: A review of the literature. *Trauma, Violence, & Abuse, 6*(2), 103–129.

Cochran, S. D. (2001). Emerging issues in research on lesbians' and gay men's mental health: Does sexual orientation really matter? *American Psychologist, 56*, 932–947.

Cochran, S. D., Sullivan, J. G., & Mays, V. M. (2003). Prevalence of mental disorders, psychological distress and mental health services use among lesbian, gay and bisexual adults in the United States. *Journal of Consulting and Clinical Psychology, 71*(1), 53–61.

Cohen, M., Deamant, C., Barkan, S., Richardson, J., Young, M., Holman, S., et al. (2000). Domestic violence and childhood sexual abuse in HIV women and women at risk for HIV. *American Journal of Public Health, 90*(4), 560–565.

Coker, A. L., Keith, E., Davis, K. E., Arias, I., Desai, S., Sanderson, M., et al. (2002). Physical and mental health effects of intimate partner violence for men and women. *American Journal of Preventive Medicine, 23*(4), 260–268.

Coker, T. R., Elliott, M. N., Kanouse, D. E., Grunmaum, J. A., Schwebel, D. C., Gilliland, M. J., et al. (2009). Perceived racial/ethnic discrimination among fifth-grade students and its association with mental health. *American Journal of Public Health, 99*(5), 878–884.

Compton, W. M., Thomas, Y. F., Stinson, F. S., & Grant, B. F. (2007). Prevalence, correlates, disability and comorbidity of DSM-IV Drug abuse and dependence in the United States. Results from the National Epidemiologic Survey on Alcohol and Related Conditions. *Archives of General Psychiatry, 64*(5), 566–576.

Cooper, H., Friedman, S. R., Tempalski, B., Friedman, R., & Keem, M. (2005). Racial/ethnic disparities in injection drug us in large US metropolitan areas. *Journal of Substance Abuse Treatment, 15*(5), 326–334.

Cooper-Patrick, C., Power, N. R., Jenckes, M. W., Gonzales, J. J., Levine, D. M., & Ford, D. E. (1997). Identification of patient attitudes and preferences regarding treatment of depression. *Journal of General Internal Medicine, 12*(7), 431–438.

Copland, V. C. (2006). Disparities in mental health service utilization among low-income African-American adolescents: Closing the gap by enhancing practitioner's competence. *Child and Adolescent Social Work Journal, 23*, 407–431.

Crawford, I., Allsion, K. W., Zamboni, B. D., & Soto, T. (2002). The influence of dual-identity development on the psychosocial functioning of African-American gay and bisexual men. *Journal of Sex Research, 39*(3), 179–189.

Crepaz, N., & Marks, G. (2002). Towards an understanding of sexual risk behavior in people living with HIV: A review of social psychological, and medical findings. *AIDS, 16*, 135–149.

Cusack, K. J., Frueh, B. C., & Brady, K. T. (2004). Trauma history screening in a community mental health center. *Psychiatric Services, 55*(2), 157–162.

Davis, R. G., Ressler, K. J., Schwartz, A. C., Stephens, K. J., & Bradley, R. G. (2008). Treatment barriers for low-income, urban African Americans with undiagnosed posttraumatic stress disorder. *Journal of Traumatic Stress, 21*(2), 218–222.

Dearwater, S. R., Cohen, J. H., Campbell, J. C., Nah, G., Glass, N., McLoughlin, E., et al. (1998). Prevalence of domestic violence in women treated at community hospital emergency departments. *Journal of the American Medical Association, 280*, 433–438.

DiClemente, R. J., Wingood, G. M., Crosby, R. A., Sionean, C., Brown, L., Rothbaum, B., et al. (2001). A prospective study of psychological distress and sexual risk behavior among Black adolescent females. *Pediatrics, 108*(5), e85.

Duncan, R. D., Saunders, B. E., Kilpatrick, T., Dean, G., Hanson, R. F., & Resnick, H. S. (1996). Childhood physical assault as a risk factor for PTSD, depression, and substance abuse: Findings from a national survey. *American Journal of Orthopsychiatry, 66*, 437–448.

Early, K. E. (1992). *Religion and suicide in the African-American community.* Westport, CT: Greenwood.

El-Bassel, N., Gilbert, L., Krishman, S., Schilling, R. F., Gaetha, T., & Purpura, S. (1998). Partner violence and HIV-risk behaviors among women in inner-city emergency department. *Violence and Victims, 13*(4), 377–393.

El-Bassel, N., Schillng, R. F., Gilbert, L., Faruque, S., Irwin, K. L., & Edlin, B. R. (2000). Sex trading and psychological distress in a street-based sample of low-income urban men. *Journal of Psychoactive Drugs, 32*, 259–267.

Felitti, V. J., Anda, R. F., Nordenberg, D., Williamson, D. F., Spitz, A. M., Edward, V., et al. (1998). Relationship of childhood abuse and household dysfunction to many of the leading causes of death in adults: The Adverse Childhood Experiences (ACD) study. *American Journal of Preventive Medicine, 14*, 245–258.

Froyum, C. M. (2007). 'At least I'm not gay': Heterosexual identify making among poor Black teens. *Sexualities, 10*(5), 603–622.

Frye, V., Latka, M. H., Wu, Y., Valverde, E. E., Knowlton, A. R., Knight, K. R., et al. (2007). Intimate partner violence perpetration against main female partners among HIV-positive male injection drug users. *Journal of Acquired Immune Deficiency Syndromes, 46*(Suppl. 2), S101–S109.

Gamble, V. N. (1993). A legacy of distrust: African Americans and medical research. *American Journal of Preventive Medicine, 9*(Suppl.), 35–38.

Gamble, V. N. (1997). Under the shadow of Tuskegee: African Americans and health care. *American Journal of Public Health, 87*(11), 1773–1778.

Gary, F. A. (2005). Stigma: Barrier to mental health care among ethnic minorities. *Issues in Mental Health Nursing, 26*, 979–999.

Gillespie, C. F., Bradley, B., Mercer, K., Smith, A. K., Connely, K., Gapen, M., et al. (2009). Trauma exposure and stress-related disorders in inner city primary care patients. *General Hospital Psychiatry, 31*(6), 505–514.

Gilmer, W. S., Trivedi, M. H., Rush, A. J., Wisniewski, S. R., Luther, J., Howland, R. H., et al. (2005). Factors associated with chronic depressive episodes: A preliminary report from the STAR-D project. *Acta Psychiatrica Scandinavica, 112*, 425–433.

Hallfors, D. D., Iritani, B. J., Miller, W. C., & Bauer, D. J. (2007). Sexual and drug behavior patterns and HIV and STD racial disparities: The need for new directions. *American Journal of Public Health, 97*, 125–132.

Hampton, R. L., & Gelles, R. J. (1994). Violence toward Black women in a nationally representative sample of Black families. *Journal of Comparative Family Studies, 25*, 105–119.

Harrison, P. M., & Beck, A. J. (2006). *Prison and jail inmates at midyear 2005*. Number of inmates in state or federal prison and local jails per 100,000 residents, by gender, race, Hispanic Origin, and age, June 30, 2005 (Tables 12 and 13). United States Department of Justice Office of Justice Programs, Bureau of Justice Statistics Bulletin (http://www.ojp.usdoj. gov/bjs/pub/pdf).

Hasin, D. S., Stinson, F. S., Ogburn, E., & Grant, B. F. (2007). Prevalence, correlates, disability, and comorbidity of DSM-IV alcohol abuse and dependence in the United States. *Archives of General Psychiatry, 64*, 830–842.

Heise, L., & Garcia-Moreno, C. (2002). Violence by intimate partners. In E. Krug, L. L. Dahlberg, J. A. Mercy, et al. (Eds.), *World report on violence and health* (pp. 87–121). Geneva, Switzerland: World Health Organization.

Herek, G. M., & Sims, C. (2008). Sexual orientation and violent victimization: Hate crimes and intimate partner violence among gay and bisexual males in the United States. In R. J. Wolitski, R. Stall, & R. O. Valdiserri (Eds.), *Unequal opportunity: Health disparities among gay and bisexual men in the United States* (pp. 35–71). New York: Oxford University Press.

Hines-Martin, V., Malone, M., Kim, S., & Brown-Piper, A. (2003). Barriers to mental health care access in an African American population. *Issues in Mental Health Nursing, 24*, 237–256.

Hoffman, J. A., Klein, H., Eber, M., & Crosby, H. (2000). Frequency and intensity of crack use as predictors of women's involvement in HIV-related sexual risk behaviors. *Drug and Alcohol Dependence, 58*, 227–236.

Holmes, W. C., & Sammel, M. D. (2005). Brief communication: Physical abuse of boys and possible associations with poor adult outcomes. *Annals of Internal Medicine, 143*, 581–586.

Hutton, H. E., Lyketos, C. G., Zenilman, J. M., Thompson, R. E., & Erbelding, E. J. (2004). Depression and HIV risk behaviors among patients in a sexually transmitted disease clinic. *American Journal of Psychiatry, 161*, 912–914.

Hutton, H. E., Treisman, G. J., Hunt, W. R., Fishman, M., Kendig, N., Swetz, A., et al. (2001). HIV risk behaviors and their relationship to posttraumatic stress disorder among women prisoners. *Psychiatric Services, 52*(4), 509–513.

Iguchi, M. Y., & Bux, D. A. (1997). Reduced probability of HIV infection among crack cocaine-using injection drug users. *American Journal of Public Health, 87*, 1081–1012.

International Society for Traumatic Stress Studies (2009). Traumatic stress and substance use problems. www.istss.org/resources/Traumatic_Stress_and_Substance_Abuse.cfm (downloaded 6-22-2009).

Kaiser Family Foundation (1998). Survey of African Americans on HIV/AIDS report (Part 2) 1998, Publication No. 1372. http://www.kff.org/hivaids/1372-afr_amerre2.cfm (accessed January 17, 2008).

Kalichman, S. C. (1999). Psychological and social correlates of high-risk sexual behavior among men and women living with HIV/AIDS. *AIDS Care, 11*, 415–428.

Kelly, B., Raphael, B., Judd, F., Perdices, M., Kernutt, G., Burnett, P., et al. (1998). Posttraumatic stress disorder in response to HIV infection. *General Hospital Psychiatry, 20*, 345–352.

Kennamer, J. K., Honnold, J., Bradford, J., & Hendricks, M. (2000). Differences in disclosure of sexuality among African American and white gay/bisexual men: Implications for HIV/AIDS prevention. *AIDS Education and Prevention, 12*, 519–531.

Kessler, R. C., Berglund, P., Demler, O., Jin, R., Koretz, D., Merikangas, K. R., et al. (2003). The epidemiology of major depressive disorder: Results for the National Comorbidity Survey Replication (NCS-R). *Journal of the American Medical Association, 289*, 3095–3105.

Kessler, R. C., Berglund, P., Demler, O., Jin, R., & Walters, E. E. (2005). Lifetime prevalence and age-of-onset distributions of DSM-IV disorders in the National Comorbidity Survey Replication. *Archives of General Psychiatry, 62*(6), 593–602.

Kessler, R. C., Demler, O., Frank, R. G., Olfson, M., Pincus, H. A., Walters, E. E., et al. (2005). Prevalence and treatment of mental disorders, 1990 to 2003. *New England Journal of Medicine, 352*, 2515–2523.

Kessler, R. C., McGonagle, K. A., Zhao, S., Nelson, C. B., Hughes, M., Eshleman, S., et al. (1994). Lifetime and 12-month prevalence of DSM-III-R psychiatric disorders in the United States: Results from the National Comorbidity Survey. *Archives of General Psychiatry, 51*, 8–19.

Kessler, R. C., Michelson, K. D., & Williams, D. R. (1999). The prevalence, distribution, and mental health correlates of perceived discrimination in the United States. *Journal of Health and Social Behavior, 40*, 208–230.

Kessler, R. C., Sonnega, A. J., Bromet, E., Hughes, M., & Nelson, C. B. (1995). Posttraumatic stress disorder in the National Comorbidity Survey. *Archives of General Psychiatry, 52*, 1048–1060.

Kisera, L. J., & Black, M. M. (2005). Family processes in the midst of urban poverty: What does the trauma literature tell us? *Aggressive Violent Behavior, 10*(6), 715–750.

Klinkenberg, W. D., & Sacks, S. (2004). Mental disorders and drug abuse in persons living with HIV/AIDS. *AIDS Care, 16*(Suppl. 1), S22–S42.

Koenig, L.J., Whitaker, D.J., Royce, R.A., Wilson, T.E., Callaham, M.R. Fernandez, I. (2002). Violence during pregnancy among women with or at risk for HIV infection. African Journal of Public Health, 92(3), 367–370.

Koenig, L. J., & Clark, H. (2004). Sexual abuse of girls and HIV infection among women: Are they related? In L. J. Koenig, L. Doll, A. O'Leary, & W. Pequegnat (Eds.), *From child sexual abuse to adult sexual risk: Trauma, revictimization, and intervention*. Washington, DC: American Psychological Association Books.

Koenig, L. J., & Moore, J. (2000). Women, violence, and HIV: A critical evaluation with implications for HIV services. *Maternal and Child Health Journal, 4*(2), 103–109.

Livingston, I. L. (2004). *Handbook of Black American health: Policies and issues behind disparities in health* (2nd ed.). Westport, CT: Praeger.

Logan, T. K., & Leukefeld, C. G. (2000). Sexual and drug use behaviors among female crack users: A multi-site sample. *Drug and Alcohol Dependence, 58*(3), 237–245.

Logan, T. K., Leukefeld, C. G., & Farabee, D. (1998). Sexual and drug use behaviors among women crack users: Implications for prevention. *AIDS Education and Prevention, 10*(4), 327–340.

Ma, G. X., & Shive, S. (2000). A comparative analysis of perceived risks and substance abuse among ethnic groups. *Addictive Behaviors, 25*(3), 361–371.

MacDonald, T. K., MacDonald, G., Zanna, M. P., & Fong, G. T. (2000). Alcohol, sexual arousal, and intentions to use condoms in young men: Applying alcohol myopia theory to risky sexual behavior. *Health Psychology, 19*(3), 290–298.

MacMillan, H. L., Fleming, J. E., Streiner, D. L., Lin, E., Boyle, M. H., Jamieson, E., et al. (2001). Childhood abuse and lifetime psychopathology in a community sample. *American Journal of Psychiatry, 158*, 1878–1883.

Maker, A. H., Kemmelmeier, M., & Peterson, C. (2001). Child sexual abuse, peer sexual abuse and sexual assault in adulthood: A multi-risk model of re-victimization. *Journal of Traumatic Stress, 14*, 351–368.

Maman, S., Campbell, J., Sweat, M. D., & Gielen, A. C. (2000). The intersections of HIV and violence: Direction of future research and interventions. *Social Science & Medicine, 50*, 459–478.

Marks, G., Bingman, C., & Duval, T. S. (1998). Negative affect and unsafe sex in HIV-positive men. *AIDS and Behavior, 2*(2), 89–99.

Martinez, A., Israelski, D., Walker, C., & Koopman, C. (2002). Posttraumatic stress disorder in women attending human immunodeficiency virus outpatient clinics. *AIDS Patient Care and STDs, 16*(6), 283–291.

Medrano, M. A., Desmond, D. P., Zule, W. A., & Hatch, J. P. (1999). Histories of childhood trauma and the effects on risky HIV behaviors in a sample of women drug users. *American Journal of Drug and Alcohol Abuse, 25*, 593–606.

Milam, J., Richardson, J. L., Espinoza, L., & Stoyanoff, C. (2006). Correlates of unprotected sex among adult heterosexual men living with HIV. *Journal of Urban Health, 83*, 669–681.

Millett, G. A., Peterson, J. L., Wolitski, R. J., & Stall, R. (2006). Greater risk for HIV infection of black men who have sex with men: A critical literature review. *American Journal of Public Health, 96*, 1007–1019.

Morrill, A., & Ickovics, J. (1996). Surviving abuse and HIV risk: How women's experience of abuse shapes their heterosexual risk for HIV. In *Poster symposium at the XI international conference on AIDS*, Vancouver, CA.

Myers, H. F., & Durvasula, R. S. (1999). Psychiatric disorders in African American men and women living with HIV/AIDS. *Cultural Diversity & Ethnic Minority Psychology, 5*(3), 249–262.

Myers, H. F., Javanbakht, M., Martinez, M., & Obediah, S. (2003). Psychosocial predictors in African American men: Implications for prevention. *AIDS Education and Prevention, 15*(Supp. A), 66–79.

Najavits, L. M., Gastfriend, D. R., Barber, J. P., Reif, S., Muenz, L. R., Blaine, J., et al. (1998). Cocaine dependence with and without PTSD among subjects in the National Institute on Drug Abuse Collaborative Cocaine Treatment Study. *American Journal of Psychiatry, 155*, 214–219.

Neff, J. A., Holamon, B., & Schluter, T. D. (1995). Spousal violence among Anglos, Blacks, and Mexican Americans: The role of demographic variables, psychosocial predictors, and alcohol consumption. *Journal of Family Violence, 10*, 1–22.

Neighbors, H. W., & Jackson, J. S. (1996). *Mental health in Black America*. Thousand Oaks, CA: Sage.

Neighbors, H. W., Jackson, J. S., Bowman, P. J., & Gurin, G. (1983). Stress, coping, and Black mental health: Preliminary findings from a national study. *Prevention in Human Services, 23*, 5–29.

Neighbors, H. W., Jackson, J. S., Campbell, L., & Williams, D. (1989). The influence of racial factors on psychiatric diagnosis: A review and suggestions for research. *Community Mental Health Journal, 25*(4), 301–311.

Ozer, E. J., Best, S. R., & Lipsey, T. L. (2003). Predictors of posttraumatic stress disorder and symptoms in adults: A meta-analysis. *Psychological Bulletin, 129*(1), 62–73.

Paradies, Y. (2006). A systematic review of empirical research on self-reported racism and health. *International Journal of Epidemiology, 35*, 888–901.

Paxton, K. C., Myers, H. F., Hall, N. M., & Javanbakht, M. (2004). Ethnicity, serostatus, and psychosocial differences in sexual risk behavior among HIV-seropositive and HIV-seronegative women. *AIDS and Behavior, 8*(4), 405–415.

Perdue, T., Hagan, H., Thiede, H., Valleroy, L. (2003). Depression and HIV risk behavior among injection drug users and young men who have sex with men. *AIDS Education and Prevention, 15*(1), 81–92.

Pence, B. W., Reif, S., Whetten, K., Leserman, J., Stangl, D., Swartz, M., et al. (2007). Minorities, the poor, and survivors of abuse: HIV-infected patients in the US deep South. *Southern Medical Association, 100*(11), 1114–1115.

Plichta, S. B. (2004). Intimate partner violence and physical health consequences: Policy and practice implications. *Journal of Interpersonal Violence, 19*(11), 1296–1323.

Purugganan, O. H., Stein, R. K., Silver, E. J., & Benenson, B. S. (2003). Exposure to violence and psychosocial adjustment among urban school-aged children. *Journal of Developmental and Behavioral Pediatrics, 24*(6), 424–430.

Radcliffe, J., Lleisher, C. L., Hawkins, L. A., Tanney, M., Kassam-Adam, N., Ambrose, C., et al. (2007). Posttraumatic stress and trauma history in adolescents and young adults with HIV. *AIDS Patient Care and STDs, 21*, 501–508.

Rennison, C. (2002). *Criminal victimization 2001: Changes 2001–2001 with trends 1993–2001.* Washington, DC: U.S. Bureau of Justice Statistics (Publication No. NCJ 194610; http://www.ojp.usdoj.gov/bjs/abstract/cv01.htm).

Rennison, C., & Planty, M. (2003). Nonlethal intimate partner violence: Examining race, gender, and income patterns. *Violence and Victimization, 18*(4), 433–443.

Rennison, C. M., & Welchans, S. (2000). *Intimate partner violence. Bureau of Justice Statistics Special Report.* Retrieved July 17, 2008, from www.ojp.usdoj.gov/bjs/pub/pdf/ipv.pdf.

Richardson, M. S., Myers, H. F., Bing, E. G., & Saltz, P. (1997). Substance use and psychopathology in African American men at risk for HIV infection. *Journal of Community Psychology, 25*, 353–370.

Richman, L. S., Kohn-Wood, L. P., & Williams, D. R. (2007). The role of discrimination and racial identity for mental health service utilization. *Journal of Social and Clinical Psychology, 286*(8), 960–981.

Riolo, S. A., Nguyen, T. A., Greden, J. F., & King, C. A. (2005). Prevalence of depression by race/ethnicity: Findings from the National Health and Nutrition Examination Survey III. *American Journal of Public Health, 95*(6), 998–1000.

Roberts, A. C., Wechsberg, W. M., Zule, W., & Burrough, A. R. (2003). Contextual factors and other correlates of sexual risk of HIV among African-American crack-abusing women. *Addictive Behaviors, 28*, 523–536.

Roberts, T. A., Auinger, P., & Klein, J. D. (2005). Intimate partner abuse and the reproductive health of sexually active female adolescents. *Journal of Adolescent Health, 36*(5), 380–385.

Roberts, T. A., Klein, J. D., & Fisher, S. (2003). Longitudinal effect of intimate partner abuse on high-risk behavior among adolescents. *Archives of Pediatrics & Adolescent Medicine, 57*(9), 875–881.

Rosenhan, D. L., & Seligman, M. P. (1995). *Abnormal psychology* (3rd ed.). New York: WW Norton.

Roth, S., Newman, E., Pelcovitz, D., van der Kolk, B., & Mandel, F. S. (1997). Complex PTSD in victims exposed to sexual and physical abuse: Results from the DSM-IV field trial for posttraumatic stress disorder. *Journal of Traumatic Stress, 10*, 539–555.

Schwartz, A. C., Bradley, R. L., Sexton, M., Sherry, A., & Ressler, K. J. (2005). Posttraumatic stress disorder among African-Americans in an inner city mental health clinic. *Psychiatric Services, 56*, 212–215.

Senn, T. E., Carey, M. P., & Vanable, P. A. (2006). Childhood sexual abuse and sexual risk behavior among men and women attending a Sexually Transmitted Disease Clinic. *Journal of Consulting and Clinical Psychology, 74*(4), 720–731.

Seth, P., Raiji, P. T., DiClemente, R. J., Wingood, G. M., & Rose, E. (2009). Psychological distress as a correlate of a biologically confirmed STI, risky sexual practices, self-efficacy and communication with male sex partners in African-American female adolescents. *Psychology, Health & Medicine, 14*, 291–300.

Sickmund, M., Sladky, T. J., & Kang, W. (2005). *Census of juveniles in residential placement databook*. Available from http://ojjdp.ncjrs.org/ojstatbbc/cjrp/ (accessed January 12, 2009).

Silverman, J. G., Raj, A., Mucci, L., & Hathaway, J. (2001). Dating violence against adolescent girls and associated substance use, unhealthy weight control, sexual risk behavior, pregnancy, and suicidality. *Journal of the American Medical Association, 286*(5), 572–579.

Snowden, L. R. (2001). Barriers to effective mental health services for African Americans. *Mental Health Service Research, 3*, 181–187.

Somervell, P. D., Leaf, P. J., Weissman, M. M., Blazer, D. G., & Bruce, M. L. (1989). The prevalence of major depression in black and white adults in five United States communities. *American Journal of Epidemiology, 130*, 725–735.

Somlai, A. M., Kelly, J. A., McAuliffe, T. L., Ksobiech, K., & Lackl, K. L. (2003). Predictors of HIV sexual risk behaviors in a community sample of injection drug using men and women. *AIDS and Behavior, 7*(4), 383–303.

Stein, M., Herman, D. S., Trisvan, E., Pirraglia, P., Engler, P., & Anderson, B. J. (2005). Alcohol use and sexual risk behavior among human immunodeficiency virus – Positive persons. *Alcoholism: Clinical and Experimental Research, 29*(5), 837–843.

Stith, S. M., Smith, D. B., Pee, C. E., Ward, D. B., & Tritt, D. (2004). Intimate partner physical abuse perpetration and victimization risk factors: A meta-analytic review. *Aggression and Violent Behavior, 10*, 65–98.

Stokes, J. P., & Peterson, J. L. (1998). Homophobia, self-esteem, and risk for HIV among African American men who have sex with men. *AIDS Education and Prevention, 10*, 278–292.

Straus, M. A., & Gelles, R. J. (1986). Societal change and change in family violence from 1975 to 1985 as revealed by two national surveys. *Journal of Marriage and the Family, 48*, 465–479.

Sullivan, P. S., Nakashima, A. K., Purcell, D., Ward, J. W., & The Supplement to HIV/AIDS Surveillance Study Group. (1998). Geographic differences in noninjection and injection substance use among HIV-seropositive men who have sex with men: Western United States versus other regions. *Journal of Acquired Immune Deficiency Syndromes and Human Retrovirology, 19*, 266–273.

Terr, L. C. (1991). Childhood traumas: An outline and overview. *American Journal of Psychiatry, 148*, 10–20.

Timpson, S. C., Williams, M. L., Bowen, A. M., & Keel, K. B. (2003). Condom use behaviors in HIV-infected African American crack cocaine users. *Substance Abuse, 24*(4), 211–291.

Tjaden, P., & Thoennes, N. (2000). *Extent, nature, and consequences of intimate partner violence: Findings from the National Violence Against Women Survey.* Washington, DC: United States Department of Justice (Publication No. NCJ 181867; www.ojp.usdoj.gov/nij/pubs-sum/181867.htm).

Tjaden, P., Thoennes, N., & Allison, C. J. (1999). Comparing violence over the life span in samples of same-sex and opposite-sex cohabitants. *Violence Victimization, 14*, 413–425.

United States Department of Health and Human Services (USDHHS). (1999a). *Mental health: A report of the surgeon general.* Rockville, MD: US Department of Health and Human Services.

United States Department of Health and Human Services (USDHHS). (1999b). *National Household Survey on drug abuse: Population estimates 1998.* Rockville, MD: US Department of Health and Human Services.

United States Department of Health and Human Services (USDHHS). (2001). *Mental health: Culture, race and ethnicity – A supplement to mental health: A report of the surgeon.* Rockville, MD: US Department of Health and Human Services.

United States Department of Justice (USDOJ). (2000). *Extent, nature, and consequences of intimate partner violence: Findings from the National Violence Against Women Survey.* Washington, DC: US Department of Justice.

United States Department of Justice (USDOJ) (2006). *A National Crime Victimization Survey, 2005* – Statistical tables (NCJ 215244): Tables 3, 4, 9, 10. Violent crime victimization rates (per 1,000), ages 12–19, by gender, race, and type of crime, 2005.

United States Department of Justice (USDOJ) (2008). *Black victims of violent crimes. Bureau of justice statistics special report (August 2007).* (Publication No. NCJ 214258)

Utsey, S. O., & Payne, Y. (2000). Psychological impacts of racism in a clinical versus normal sample of African American men. *Journal of African American Men, 5*(3), 570–572.

Viosin, D. R. (2002). Family ecology and HIV sexual risk behaviors among African Americans and Puerto Rican adolescent males. *American Journal of Orthopsychiatry, 72*, 294–303.

Viosin, D. R. (2005). The relationship between violence exposure and HIV sexual risk behaviors: Does gender matter? *American Journal of Orthopsychiatry, 75*(4), 497–506.

Vlahov, D., Weintge, D., Moore, J., Flynn, C., Schuman, P., Schoenbaum, E., et al. (1998). Violence among women with or at risk for HIV infection. *AIDS and Behavior, 2*, 53–60.

Voisin, D. R. (2003). Victims of community violence and HIV sexual risk behaviors among African American adolescent males. *Journal of HIV/AIDS Prevention & Education for Adolescents & Children, 5*(3/4), 87–110.

Warheit, G. J., Holzer, C. D., & Arey, S. A. (1975). Race and mental illness: An epidemiologic update. *Journal of Health and Social Behavior, 16*, 243–256.

Whaley, A. L. (2004). Ethnicity/race, paranoia, and hospitalization for mental health problems among men. *American Journal of Public Health, 94*(1), 78–81.

Whetten, K., Leserman, J., Lowe, K., Stangl, D., Thielman, N., Swartz, M., et al. (2006). Prevalence of childhood sexual abuse and physical trauma in an HIV-positive sample from the deep south. *American Journal of Public Health, 96*(6), 1028–1030.

Widom, C. S. (1999). Posttraumatic stress disorder in abused and neglected children grown up. *American Journal of Psychiatry, 156*, 1223–1229.

Williams, C. T., & Latkin, C. A. (2005). The role of depressive symptoms in predicting sex with multiple and high-risk partners. *Journal of Acquired Immune Deficiency Syndromes, 38*, 69–73.

Williams, D. H. (1986). The epidemiology of mental illness in Afro-Americans. *Hospital & Community Psychiatry, 37*(1), 42–49.

Williams, D. R. (1998). African-American health: The role of the social environment. *Journal of Urban Health, 75*(2), 300–321.

Williams, D. R., Gonzalez, H. M., Neighbors, H., Nesse, R., Abelson, J. M., Sweetman, J., et al. (2007). Prevalence and distribution of major depressive disorder in African Americans, Caribbean Blacks, and Non-Hispanic Whites – Results from the National Survey of American Life. *Archives of General Psychiatry, 64*, 305–315.

Williams, D. R., Neighbors, H. W., & Jackson, J. S. (2003). Racial/Ethnic discrimination and health: Findings from community studies. *American Journal of Public Health, 93*, 200–208.

Williams, D. R., & Williams-Morris, R. (2000). Racism and mental health: The African American experience. *Ethnicity & Health, 5*(34), 243–268.

Willis, L. A., Coombs, D., Cockerham, W. C., & Frison, S. L. (2002). Ready to die: A postmodern interpretation of the increase of African-American adolescent male suicide. *Social Science & Medicine, 55*(6), 907–920.

Wilson, J. W. (1987). *The truly disadvantaged: The inner city, the underclass, and public policy.* Chicago, IL: The University of Chicago Press.

Windle, M. (1997). The trading of sex for money or drugs, sexually transmitted diseases (STDs), and HIV-related risk behaviors among multisubstance using alcoholic inpatients. *Drug and Alcohol Dependence, 49*(1), 33–38.

Wolitski, R. J., Bailey, C. J., O'Leary, A., Gomez, C. A., & Parsons, J. T. (2003). Self-perceived responsibility of HIV-seropositive men who have sex with men for preventing HIV transmission. *AIDS and Behavior, 7*(4), 363–372.

Wu, E., El-Bassel, N., Witte, S. S., Gilbert, L., & Chang, M. (2003). Intimate partner violence and HIV risk among urban minority women in primary health care settings. *AIDS and Behavior, 7*(3), 291–301.

Wyatt, G. E., Axelrod, J., Chin, D., Carmona, J. V., & Loeb, T. B. (2000). Examining patterns of vulnerability to domestic violence among African American women. *Violence Against Women, 6*(5), 495–514.

Wyatt, G. E., Guthrie, D., & Norgrass, C. M. (1992). Differential effects of women's child sexual abuse and subsequent sexual revictimization. *Journal of Consulting and Clinical Psychology, 60*(2), 167–173.

Wyatt, G. E., Myers, H. F., Williams, J. K., Kitchen, C. R., Loeb, T., Vargas Carmona, J., et al. (2002). Does a history of trauma contribute to HIV risk for women of color? Implications for prevention and policy. *American Journal of Public Health, 92*, 60–65.

Wynia, M. K., & Gamble, V. N. (2006). Mistrust among minorities and the trustworthiness of medicine. *PLoS Medicine, 3*(5), e244.

Zierler, S., Witbeck, B., & Mayer, K. (1996). Sexual violence against women living with or at risk for HIV infection. *American Journal of Preventive Medicine, 12*, 304–310.

Zweig, J. M., Naser, R., Blackmore, J., & Schaffer, M. (2006). *Addressing sexual violence in prisons – A national snapshot of approaches and highlights of innovative strategies.* Washington, DC: Urban Institute (http://www.urban.org/UploadedPDF/411367_psv_programs.pdf).

Chapter 7
Countering the Surge of HIV/STIs and Co-occurring Problems of Intimate Partner Violence and Drug Abuse Among African American Women: Implications for HIV/STI Prevention

Nabila El-Bassel, Louisa Gilbert, Susan Witte, Elwin Wu, and Danielle Vinocur

Hardest Hit: HIV Among African American Women

For the past quarter century, HIV/AIDS has had a devastating impact on African American women in the United States. According to the Centers for Disease Control (CDC), Black women represent 68% of new HIV cases among women in the United States. HIV/AIDS is now the leading cause of death for African American women aged 25–34 years (CDC, 2004a). Between 2000 and 2003, rates of HIV/AIDS among African American women were 19 times the rates among non-Hispanic white women and 5 times the rates among Hispanic women (CDC, 2004b). Furthermore, 2004 CDC statistics show that the rates of gonorrhea among African American women were 15 times higher than among white women, while the rates of chlamydia were more than 7 times higher than the rates among white women (CDC, 2004b). These alarming racial discrepancies raise several questions: Why do African American women continue to be hit the hardest by HIV and other sexually transmitted infections (STIs) in comparison to other ethnic groups in the United States? What are the unique forces that are driving the pandemic among the African American women and their partners?

Substantial evidence indicates that the staggering rates of HIV and other STIs found among African American women have been fueled by this population's greater likelihood of experiencing co-occurring problems of drug use and intimate partner violence (IPV). This chapter focuses on: (1) the rates of IPV among drug-involved, African American women; (2) the interpersonal contexts that link experiencing IPV and engaging in HIV/STI transmission risks among African American, drug-involved women; (3) drug involvement as a cause and correlate of IPV and HIV/STI transmission risks; (4) community-level factors influencing HIV/STIs

N. El-Bassel (✉)
Social Intervention Group, Columbia University School of Social Work,
1255 Amsterdam Avenue, New York, NY 10027, USA
e-mail: ne5@columbia.edu

D.H. McCree et al. (eds.), *African Americans and HIV/AIDS,*
DOI 10.1007/978-0-387-78321-5_7, © Springer Science+Business Media, LLC 2010

among African American women; (5) macro-structural level risk factors, which influence the co-occurring problems of IPV, HIV/STI risk, and drug use among African American women; and (6) implications for HIV/STI prevention addressing the co-occurring problems of HIV, STIs, drug use and IPV among African American women.

Intimate Partner Violence: A Co-occurring Problem Among African American Women

For the purpose of this paper, IPV refers to violent or abusive behavior perpetrated against women by men who may be considered their boyfriends, spouses, former boyfriends, or former spouses. Relationships between intimate partners do not necessarily involve sexual activity or living together. The American Medical Association (American Medical Association [AMA], 2000) defines IPV on a continuum that may include the following patterns of coercive behaviors:

- Physical assaults, such as hits, slaps, kicks and beatings.
- Psychological abuse, such as constant belittling, name calling, intimidation, threatening and controlling behaviors, like isolating women from family and friends and restricting their access to money and resources.
- Sexual coercion, which may include threats or physical force used to coerce women into having unwanted sexual activity.

These behaviors often co-occur together in the same episode and such episodes may be rare events or take place in established daily threatening and controlling patterns (AMA, 2000).

Research suggests that African American women are at elevated risk for IPV (Hampton, Oliver, & Magarian, 2003; Rennison & Welchans, 2000). A National Crime Victimization Survey conducted from 1993 to 1998 found that African American women reported experiencing IPV at a rate 35% higher than white women and at a rate twice that of women from other racial categories (Rennison & Welchans). Moreover, IPV disproportionately affects drug-involved African American women. Past year prevalence rates of physical and sexual IPV among drug-dependent women have been found to range between 25 and 57%, rates two to ten times higher than prevalence rates found in community-based samples (Brewer, Fleming, Haggerty, & Catalano, 1998; El-Bassel, Gilbert, Schilling, & Wada, 2000; El-Bassel, Gilbert, Wu, Go, & Hill, 2005b). In a recent study among a random sample of 100 African American women recruited from different methadone treatment programs, over half (55%) of the women reported experiencing some type of IPV (sexual, physical and injury-related IPV) combining both minor and severe degree in the past 6 months (El-Bassel, Gilbert, & Wu, 2007); in addition, rates of severe acts of IPV were relatively high with 18% of the women reporting any form of severe IPV, 17% reporting severe physical and/or injury-related IPV, and 4% reporting severe sexual IPV (e.g., rape) in the past 6 months.

The Multifaceted, Bi-directional Relationships Between IPV and HIV/STI Risks

While accumulating research conducted with samples that include African American, heterosexual women has found that experiencing IPV is associated with sexual HIV/STI transmission risks and sexual risk reduction behaviors, to date, possible temporal relationships between sexual HIV/STI transmission risks and experiencing IPV among drug-involved women have yet to be elucidated. Researchers have begun to explore whether sexual HIV/STI transmission risks and/ or sexual risk reduction behaviors, such as requesting that a partner use condoms, lead to IPV; and alternatively, whether experiencing IPV leads to an increase in a woman's risk of sexual HIV/STI transmission and/or to a decrease in sexual risk reduction behaviors. Growing evidence suggests that the relationship between experiencing IPV and HIV/STI risk is multi-faceted and bidirectional, leading to a vicious cycle of relationship dynamics and power imbalance that increases the likelihood of HIV/STI transmission among women (El-Bassel, Gilbert, Wu, Go, & Hill, 2005a; El-Bassel et al., 2005b). The myriad interpersonal contexts linking IPV and HIV/STI risk behaviors among African American women are detailed below.

Interpersonal Contexts Linking IPV and HIV Risks Among African American Women

Sexual Coercion, Fear of Violence and HIV/STIs

Quantitative and qualitative research has elucidated several interpersonal contexts accounting for the multiple relationships between experiencing IPV and different HIV/STI transmission risks. The first direct pathway between IPV and HIV/STI transmission risks is through sexual coercion. Studies conducted among predominantly African American women have demonstrated that experiencing physical IPV increases the likelihood of experiencing sexual coercion and leads to HIV and other STIs (Beadnell, Baker, Morrison, & Knox, 2000; Wingood & DiClemente, 1998). According to a qualitative study of 50 HIV-positive, African American women, HIV/STI risks occurred in the context of women being beaten and raped into sexual ownership, that is, by becoming a "captive body" (Mermelstein, Cohen, Lichtenstein, Baer, & Kamarck, 1986). The increased likelihood of HIV/STI transmission associated with forced sex is a result of vaginal, anal, and urethral trauma, which facilitates direct transmission of microorganisms into the bloodstream or via back flow into the urethra (Jenny et al., 1990).

Sexual coercion has also been linked to a decreased likelihood of condom use (El-Bassel, Gilbert, Rajah, Foleno, & Frye, 2000). Women often will forgo requesting condoms when sexually coerced by an intimate partner out of fear that such requests may further provoke their partners and jeopardize their safety (Gilbert, El-Bassel, Rajah et al., 2000). Dovetailing with these findings, a cross sectional study of 125 African American women in low income housing found that women who experienced sexual IPV were more likely than their non-abused counterparts to report being "afraid to ask a man to wear a condom because he might strike her" (Kalichman, Williams, Cherry, Belcher, & Nachimson, 1998). Thus, the goal of women in such encounters is to avoid or minimize physical harm and to ensure that the experience is over as quickly as possible (El-Bassel et al., 2000). In sum, these studies suggest that sexual coercion creates a context of male dominance, fear and control that strips women of power or agency to negotiate their sexual health needs, often forcing women to choose between protecting themselves from HIV/STIs or IPV.

Negotiation of Safe Sex and Attempt of Women Protect Themselves from HIV and IPV

According to research findings based on samples of predominantly African American, drug-involved women, those who negotiate condom use in order to protect themselves from HIV/STIs experience higher rates of IPV (El-Bassel et al., 2005a; Gilbert, El-Bassel, Schilling, Wada, & Bennet, 2000). In addition to asking their partners to use condoms, some women may try to safeguard themselves from HIV/STI transmission by refusing sex, or at least, refusing unprotected sex. In retaliation to the refusal, the partner may react violently towards his female partner (El-Bassel et al., 1998, 2000; Gilbert, El-Bassel, Rajah et al., 2000). Requesting partners to use condoms may also lead to verbal abuse, as well as threats of physical IPV and abandonment (Wingood & DiClemente, 1997). Qualitative research further confirms that for both men and women in committed relationships, condom use is often synonymous with infidelity or casual sex, and thus, condom requests threaten to reduce the couple's intimate relationship status of intimacy to a cheap encounter (El-Bassel et al., 2000).

If a woman suspects infidelity, injection drug use, or other risky behaviors, requesting her partner to use condoms or get tested for HIV/STIs may signal a lack of trust in him (El-Bassel et al., 2000; Gilbert et al., 2000; Kelly & Kalichman, 1995). Alternatively, such requests may incite relationship conflict that leads to IPV if the male partner feels accused of having extra-dyadic sex or engaging in other risky behaviors like injecting drugs. Condom request may even imply to some men that *she has engaged* in risky behaviors or extra-dyadic sex, activities which breach gender role expectations (El-Bassel et al.). Such perceptions threaten the stability of the couple and increase the likelihood of abuse (O'Leary & Wingood, 2000), as some men resort to using physical and/or sexual IPV as a mechanism to repair their masculine self-esteem and maintain or reestablish male power.

Disclosure of HIV/STIs and IPV

Although the relationship between HIV/STI disclosure and IPV is inconsistent, research among women has documented that disclosure of an STI or HIV status is associated with IPV (Gielen, O'Campo, Anderson, Keller, & Faden, 2000; Gielen, O'Campo, Faden, & Eke, 1997; North & Rothenberg, 1993). Qualitative research with a sample of women on methadone (38% were African American) showed that abused women who test positive for HIV or other STIs were more reluctant to disclose their positive status knowing that it may incite IPV (El-Bassel et al., 2000). However, according to the results of a study of 50 HIV-positive, mostly African American women, disclosure carried both positive (acceptance, understanding) and negative consequences (rejection, abandonment, physical abuse) (Gielen et al., 1997).

IPV and HIV/STIs

Accumulating research, based on samples that include African American, hetero-sexual women, has shown that experiencing IPV is associated with: (1) engaging in unprotected sex (Amaro, 1995; Cunningham, Stiffman, Dore, & Earls, 1994; El-Bassel et al., 2005a; Gielen, McDonnell, & O'Campo, 2002; Wingood & DiClemente, 1997; Wyatt, 1991); (2) higher rates of STIs (El-Bassel et al., 1998; El-Bassel et al., 2000; Hogben et al., 2001; Rodriguez, Szkupinski Quiroga, & Bauer, 1996); (3) sex with multiple sexual partners (Gilbert et al., 2000); and (4) trading sex for drugs or money (Beadnell et al., 2000).

IPV and Unprotected Sex

Significant associations between unprotected sex and experiencing IPV were found in a longitudinal study of 416 (40% African American) women followed for 12 months (El-Bassel et al., 2005a). Among those women who were sexually active, those who always requested that their partner use condoms were one-fifth as likely to report subsequent IPV compared to women who did not always request condoms. Furthermore, in a cross-sectional study of 100 African American women recruited from different methadone treatment programs (El-Bassel et al., 2007), 9% of the women who experienced any form of physical and sexual IPV reported always using condoms compared to 27% of the non-abused in the past 6 months. These findings can be understood in light of qualitative research, which found that women who always use condoms do not need to repeatedly negotiate condom use as a norm of condom use has already been established within that partnership (El-Bassel et al., 2000). Thus, it appears that the risks of IPV tend to be lower with established, consistent condom use ("always"), while negotiation of condom use and inconsistent condom use ("not always") carry higher IPV risks.

IPV and Multiple Sex Partners

The significant association between IPV and multiple sex partners also emerged in the above-mentioned cross-sectional study of African American on methadone (El-Bassel et al., 2007). Among the abused women in this sample, 31% of the women had more than one sexual partner in the past 6 months, a rate that was significantly higher than 11% of the non-abused women. Other studies have also documented a link between intimate partner victimization among heterosexual women and engagement in concurrent relationships with other intimate, casual or sex exchanging partners (Gilbert, El-Bassel, Schilling et al., 2000; Raj, Silverman, & Amaro, 2004). The relationship instability associated with IPV may increase the likelihood that one or both partners will engage in outside relationships as an exit strategy.

IPV and Risky Sexual Partners

Research conducted with samples including African American women indicates that having a risky partner (e.g., one who injects drugs, is HIV positive and/or has had sex with multiple partners) is associated with HIV risks (Beadnell et al., 2000; El-Bassel et al., 1995, 2000, 2001; Gielen et al., 2002; Gilbert, El-Bassel, Schilling et al., 2000; Raj et al., 2004). Some research has suggested that men who perpetrate IPV, particularly drug-involved men, are more likely to engage in these co-occurring risky behaviors (El-Bassel et al., 2001). A partner's HIV positive status, closeted sex with other men or injection behaviors may create or exacerbate relationship conflict that could escalate into IPV. Alternatively, as relationship conflict escalates into IPV, male partners may engage in extra-dyadic sex as a strategy to exit the relationship or to retaliate with the explicit purpose of creating jealousy and a desire in a female partner to compete for reconnection. In instances where women fear losing their partners to other women, it is unlikely that they will insist on using condoms even if they know that their partners have engaged in outside affairs (Beadnell et al., 2000).

Trauma, PTSD, HIV/STIs and Drug Abuse

Beyond current experiences of interpersonal violence, research also indicates that women with a past history of interpersonal trauma are more likely to engage in risky sexual behaviors. For example, one study documented that women with past histories of sexual IPV report having more sexual partners and using condoms less consistently than women without histories of sexual IPV (Maman, Campbell, Sweat, & Gielen, 2000). Furthermore, based on study findings among predominantly African American, drug-involved women, it appears that Post Traumatic Stress Disorder (PTSD) may mediate IPV and engaging in risky sexual behavior (Hutton et al., 2001; Stiffman et al., 1992). PTSD, which may stem from a range of interpersonal trauma, such as sexual coercion, childhood sexual abuse (CSA), physical IPV and/or sex trading, is more common among women with abuse histories than among the general population, with rates among abused women ranging between 50 and 64% (Hutton et al., 2001; Lewis, 2005; Zlotnick, 1997). Moreover, there is evidence that women with a PTSD diagnosis and/or other trauma-related symptoms often abuse substances in order to cope, albeit unsafely, with aversive, distressing emotional and physiological states (Najavits et al., 1998). A pernicious cycle among the co-occurring problems of current IPV, past interpersonal trauma, substance abuse and HIV/STI risk can frequently be seen as women attempt to cope with the after-effects of past and current violence through drug use, which in turn renders them more vulnerable to future risk of experiencing IPV and engaging in HIV/STI risk behaviors.

Drug Abuse as a Cause of HIV/STIs Among African American Women

According to CDC reports, following sexual risk behaviors, injection drug use is the second leading transmission route of new HIV infections among African American women with one report indicating that African American women represented 66% of all injection drug use-related HIV cases (Blankenship, Smoyer, Bray, & Mattocks, 2005). Furthermore, non-injection drug use–which has also fueled the HIV/AIDS epidemic among low income, African American women–has been linked to heterosexual transmission of HIV (Chaisson, Stoneburner, Hildebrandt, Telzak, & Jaffe, 1990; Holmberg, 1996) and other STIs among women (Chirgwin, DeHovitz, Dillon, & McCormack, 1991). For example, in several studies of drug-involved, mostly African American women, the vast majority of women were sexually active, 45–55% reported multiple sexual partners, 20–50% stated exchanging sex for money or drugs, and 15–30% noted injection drug use (Belenko, Langley, Crimmins, & Chaple, 2004; Grella, Stein, & Greenwell, 2005).

In addition to the above-discussed multiple direct pathways linking drug abuse to HIV/STI risk among African American women, qualitative research has elucidated multiple ways in which substance use by the woman and/or her partner may mediate the relationship between IPV and HIV/STI transmission. First, substance use by the woman or her partner may increase her partner's expectations for unwanted and unprotected sex (El-Bassel et al., 2000; Sterk, 1999). Second, victims and perpetrators both tend to believe that perpetrators under the influence of drug or alcohol may not be held accountable for sexual coercion. Such social expectations may enable partners to continue perpetrating sexual IPV (Gelles, 1993; Gilbert, El-Bassel, Rajah, Foleno, & Frye, 2001). Third, drug and alcohol use of perpetrators intensify paranoia, jealousy and irritability as well as impair judgments; these psychopharmacological effects may increase the likelihood of IPV and decrease ability to use condoms (Gelles, 1993; Gilbert et al., 2001). Fourth, women under the influence of drugs or alcohol are less likely to identify risky situations, to pick up on cues of impending sexual coercion, and are less able to negotiate condom use in such encounters. A substance-induced compromise in ability to anticipate and/or read signs of imminent sexual coercion may account for research findings indicating that women's use of different drugs increases the likelihood of sexual coercion (El-Bassel et al., 1998, 2000; Gilbert, El-Bassel, Rajah et al., 2000; Kalichman et al., 1998; Sterk, 1999). Fifth, psychological abuse, which is often aimed at the perceived low social status, sexual promiscuity and stigma of being a drug-dependent woman, may further disempower drug-involved women from negotiating safer sex (Gilbert, El-Bassel, Rajah et al., 2000; Gilbert et al., 2001; Sterk, 1999).

Lastly, drug dependency, in addition to possible pressure to sell sex to supply their addicted partners with drugs, may lead women to exchange sex for money in risky unprotected encounters (El-Bassel et al., 2000; Sterk, 1999). Several studies have documented the perilous and degrading circumstances–where coercive sex is common and condom use is infrequent– under which women exchange sex for money or drugs (El-Bassel et al., 1996; Fullilove, Lown, & Fullilove, 1992). Furthermore, because drug dependent women are often considered "sexually promiscuous" or "damaged goods," they are perceived by men in society as violating traditional gender role norms, and thus, are deemed more deserving of abuse (Miller, 1990).

Community-Level Factors Influencing HIV/STIs Among African American Women

Community-level factors related to urban development and gentrification, destruction of housing and neighborhood displacement have dismantled social networks and have undercut the social capital and prosocial norms of low income African American communities. African American women who live in poor neighborhoods with high levels of substance abuse, HIV/STI and violence also have more limited access to health care and social services. Poor residents are more likely to rely on their neighborhood for material and social resources but are less likely to receive such support (James, Johnson, & Raghavan, 2004). Multiple environmental stressors related to poverty, persistent residential mobility, and inadequate access to resources continue to constrain HIV/AIDS prevention and treatment efforts, limit the sources of support for recovery from substance abuse and undermine sources of resistance against IPV in poor African American communities.

This disruption of the social fabric in these communities has also created risk and mixing patterns of sexual and drug using networks that have facilitated the spread of HIV/STIs among African Americans (Rhodes, Singer, Bourgois, Friedman, & Strathdee, 2005). Previous research suggests that African American, drug-involved women who live in poor urban neighborhoods have a greater likelihood of having sex with a "risky" partner by virtue of the higher prevalence of injection drug users and HIV-positive men in their sexual networks and communities (McNair & Prather, 2004). Among Blacks, one in five (19%) new HIV infections is attributed to the sharing of contaminated needles through injection drug use, a rate notably higher than for Whites or Latinos (CDC, 2004b). Moreover, African American women are at a disproportionately high risk of having partners on the down low (i.e., male partners who are in committed heterosexual relationships, but who have closeted extra-dyadic sex with men) (Mays, Cochran, & Zamudio, 2004). African American men who have sex with men (MSM) have HIV diagnosis rates twice that among white MSM (Fullilove, 2006).

Macro and Structural Level Factors Influencing HIV/STI Risks

The social status of African American women based on social constructions of gender, race and class are central to understanding the nature of macro and structural level risk factors in which HIV/STI, IPV and drug abuse co-occur (Wingood & Diclemente, 1992). Gender as a social construct reinforces fundamental power imbalances by assigning to women inferior status and roles, which limit their control over all aspects of their economic, social, family and reproductive life (Amaro, 1995). Such gender inequalities are critical to understanding the dynamics and nature of IPV as well as the interpersonal HIV/STI risk contexts that leave women powerless to negotiate condom use (El-Bassel et al., 1998, 2005a; Amaro, 1995, Wingood & Diclemente, 1992). Similarly, the social constructions of race carry implicit and explicit beliefs that form the basis of domination of one group over another through denial of equal opportunity, access to power and resources (Bruce, Takeuchi, & Leaf, 1991).

For African American women, the intersection of gender, racism and social class fuels conditions of stress, poverty, violence and poor health status which facilitate the co-occurring problems of IPV, drug abuse and HIV/STI risk (McNair & Prather, 2004, Wingood & Diclemente, 1997). Conditions of stress, poverty, violence and poor health status for low income, urban African American women have also been generated by the interplay of wider cultural beliefs and social constructions of race, gender and class with structural factors such as laws, policies, economic conditions and social inequalities (Rhodes et al., 2005).

First, the War on Drugs and changes in sentencing laws related to illicit drug use have spurred a dramatic increase in the number of African American men and women in the criminal justice system in the United States. The large scale incarceration of African American men and women has disrupted social networks in low-income, African American neighborhoods, shifted population mixing patterns and played an important role in driving the HIV/AIDS epidemic in African American communities (Rhodes et al., 2005). The HIV/AIDS cases among incarcerated persons are more than three times that of the general population and African Americans are disproportionately represented in U.S. prisons (Maruschak, 2004, 2005). Moreover, about one in five African American men are incarcerated at some point between the ages of 18–29, and, in 2004, African American women were five times more likely than white women to be incarcerated (Statistics, 2005). The disproportionate incarceration of African Americans due to draconian drug laws has

reinforced African Americans' perceptions of racial oppression and increased their
mistrust of a government, which is seen as inhibiting African Americans from seeking
help for substance abuse, HIV/STIs and IPV. African Americans' fear of systematic
mistreatment has led researchers to suggest that African American women experiencing
IPV may be more likely to protect their abusers from involvement with the law
(Yoshioka, Gilbert, & El-Bassel, 2003) and more likely to stay in abusive relationships that increase their risk of HIV/STIs and drug use (El-Bassel et al., 2003).

Second, the loss of African American men to incarceration and to violent
deaths has resulted in a sex ratio imbalance that is estimated to be 75 men to 100
females among African American adults (Mize, Robinson, Bockting, & Scheltema,
2002). Research has suggested that this sex ratio imbalance exacerbates gender
inequalities and power imbalances within intimate relationships, rendering
African American women less powerful and in control to negotiate safer relationships (Mize et al., 2002). Moreover, in a social context where men are frequently
"lost" to incarceration and death, women may alter their self-protective behaviors
in ways that are driven by a fear of losing their partner. For instance, a study of
low income, African American women found that fear of a negative partner
reaction–and presumably fear of losing the partner as a result–is associated with
lower levels of effectiveness in negotiation and lower levels of condom use
(Amaro & Raj, 2000). El-Bassel, Gilbert, Rajah et al., (2000) suggest that the fear
of disrupting a partnership when alternative partners may not be available plays
an important role in determining whether or not women are willing to insist on
condom use. Moreover, the fear of losing a partner may not only inhibit African
American women from requesting or insisting on condom use, but may also prevent them from resisting IPV or refusing drug use within an intimate partnership
(Mize et al.).

Finally, the internalized oppression and stigmatization that African American
experience as a result of sexism, racism and class exploitation may inhibit disclosure
of HIV status, IPV or risky behaviors associated with HIV/STIs out of fear of compounding layers of additional stigma. The fear of compounding stigma has also
been cited as a major driving force in the widespread closeted risky down low
behaviors among African an men who have long term, heterosexual intimate partners,
but who have undisclosed extra-dyadic sex with men (Fullilove, 2006). The stigma
and discrimination against MSM within the African American community may in
part explain why African American MSM continue to be hard hit by HIV/STIs,
with diagnosis rates twice that among white MSM (Fullilove).

Implications for HIV/STI Prevention Intervention
for Co-occurring Problems of HIV/STIV, IPV and Drug Abuse

The myriad mechanisms and macro-structural risk factors linking the co-occurring
problems of HIV/STI, drug abuse and IPV among African American women suggest
the need for multi-level HIV/STI prevention interventions (intrapersonal/individuals,

interpersonal/micro, community, macro and structural) that synergistically address the different facets of these co-occurring problems. To date, there is a paucity of empirically tested HIV prevention interventions designed to specifically address the problem of concurrent of HIV/STIs, IPV, and drug abuse among African American women. A growing number of researchers along with a recent policy report from the World Health Organization (World Health Organization, 1997) have emphasized the need for HIV/STI prevention interventions that incorporate IPV prevention, particularly for drug-involved, abused women (El-Bassel et al., 2005a; Gilbert, El-Bassel, Schilling et al., 2000; Kalichman et al., 1998; Raj et al., 2004; Wingood & DiClemente, 1997).

Additionally, the need to develop and implement culturally-congruent, gender-specific approaches that concurrently address IPV and HIV/STI is underscored by the findings of a meta-analysis of HIV/STI prevention interventions for women, which showed that most HIV preventions strategies were consistently less effective for African American women (Mize et al., 2002). Findings from a few recent randomized clinical trials (RCTs) testing culturally-congruent HIV prevention interventions for African American women, primarily based on social cognitive principles and an empowerment-based approach, found these interventions to be efficacious in increasing condom use, reducing risk behaviors and/or decreasing STIs among African American women (DiClemente et al., 2004; Kalichman, Kelly, Hunter, Murphy, & Tyler, 1993; St. Lawrence, Wilson, Eldridge, Brasfield, & O'Bannon, 2001; Wyatt et al., 2004). Although these culturally congruent HIV/STI prevention interventions represent an important advance in developing effective strategies to stem the spread of HIIV/STIs among African American women, these interventions have not specifically addressed the co-occurring risk factors of IPV and drug abuse.

In order to address this gap, the authors of this chapter designed and tested an integrated drug abuse, HIV/STIs and IPV intervention prevention consisting of 12 group sessions to reduce the co-occurring problems of IPV, drug abuse and HIV/STI risk among abused women in drug treatment. The intervention, guided by the empowerment theory (Rappaport, 1987; Zimmerman, Israel, Schulz, & Checkoway, 1992) and social cognitive theory (Bandura, 1986), was tested in a pilot RCT with 36 women on methadone who experienced IPV in the past 90 days. In the pilot RCT, women were randomly assigned to either 12 sessions of an integrated HIV/STIs, IPV and drug abuse intervention or to a single session consisting of a didactic presentation on a wide range of local, accessible community services (i.e., employment services, job training, housing, domestic violence programs, legal services, mental health services, low-cost dental services).

All 12 sessions of the integrated, culturally congruent HIV/STIs prevention intervention addressed multi-level risk factors (intrapersonal/individual, interpersonal/micro, community and macro levels) impacting African American and Latina women at risk for HIV, IPV and drug abuse. Intrapersonal components (e.g., previous history of childhood sexual abuse, trauma history and PTSD, history of substance abuse, IPV) focused on: (1) raising awareness about the co-occurrence of HIV/STIs, CSA, IPV, PTSD, and drug use, and informing women how to cope with IPV, trauma with drugs; and (2) teaching skills such as self-soothing, coping, and grounding techniques. During the first session, the facilitator assessed the level of danger in a woman's intimate relationships and provided the woman with the opportunity to disclose more sensitive, confidential information that may have been pertinent to safety planning.

Interpersonal/micro components (e.g., power imbalances in intimate relationships, sexual negotiation skills, sexual communication skills, financial dependency, relationship commitment) aimed to: (1) raise awareness about economic, social and drug dependencies, and explore ways of reducing relationship dependencies; (2) increase negotiation skills and perceived efficacy to handle potential IPV and HIV/STI risk situations (e.g., deciding when and how to have sex, managing reactions to condom request and sex refusal, etc.); (3) increase condom negotiation self-efficacy and negotiation skills for HIV/STI risk reduction with an emphasis on how to deal with abuse situation and increase safety; and (4) identify ways to avoid involvement in relationships that place women at risk for IPV and HIV/STIs, as well as to develop strategies to optimize women's control in their current relationships.

Community level components (e.g., social support, access to services, peer norms about HIV/STIs and IPV) focused on: (1) assisting women in creating supportive networks to reduce exposure to HIV/STIs, IPV and to decrease drug use; (2) helping women to access community resources in order to reduce HIV/STIs, IPV, and drug use; and (3) creating social networks that facilitate reciprocity and trust, and providing women with social support and mutual aid for reducing HIV risk and drug use as well as resisting IPV.

Macro components (e.g., gender norms, attitudes and stigma towards drug-involved women) focused on raising awareness about: (1) gender norms around sex and the meaning of having a relationship with men; (2) gender differences with respect to meaning of forced sex; and (3) attitudes towards drug-involved women, stigma and sexism that increase women risk for HIV/STIs, IPV and other co-occurring problems and identify strategies women can apply to avoid unhealthy relationships. Furthermore, this integrated intervention was tailored to the realities of low-income, African American and Latina women and focused on the enhancement of positive evaluations of self-worth, ethnic pride and risk avoidance as an investment in the future of their communities. Sessions included traditional and contemporary African American and Latina references that further enhanced cultural specificity and pride. While the cultural content primarily targeted African–American or Latina women, the content was also relevant to other low-income, urban, drug-involved women experiencing IPV and included IPV safety planning.

This pilot RCT study had several limitations, which included: (1) a small sample size, underlying threats to both internal and external validity; (2) a short time frame of follow-up; and (3) failure to address structural-level risk factors for HIV/STIs such as changes in drug-related sentencing laws, incarceration and fatality rates of African American men and the impact of sexism, racism and gender inequalities on the co-occurring problems of drug abuse, IPV and HIV/STI risk behaviors. Nonetheless, the findings demonstrated preliminary effects of the intervention in reducing IPV, drug use and HIV/STIs. Specifically, compared to women assigned to the control group of one information session, women who were assigned to the 12 session intervention were approximately 7 times more likely to report a decrease in experiencing minor physical, sexual and/or injurious IPV as well as a decrease in severe physical IPV in the past 90 days at the 3 month follow-up assessment. Furthermore, women who were assigned to the 12 session intervention compared to the control group were approximately 3 times more likely to report a decrease in any drug use, 5.7 times more likely to report a decrease in their level of depression, 4.6 times more likely to report a decrease in avoidance PTSD symptoms, about 6 times more likely to report a decrease in having sex while high on illicit drugs, 3 times more likely to report a decrease in having multiple sex partners and 3 times more likely to report unprotected acts in the past 90 days at the 3 month follow-up assessment (Gilbert et al., 2006). Thus, despite its limitations, this pilot RCT may serve as a building block for further development and testing of culturally-congruent, integrated intervention approaches that will stem the co-occurring problems of IPV, continued drug use, and HIV/STI risk among different populations of drug-involved, abused women.

Conclusion

Ample evidence indicates that the overwhelming rates of HIV and other STIs found among African American women have increased as a result of this population's greater likelihood of experiencing the co-occurring problems of HIV/STIs, drug use and IPV. In considering the unique forces that disproportionately drive this pandemic among African American women, this chapter highlighted several interpersonal contexts that link HIV/STIs, IPV, and drug use, namely (1) sexual coercion and fear of sexual and physical IPV (e.g., women acquiesce to unprotected sex because of fear of IPV); (2) self-protection from HIV/STIs by negotiating condom or refusing sex and unprotected sex; and (3) disclosure of HIV/STIs. This chapter also presented empirical data linking IPV to three HIV/STI risk indicators: unprotected sex, multiple partners, and risky partners. Following an introduction of drug abuse as a coping tool to manage PTSD symptoms associated with current and past IPV, the chapter examined drug abuse among African American as a direct cause of HIV/STIs and as a mediator between IPV and HIV/STI risks. Furthermore, this chapter discussed specific community-level, macro and structural factors that function as a breeding ground within which HIV/STIs and IPV and other co-occurring problems among African American women can thrive. These factors include poverty, discrimination, racism and low social status of women based on social constructions of gender, race and class. Moreover, the wider cultural beliefs and social constructions of race, gender and class were discussed in terms of their interplay with structural factors such as laws, policies, economic conditions and social inequalities. In addition, the chapter included a discussion of environmental stressors related to poverty, racial discrimination and inadequate access to resources as they continue to constrain HIV/AIDS prevention and treatment efforts, limit the sources of support for recovery from substance abuse and undermine the battle against IPV in poor African American communities.

Building on our discussion of these interpersonal contexts and macro-structural factors, the authors advocate for multi-level HIV/STI prevention interventions addressing the intersecting problems of HIV, STIs, IPV and drug abuse among African American women. This chapter presented an efficacious, multi-level HIV/STI prevention intervention designed to address this nexus of problems among drug-involved African American and Latina women by targeting intrapersonal, interpersonal, social support and community level factors. Finally, the chapter acknowledged progress in the design of effective HIV strategies to stem the spread of HIIV/STIs among African American women, but also underscored that these interventions have not specifically addressed the co-occurring risk factors of IPV and drug involvement.

Future Research Directions

While the past decade has seen a proliferation of research on the intersecting pandemic of HIV/STIs, IPV and drug abuse among women, this area of research applied specifically to African American women remains scarce despite their alarming rates of HIV/AIDS infections. Of the studies that examine the intersecting problems among African American women, small sample sizes and cross sectional designs limit the examination of temporal relationships between HIV/STIs and other co-occurring problems (e.g., IPV, drug use). The paucity and design of existing studies underscore the need for longitudinal studies that explore the intersecting pandemic of HIV, STIs, IPV and drug abuse specifically among a sample of African women. Moreover, HIV researchers designing prevention interventions should pay more attention to the multi-level systems (intrapersonal, interpersonal, community, macro, and structural) fuelling this nexus of problems, and multi-level HIV/STI prevention interventions must be tested for efficacy among samples of African American women. Without addressing the macro and structural risk factors, African American women will continue to be disproportionately affected by the co-occurring problems of IPV, drug use and HIV/STIs.

References

Amaro, H. (1995). Love, sex and power: Considering women's realities in HIV prevention. *American Psychologist, 50*, 437–447.

Amaro, H., & Raj, A. (2000). On the margin: The realities of power and women's HIV risk reduction strategies. *Journal of Sex Roles, 42*(7/8), 723–749.

American Medical Association. (2000). *Data on violence between intimates: CSA Report 7*. San Diego: Paper presented at the American Medical Association Council on Scientific Affairs.

Bandura, A. (1986). *Social foundations of thought and action: A social and cognitive theory*. Englewood Cliffs, New Jersey: Prentice-Hall.

Beadnell, B., Baker, S. A., Morrison, D. M., & Knox, K. (2000). HIV/STD risk factors for women with violent male partners. *Sex Roles, 42*, 661–690.

Belenko, S., Langley, S., Crimmins, S., & Chaple, M. (2004). HIV risk behaviors, knowledge, and prevention education among offenders under community supervision: A hidden risk group. *AIDS Education and Prevention, 16*(4), 367–385.

Blankenship, K. M., Smoyer, A. B., Bray, S. J., & Mattocks, K. (2005). Black-white disparities in HIV/AIDS: The role of drug policy and the corrections system. *Journal of Health Care for the Poor and Underserved, 16*, 140–156.

Brewer, D. D., Fleming, C. B., Haggerty, K. P., & Catalano, R. F. (1998). Drug use predictors of partner violence in opiate dependent women. *Violence and Victims, 13*(2), 107–115.

Bruce, M. L., Takeuchi, D. T., & Leaf, P. J. (1991). Poverty and psychiatric status: Longitudinal evidence from the New Haven Catchment Area Study. *Archives of General Psychiatry, 48*(5), 470–474.

Bureau of Justice Statistics. (2005). *Criminal Offender Statistics.* http://ojp.usdoj.gov/bjs/crimoff. htm#women. Accessed 1 Oct 2006.

Centers for Disease Control and Prevention. (2004a). Diagnosis of HIV/AIDS – 32 states, 2000–2003. *MMWR. Morbidity and Mortality Weekly Report, 53*, 1106–1110.

Centers for Disease Control and Prevention. (2004b). Racial and ethnic minorities: STD surveillance 2004. http://www.cdc.gov/std/stats04/minorities.htm. Accessed 16 Jul 2010.

Chaisson, R. E., Stoneburner, R. L., Hildebrandt, D. S., Telzak, E. E., & Jaffe, H. W. (1990). Heterosexual transmission of HIV associated with the use of smokable freebase cocaine (crack). *AIDS, 5*(9), 1121–1126.

Chirgwin, K., DeHovitz, J. A., Dillon, S., & McCormack, W. M. (1991). HIV infection, genital ulcer disease, and crack cocaine use among patients attending a clinic for sexually transmitted diseases. *American Journal of Public Health, 81*, 1576–1579.

Cunningham, R. M., Stiffman, A. R., Dore, P., & Earls, F. (1994). The association of physical and sexual abuse with HIV risk behaviors in adolescence and young adulthood: Implications for public health. *Child Abuse & Neglect, 18*(3), 233–245.

DiClemente, R. J., Wingood, G. M., Harrington, K. F., Lang, D. L., Davies, S. L., Hook, E. W., III, et al. (2004). Efficacy of an HIV prevention intervention for African American adolescent girls: A randomized controlled trial. *JAMA, 292*(2), 171–179.

El-Bassel, N., Fontdevila, J., Gilbert, L., Voisin, D., Richman, B., & Pitchell, P. (2001). HIV risks of men in methadone maintenance treatment programs who abuse their intimate partners: A forgotten issue. *Journal of Substance Abuse, 13*, 1–15.

El-Bassel, N., Gilbert, L., Ivanoff, A., Schilling, R. F., Borne, D., & Safyer, S. F. (1996). Correlates of crack abuse among incarcerated women: Psychological trauma, social support and coping behavior. *American Journal of Drug and Alcohol Abuse, 22*, 41–56.

El-Bassel, N., Gilbert, L., Krishnan, S., Schilling, R. F., Gaeta, T., Purpura, S., et al. (1998). Partner violence and sexual HIV-risk behaviors among women in an inner-city emergency department. *Violence and Victims, 13*(4), 377–393.

El-Bassel, N., Gilbert, L., Rajah, V., Foleno, A., & Frye, V. (2000). Fear and violence: Raising the HIV stakes. *AIDS Education and Prevention, 12*(2), 154–170.

El-Bassel, N., Gilbert, L., Schilling, R. F., & Wada, T. (2000). Drug abuse and partner violence among women in methadone treatment. *Journal of Family Violence, 15*(3), 209–225.

El-Bassel, N., Gilbert, L., Wu, E., Go, H., & Hill, J. (2005a). HIV and intimate partner violence among women on methadone. *Social Science & Medicine, 61*(1), 171–183.

El-Bassel, N., Gilbert, L., Wu, E., Go, H., & Hill, J. (2005b). The temporal relationship between drug abuse and intimate partner violence: A longitudinal study among women on methadone. *American Journal of Public Health, 95*(3), 465–470.

El-Bassel, N., Gilbert, L., & Wu, E. (2007). The intersecting problems of HIV and IPV among African American women on methadone. Manuscript in preparation.

El-Bassel, N., Ivanoff, A., Schilling, R. F., Gilbert, L., Borne, D., & Chen, D. (1995). Preventing HIV/AIDS in drug-abusing incarcerated women through skills-building and social support enhancement: Preliminary outcomes. *Social Work Research, 19*, 131–141.

El-Bassel, N., Witte, S. S., Gilbert, L., Wu, E., Chang, M., Hill, J., et al. (2003). The efficacy of a relationship-based HIV/STD prevention program for heterosexual couples. *American Journal of Public Health, 93*(6), 963–969.

Fullilove, M. T., Lown, A., & Fullilove, R. E. (1992). Crack "hos and skeezers": Traumatic experiences of women crack users. *Journal of Sex Research, 29*, 257–287.

Fullilove, R. (2006). African Americans, health disparities and HIV/AIDS: Recommendations for confronting the epidemic in Black America. Washington, DC: National Minority AIDS Council.

Gelles, R. (1993). Through a sociological lens: Social structure and family violence. In R. Gelles & D. Loseke (Eds.), *Current controversies on family violence* (pp. 31–46). Newbury Park, CA: Sage Publications.

Gielen, A. C., McDonnell, K. A., & O'Campo, P. J. (2002). Intimate partner violence, HIV status, and sexual risk reduction. *AIDS and Behavior, 6*(2), 107–116.

Gielen, A. C., O'Campo, P., Anderson, J., Keller, J., & Faden, R. (2000). Women living with HIV: Disclosure, violence, and social support. *Journal of Urban Health, 77*, 480–491.

Gielen, A. C., O'Campo, P., Faden, R. R., & Eke, A. (1997). Women's disclosure of HIV status: Experiences of mistreatment and violence in an urban setting. *Women and Health, 25*(3), 19–31.

Gilbert, L., El-Bassel, N., Manuel, J., Wu, E., Go, H., Golder, S., et al. (2006). An integrated relapse prevention and relationship safety intervention for women on methadone: testing short-terms effects on intimate partner violence and substance use. *Violence and Victims, 21*(5), 657–672.

Gilbert, L., El-Bassel, N., Rajah, V., Foleno, A., Fontdevila, J., Frye, V., et al. (2000). The converging epidemics of mood-altering-drug use, HIV, HCV, and partner violence: A conundrum for methadone maintenance treatment. *Mount Sinai Journal of Medicine, 67*(5–6), 452–464.

Gilbert, L., El-Bassel, N., Rajah, V., Foleno, A., & Frye, V. (2001). Linking drug related activities with experiences of partner violence: A focus group study of women in methadone treatment. *Violence and Victims, 16*(5), 517–536.

Gilbert, L., El-Bassel, N., Schilling, R., Wada, T., & Bennet, B. (2000). Partner violence and sexual HIV risk behaviors among women in methadone treatment. *AIDS and Behavior, 4*(3), 261–269.

Grella, C. E., Stein, J. A., & Greenwell, L. (2005). Associations among childhood trauma, adolescent problem behaviors, and adverse adult outcomes in substance-abusing women offenders. *Psychology of Addictive Behaviors, 19*(1), 43–53.

Hampton, R., Oliver, W., & Magarian, L. (2003). Domestic violence in the African American community: An analysis of social and structural factors. *Violence Against Women, 9*(5), 533–551.

Hogben, M., Gange, S. J., Watts, D. H., Robison, E., Young, M., & Richardson, J. (2001). The effect of sexual and physical violence on risky sexual behavior and STDs among a cohort of HIV seropositive women. *AIDS and Behavior, 5*, 353–361.

Holmberg, S. D. (1996). The estimated prevalence and incidence of HIV in 96 large US metropolitan areas. *American Journal of Public Health, 86*(5), 642–654.

Hutton, H. E., Treisman, G. J., Hunt, W. R., Fishman, M., Kendig, N., Swetz, A., et al. (2001). HIV risk behaviors and their relationship to posttraumatic stress disorder among women prisoners. *Psychiatric Services, 52*(4), 508–513.

James, S. E., Johnson, J., & Raghavan, C. (2004). "I couldn't go anywhere" contextualizing violence and drug abuse: A social network study. *Violence Against Women, 10*(9), 991–1014.

Jenny, C., Hooton, T., Bowers, A., Copass, M., Krieger, J., Hillier, S., et al. (1990). Sexually transmitted diseases in victims of rape. *The New England Journal of Medicine, 322*(11), 713–716.

Kalichman, S. C., Kelly, J. A., Hunter, T. L., Murphy, D. A., & Tyler, R. (1993). Culturally-tailored HIV/AIDS risk reduction messages targeted to African American urban women: Impact on risk sensitization and risk reduction. *Journal of Consulting and Clinical Psychology, 61*, 291–295.

Kalichman, S. C., Williams, E. A., Cherry, C., Belcher, L., & Nachimson, D. (1998). Sexual coercion, domestic violence, and negotiating condom use among low-income African American women. *Journal of Women's Health, 7*, 371–378.

Kelly, J. A., & Kalichman, S. C. (1995). Increased attention to human sexuality can improve HIV-AIDS prevention efforts: Key research issues and directions. *Journal of Consulting and Clinical Psychology, 63*, 907–918.

Lewis, C. F. (2005). Post-Traumatic Stress Disorder in HIV positive Incarcerated Women. *Journal of American Academy of Psychiatry and Law, 33*, 455–464.

Maman, S., Campbell, J., Sweat, M., & Gielen, A. (2000). The intersections of HIV and violence: Directions for future research and interventions. *Social Science & Medicine, 50*, 459–478.

Maruschak, L. M. (2004). HIV in prisons and jails, 2002. *Bureau of Justice Statistics Bulletin, NCJ, 205333*, 1–11.

Maruschak, L. M. (2005). HIV in prisons, 2003 (NCJ 210344). Washington, DC: Bureau of Justice Statistics.

Mays, V. M., Cochran, S., & Zamudio, A. (2004). HIV prevention research: Are we meeting the needs of African American men who have sex with men. *Journal of Black Psychology, 30*, 78–105.

McNair, L. D., & Prather, C. M. (2004). African American women and AIDS: Factors influencing risk and reaction to HIV disease. *Journal of Black Psychology, 30*(1), 106–123.

Mermelstein, R., Cohen, S., Lichtenstein, E., Baer, J. S., & Kamarck, T. (1986). Social support and smoking cessation and maintenance. *Journal of Consulting and Clinical Psychology, 54*, 447–453.

Miller, B. A. (1990). The interrelationships between alcohol and drugs and family violence. *National Institute on Drug Abuse Research Monographs, 103*, 177–207.

Mize, S. J. S., Robinson, B. E., Bockting, W. O., & Scheltema, K. E. (2002). Meta-analysis of the effectiveness of HIV prevention interventions for women. *AIDS Care, 14*(2), 163–180.

Najavits, L., Gastfried, D., Barber, J., et al. (1998). Cocaine dependence with and without PTSD among subjects in the National Institute on Drug Abuse Collaborative Cocaine Treatment Study. *American Journal of Psychiatry, 149*, 664–670.

North, R. L., & Rothenberg, K. H. (1993). Partner notification and the threat of domestic violence against women with HIV infection. *The New England Journal of Medicine, 329*(16), 1194–1196.

O'Leary, A., & Wingood, G. M. (2000). Interventions for sexually active heterosexual women. In J. L. Peterson & R. J. DiClemente (Eds.), *Handbook of HIV prevention* (pp. 179–197). New York: Plenum Publishing Corp.

Raj, A., Silverman, J. G., & Amaro, H. (2004). Abused women report greater male partner risk and gender-based risk for HIV: Findings from a community-based study with Hispanic women. *AIDS Care, 16*(4), 519–529.

Rappaport, J. (1987). Terms of empowerment/exemplars of prevention: Toward a theory for community psychology. *American Journal of Community Psychology, 15*(2), 121–148.

Rennison, C. M., & Welchans, S. (2000). *Bureau of Justice Statistics special report: Intimate partner violence*. Bureau of Justice Statistics Special Report. NCJ 178247. http://www.ojp.usdoj.gov/bjs. Accessed 1 Oct 2006.

Rhodes, T., Singer, M., Bourgois, P., Friedman, S. R., & Strathdee, S. A. (2005). The social structural production of HIV risk among injecting drug users. *Social Science & Medicine, 61*(5), 1026–1044.

Rodriguez, M. A., Szkupinski Quiroga, S., & Bauer, H. M. (1996). Breaking the silence: Battered women's perspective on medical care. *Archives of Family Medicine, 5*, 153–158.

St. Lawrence, J. S., Wilson, T. E., Eldridge, G. D., Brasfield, T. L., & O'Bannon, R. E. (2001). Community based interventions to reduce low income, African American women's risk of sexually transmitted diseases: A randomized controlled trial of three theoretical models. *American Journal of Community Psychology, 29*(6), 637–664.

Sterk, C. E. (1999). *Fast lives: Women who use crack cocaine*. Philadelphia, PA: Temple University Press.

Stiffman, A., Dore, P., Earls, F., et al. (1992). The influence of mental health problems on AIDS-related risk behaviors in young adults. *Journal of Nervous and Mental Disease, 180*, 314–320.

Wingood, G. M., & DiClemente, R. J. (1992). Cultural, gender and psychosocial influences on HIV related behavior of African American female adolescents: Implications for the development of tailored prevention programs. *Ethnicity and Disease, 2*, 381–388.

Wingood, G. M., & DiClemente, R. J. (1997). The effects of an abusive primary partner on the condom use and sexual negotiation practices of African–American women. *American Journal of Public Health, 87*(6), 1016–1018.

Wingood, G. M., & DiClemente, R. J. (1998). Partner influences and gender-related factors associated with non-condom use among young adult African American women. American Journal of Community Psychology, 26(1), 29–51.

World Health Organization. (1997). *The female condom: A review.* Geneva, Switzerland: World Health Organization.

Wyatt, G. E. (1991). Child sexual abuse and its effects on sexual functioning. *Annual Review of Sex Research, 2,* 249–266.

Wyatt, G. E., Longshore, D., Chin, D., Carmona, J. V., Loeb, T. B., Myers, H. F., et al. (2004). The efficacy of an integrated risk reduction intervention for HIV-positive women with child sexual abuse histories. *AIDS & Behavior, 8*(4), 453–462.

Yoshioka, M., Gilbert, L., & El-Bassel, N. (2003). Social support and disclosure of abuse: A comparison of African American, Hispanic, and South Asian battered women. *Journal of Family Violence, 18*(3), 171–179.

Zimmerman, M. A., Israel, B. A., Schulz, A., & Checkoway, B. (1992). Further explorations in empowerment theory: An empirical analysis of psychological empowerment. *American Journal of Community Psychology, 20*(6), 707–727.

Zlotnick, C. (1997). Post-Traumatic Stress Disorder (PTSD), PTSD comorbidity, and childhood abuse among incarcerated women. *Journal of Nervous and Mental Disease, 185,* 761–763.

Chapter 8
Childhood Sexual Abuse, African American Women, and HIV Risk

Lekeisha A. Sumner, Gail E. Wyatt, Dorie Glover, Jennifer V. Carmona, Tamra B. Loeb, Tina B. Henderson, Dorothy Chin, and Rotrease S. Regan

Child sexual abuse (CSA) is defined as unwanted or coerced sexual contact prior to the age of 18 (Wyatt, 1985; Wyatt, Newcomb, & Riederle, 1995). Once thought to rarely occur, conservative estimates suggest that at least 20% of women and 5–10% of men worldwide report being sexually abuse as children (World Health Organization, 2002). Within the United States, the prevalence of CSA among women is approximately 33% (Briere & Elliott, 1993; Loeb et al., 2002a; Wyatt, Guthrie, & Notgrass, 1992). A large body of epidemiological evidence suggests that the impact of childhood sexual abuse is varied and wide-reaching. Further, a history of childhood sexual abuse is linked to increased risks for psychosocial, behavioral, and physical health problems, including HIV (Chin, Wyatt, Carmona, Loeb, & Myers, 2004).

This chapter holds the assumption that the reader has little knowledge of CSA. We focus exclusively on those aspects of CSA that influence high-risk behaviors. We present the rationale for examining the role of CSA in HIV risk followed by a brief questionnaire to assess adults for CSA histories. We then review the impact of CSA within the domains most commonly associated with high-risk behaviors – namely, sexual health, emotional and social functioning, and biological dysfunction. We examine these problems within a sociocultural context relevant to a group disproportionately affected by HIV/AIDS in the United States – African American women. In addition, we discuss the importance as well as the challenges in implementing community interventions that integrate HIV-risk reduction and CSA. Finally, in our concluding remarks, we recommend that findings from across disciplines be extrapolated to inform future interventions.

L.A. Sumner (✉)
Department of Psychiatry and Biobehavioral Sciences,
UCLA, Los Angeles, CA 90034, USA
e-mail: lsumner@mednet.ucla.edu

D.H. McCree et al. (eds.), *African Americans and HIV/AIDS*,
DOI 10.1007/978-0-387-78321-5_8,

Overview: Why Examine CSA and HIV Risk?

The rate of AIDS among African American women is approximately 24 times the rate of Caucasian women (Centers for Disease Control and Prevention, 2007). In 2005, African American women accounted for 66% of all HIV/AIDS diagnoses among women and was the leading cause of death of African American women between the ages of 24–34 (Centers for Disease Control and Prevention, 2007). Among African American women, unprotected sex with an HIV positive male is the primary mode of transmission followed by injection drug use (Center for Disease Control and Prevention, 2005). Although the prevalence of childhood sexual abuse does not differ across ethnicities or socio-economic backgrounds in the United States, the presentation of its effects are influenced by cultural factors.

HIV-related high risk behaviors, such as risky sexual practices and drug use, increase the likelihood of a woman contracting HIV (Bensley, Eenwyk, & Simmons, 2000; Johnsen & Harlow, 1996; Wyatt et al., 1997). Studies using community samples of ethnic women have found that women with histories of childhood sexual abuse have a sevenfold increase in HIV-related risk behaviors compared with women without abuse histories (Wyatt et al., 2002). Moreover, these women are at increased risk for subsequent revictimization and higher rates of sexually transmitted infections (STIs) (Bensley et al., 2000; Johnsen & Harlow, 1996; West, Williams, & Siegel, 2000; Wyatt et al., 1992). CSA has been reported as an antecedent to prostitution, low self-esteem, and turbulent interpersonal relationships (Blankertz, Cnann, & Freedman, 1993; Freshwater, Leach, & Aldridge, 2001).

Sexual Health

The degree to which women are unaware of how to protect and control their bodies and reproductive health and do not participate in sexual decision-making are influenced by early non-consensual sexual experiences, cultural beliefs, and economic dependence. These factors increase the chances of unwanted sexual outcomes, specifically unintended pregnancies, HIV, and other STIs.

Female survivors of childhood sexual abuse report higher rates of high-risk sexual behaviors than those without histories (Polusny & Follette, 1995). Perhaps due to lower self-efficacy for condom use, African American women with histories of CSA are less likely to use contraceptives, including condoms, thereby increasing their vulnerability to HIV infection (Harlow et al., 1998; Heise, Moore, & Toubia, 1995; Thompson, Potter, Sanderson, & Maibach, 1997; Wyatt, Notgrass, & Gordon, 1995). Female survivors of childhood sexual abuse appear to engage in anal sex without condoms more often than women without childhood sexual abuse histories

(Bensley et al., 2000). These women also report higher rates of unintended pregnancy (Wyatt et al., 1995).

Sexual problems in adulthood have also been associated with childhood sexual abuse. Sexually abused women are more likely to report sexual arousal problems, higher sexual dissatisfaction, and have an aversion to sex as well as to their own and/or their partner's bodies (Laumann, Paik, & Rosen, 1999; Mullen, Martin, Anderson, Romans, & Herbison, 1994). Compulsive sexual behavior has also been noted and an inability to distinguish affection from sex (Briere & Runtz, 1988). Women may differ on a continuum of sexual health and risk taking, including being socialized to be passive partners, having unprotected sex, engaging in minimal communication about sex and engaging in less body touching (Wyatt & Riederle, 1994a, b)

Assessing Histories of Childhood Sexual Abuse

Given the increased psychosocial, behavioral and physical vulnerability of women with histories of childhood sexual abuse, screening for abuse history is critical. To address the clinical and research needs in identifying adults with histories of childhood sexual abuse, Dr. Gail Wyatt developed two assessment tools. The first is the Wyatt Sex History Questionnaire (WSHQ-R), a 478-item, face-to-face structured interview that utilizes open- and closed-ended items (Wyatt, 1985, 1992). The WSHQ-R asks about demographic characteristics, incidents of non-consensual sexual abuse, consensual sex, psychological status, substance abuse, medication adherence, and sexual decision making. The WSHQ-R was created for use with multi-ethnic populations and has been used worldwide. Test–retest reliability on closed-ended items ($r = 0.90$) and interrater reliability on open-ended items were established on a weekly basis ($r = 0.95$). For a brief screen, Wyatt recommends using the following screening questions:

It is generally realized that many women, while they were children or adolescents have had a sexual experience with an adult or someone older than themselves. By sexual, I mean behaviors ranging from someone exposing themselves (their genitals) to you, to someone having intercourse with you. These experiences may have involved a relative, a friend of the family, or a stranger. Some experiences are very upsetting and painful while others are not, and some may have occurred without your consent.

Now I'd like you to think back to your childhood and adolescence and remember if you had any sexual experiences with a relative, a family friend, or stranger. Describe each experience completely and separately.

1. During childhood and adolescence, did anyone ever expose themselves (their sexual organs) to you?
2. During childhood and adolescence, did anyone masturbate in front of you?
3. Did a relative, family friend or stranger ever touch or fondle your body, including your breasts or genitals, or attempt to arouse you sexually?
4. During childhood and adolescence, did anyone try to have you arouse them, or touch their body in a sexual way?
5. Did anyone rub their genitals against your body in a sexual way?
6. During childhood and adolescence, did anyone attempt to have intercourse with you?
7. Did anyone have intercourse with you?
8. Did you have any other sexual experiences involving a relative, family friend, or stranger?

Socio-Cultural Factors and High-Risk Behavior

Complicating the study of childhood sexual abuse and HIV risk behaviors among African American women are cultural norms of sexual behavior within the African American community as well as gender stereotypes and expectations. Such norms often influence the manner in which African American women respond to and cope with CSA. For instance, due to distrust with the legal and medical system, African American families are less likely to report childhood sexual abuse (Cargill, Stone, & Robinson, 2004; Wyatt, 1997). Being a part of a collectivistic culture, African American victims may choose the maintenance of the family unit over disclosing familial abuse and thereby risk fracturing close relationships. . Moreover, as a result of the disproportionate availability of African American men relative to women, African American women may feel less empowered to demand condom use due to fear of losing their mate (Wyatt, 1994a, b). It is therefore critical that CSA and HIV risk among African American women are examined through a historical and cultural frame of reference. As such, investigators have recently begun to urge researchers to utilize theoretical frameworks that integrate theories of power, specifically, as it relates to culture, gender, race, and class in HIV behavioral studies (Amaro, 1995; Amaro & Raj, 2000). For example, Wyatt has developed the Sexual Health Model, a framework to further the understanding of African American female sexuality. Its components include cultural values (e.g. connectedness), behaviors (e.g. body touching), and social cognition (e.g., empowerment) relevant to African American women.

Attitudes, Beliefs, and Emotional Consequences

There are emotional effects of sexual abuse that can also increase HIV-related risks for individuals and couples. The attitudes and beliefs developed in childhood as a result of sexual abuse impacts a woman's attitude and beliefs in adulthood contributing to poor decision-making in characterizing people and social situations (Smith, 1992).

For instance, women with histories of childhood sexual abuse often engage in self-blame for the assault, leading to social impairment such as social isolation, poor qualities of social support, difficulties with assertiveness, and being overly responsible (Gibson & Hartshorne, 1996; Koopman, Gore-Felton, Classen, Kim, & Spiegel, 2001). These characteristics, along with maladaptive beliefs, may explain why some women may accept unwanted sexual invitations (Cloitre, Scarvalone, & Difede, 1997).

Childhood sexual abuse is also associated with psychological distress, with a third of all victims reporting symptoms of depression and anxiety as well as self-destructive behaviors, including patterns of substance abuse and sexual risk behaviors (Bensley et al., 2000; McCauley, Kern, Kolodner, Derogatis, & Bass, 1998; Wyatt, Carmona, Loeb, Ayala, & Chin, 2002). Adults with histories of childhood sexual abuse are four times more likely to receive a diagnosis of major depression than those without (Boudewyn & Liem, 1995). Women with a history of early sexual abuse are more likely to receive a diagnosis of posttraumatic stress disorder (PTSD), with some estimating at a rate of up to 48% among both sexes (Simpson, 2002). While most survivors of childhood sexual abuse do not meet diagnostic criteria for PTSD, up to 80% have posttraumatic stress symptoms including repetitive, instructive thoughts of sexual abuse, hyperarousal, and nightmares that are centered around guilt, humiliation, and sexual abuse (Zlotnick, Mattia, & Zimmerman, 2001). Given that African Americans are at increased risk for exposure to traumatic events and women are more likely than men to develop PTSD, African American women may be particularly vulnerable to symptoms of trauma.

Mounting evidence indicates that childhood trauma increases an individual's vulnerability to substance use and abuse (Molnar, Buka, & Kessler, 2001; Myers et al., 2009). Given that women with histories of childhood sexual often have limited coping strategies, alcohol and/or recreational drugs is commonly utilized as a coping strategy, particularly by younger women. Substance use, while temporarily numbing emotional pain, often impairs sexual decision-making, encourages sexual risk-taking and may lead to substance dependence. Several studies have found associations between childhood sexual abuse and heavy drinking among women (Vogeltanz et al., 1999; Downs, 1993). African American women with childhood sexual abuse histories are more likely to consume three or more glasses of alcohol at one sitting than those without histories of childhood sexual abuse (Wingood & DiClemente, 1997a). In a study of 75 African American HIV-positive women with histories of childhood sexual abuse, over 80% used at least one illicit substance regularly and 28% engaged in injection drug use (Wyatt, Carmona, Loeb, & Williams, 2005). This finding is particularly relevant to African American female injection drug users as IDU-associated AIDS account for a large proportion of cases among this ethnic group.

Intimate Relationships, Revictimization and High-Risk Behavior

Intimate relationships are an important aspect of women's lives. However, traumatic experiences such as early sexual abuse and HIV infection can have detrimental affects on relationships. Sexual abuse is associated with negative long-term effects on intimate relationships including deficits in the ability to communicate and negotiate with others (Smith, 1992). Also, given that childhood sexual abuse often takes place with familiar or related perpetrators, betrayal and distrust develops at an early age that can result in intimacy disturbances, fear and distrust of others, including sexual partners (Gorcey, Santiago, & McCall-Perez, 1986). For both women with histories of childhood sexual abuse and women infected with HIV, a resistance to disclosing these histories may be due to continued fear of rejection by others and feelings of shame and guilt associated with childhood sexual abuse and HIV (Chin & Kroesen, 1999; Smith et al., 2000). Thus, feelings of loneliness and isolation resulting from these patterns of secrecy are common among HIV-positive sexually abused women.

Early traumatic sexual experiences can often result in experience of other types of trauma because women with these histories are less likely to be able to protect themselves from future abuse (Wyatt, Axelrod, Chin, Carmona, & Loe, 2000). Considerable evidence suggests that victims of childhood sexual abuse are at elevated risk of experiencing adult interpersonal violence, specifically domestic violence (Cohen et al., 2000). CSA is associated with a lifetime of domestic violence, poor social relationships, drug abuse and high-risk drug-related behaviors, high number of sexual partners or risky having male partners (Cohen et al., 2000).

Women in abusive relationships are less able to negotiate sexual practices, including condom use, due to fear and limited negotiation skills in sexual relationships (Wyatt, 1994a). It is suggested that HIV-positive women have higher rates of intimate partner violence (IPV) compared to HIV-negative women, and HIV-positive African American women experienced the highest rates of IPV compared to European Americans and Latinas (Axelrod, Myers, Durvasula, Wyatt, & Cheng, 1999). Women in abusive relationships are less likely to use condoms and are more likely to experience verbal, emotional, and threats of physical abuse when they discuss condom use with their partners. Wingood & DiClemente (1997a) found that African American women with histories of CSA reported a five-fold increase in physical abuse from their partners in the past 3 months. One study found African American women in abusive relationships worried about becoming infected with HIV more than women not in abusive relationships (Wingood & DiClemente, 1997b). This finding has been supported by those from more recent studies of adult sexual revictimization among African American women with histories of sexual abuse. Compared to women with childhood sexual abuse only, women with both childhood sexual abuse and adult partner violence are more likely to be involved in prostitution and have increased gynecological problems such as sexually transmitted diseases (Fleming & Wasserheit, 1999; West, Williams, & Siegel, 2000).

Being in an abusive relationship also increases a women's risk of being sexually active with a partner with high-risk behaviors (Baker et al., 2003). In one study, low income African American women who were revictimized were not involved in monogamous relationships but were four times less likely to use condoms on a consistent basis. While one study, controlling for income, did not find ethnic differences in increased revictimizations (Wyatt, Carmona, Loeb, Ayala, & Chin, 2002), other studies have found that limited-income African American women with CSA were more likely to be raped as adults when compared to women with CSA from other ethnic backgrounds (Urquiza & Goodlin-Jones, 1994; Wyatt et al., 1995; West, Williams, & Siegel, 2000).

Biological Impact of Childhood Sexual Abuse

There are also biological effects of early abuse and trauma. Recent findings suggest that the severe stress of childhood sexual abuse is associated with increased risk for mental health disorders and associated biological vulnerabilities (Stein, Koverola, Hanna, Torchia, & McClarty, 1997; Heim et al., 2000). Beyond the negative psychiatric and behavioral outcomes, there are substantial biological consequences of severe stress exposure and these can directly alter brain structure or function (Schiffer et al., 2007). Changes in brain structure or function have widespread implications for health; neurological changes ultimately may impact vulnerability to infection upon exposure to HIV and also accelerate disease progression once infected (Kumar, Kumar, Walididrop, Antoni, & Eisdorfer, 2003; Kopnisky, Stoff, & Rausch, 2004). The post-CSA biological response can be seen as triggering a cascade of negative psychological and social sequelae that in turn contribute to HIV rates in African American women. Research is beginning to track the complex interplay of the reciprocal interactions between psychological stress and immune, endocrine, central and peripheral nervous systems in HIV (Kopnisky et al., 2004). The objective of this section is to provide a general overview of the systems involved in response to threat (the reader is referred to the references in this section for a details).

The Initial Response to Threat

Stressful experiences bring about a complex and counterbalancing set of hormonal responses in biological systems designed to maintain bodily functions as basic as heart rate and breathing. Three such systems related to stress are: the sympathetic-adrenomedulary (SAM) system, the hypothalamic-pituitary–adrenal (HPA) axis, and the immune system. The basic components of these systems have been mapped out through animal studies which allow for scientific control over the timing, frequency, type and severity of the stress (Friedman, Charney, & Deutch, 1995). Faced with an immediate threat, the SAM system releases neurohormones called "catecholamines" (*adrenaline/epinephrine* (EPI) and *noradrenaline/norepinephrine* (NE). The catecholamines facilitate subsequent processes that increase the heart rate, blood pressure and blood glucose levels in muscles and vital organs in order to allow the body to adapt to the increased demand of a stressor. An immediate threat also triggers the HPA axis to release a sequence of brain substances from different parts of the brain. Neuropeptides stimulate release of *corticotrophin-releasing hormone (CRH)* from the hypothalamus. CRH then stimulates release of *adrenocorticotropic hormone (ACTH)* from the pituitary and in turn the adrenal glands release *glucocorticoids* (in humans, glucocorticoids are commonly called "cortisol") and *dehydroepiandosterone (DHEA)*. These hormones further act on the immune system, which results in changes in the levels and activity of immune system substances such as *cytokines* that are especially relevant for host protection against viral infections like HIV (i.e., CD4 and CD8 T cells) (Coe & Laudenslager, 2007; Kiecolt-Glaser & Glaser, 1992).

Under normal circumstances, specialized feedback systems are designed to ensure a return to normal functioning or "allostasis" once the threat is gone. Cortisol has an important role in shutting down the SAM system and suppressing the HPA axis by a negative feedback mechanism acting on brain structures of the pituitary, hippocampus, hypothalamus and amygdala. The anti-corticoid properties of DHEA are also believed to help counter the possible negative effects of high cortisol levels on the brain (Rasmusson, Vythilingam, & Morgan, 2003). Once the perception of threat recedes, the negative feedback mechanisms help restore hormone levels to allostasis.

Results of Biomarker Studies in Humans

Emerging studies of abused children (childhood sexual abuse and other types of child abuse) demonstrate that abuse is associated with abnormalities at rest or in response to a challenge. Most recently, Carrion, Weems, Garret, Mennon, & Reiss (2007) reported brain changes associated with cortisol and PTSD symptoms in 15 children exposed to at least one traumatic event. Most had experienced multiple traumatic events, including sexual, physical and emotional abuse as well as witnessing violence. The sample included 6 boys and 9 girls ages 8 to 14 (mean = 10.4), and a mixed ethnic composition of primarily Caucasian ($n = 7$) or African Americans ($n = 6$). The children were assessed twice, with assessments separated by 12–18 months. Brain imaging techniques were used to evaluate changes in hippocampal size over time in relation to PTSD symptoms and home-collected cortisol levels across the day. Results showed that participants with the highest severity of PTSD symptoms at Time 1 showed the greatest reductions in the right hippocampus from the first to the second assessment. Elevated evening (pre-bed) salivary cortisol at Time 1 was also related to reductions in hippocampal size at the next assessment. As the hippocampus is associated with the encoding and retrieval of autobiographical memory, these results are consistent with clinical findings of amnesia as one component of PTSD.

Contextual and Social Factors

Feelings of isolation and shame may be especially pronounced for women facing the double stigma of childhood sexual abuse and HIV. As a consequence women may fear being rejected, and therefore may avoid disclosing their seropositive status with partners, friends or family. They are often worried about burdening or worrying family members and disrupting relationships (Chin & Kroesen, 1999; Hays et al., 1993; Simoni, Mason, Marks, & Ruiz, 1995a, b).

An adverse family context not only may contribute directly to childhood sexual abuse, but may also increase the odds that revictimization may occur (Briere, 2004). Poor family functioning, operationalized as a lack of autonomy and intimacy, has been noted to influence the trauma severity of early sexual abuse experiences, regardless of whether or not they occurred within the family (Draucker, 1997). Other adverse family patterns include inconsistency and unpredictability, denial, lack of empathy, lack of clear boundaries, role reversal, incongruent communication, too much or too little conflict and a closed family system (Briere, 2004). Among African American adolescent females it has been reported that low family support and infrequent mother-daughter communication were associated with STIs (Crosby, Wingood, DiClemente, & Rose, 2002).

The Cultural Context

There is often confusion about the role and importance of examining cultural values and histories of CSA in HIV prevention research. Cultural and religious values related to sexuality mirror histories of CSA and the trauma experienced in the aftermath of these experiences (see Table 8.1). In other words, cultural or religious

Table 8.1 The mimic effect

Effects of child sexual abuse (CSA)	Cultural and religious messages	HIV risk behaviors
Poor personal boundaries	Externalized control of the body (limited sexual ownership) "My partner will please me"	Inadvertent selection of high-risk, controlling sexual partner
Lack of trust		
Avoidance of health seeking, physical exams, questions about sexual history	Lack of body awareness, knowledge of health/STD/ HIV status. health paranoia (body awareness) *carnal knowledge is not*	Avoidance of being tested for STD/HIV multiple partners
Poor assessment of risks		
Self-medication to avoid PTSD, depression, or anxiety	Value of relationships to enhance self-worth. interconnectedness procreational rather than recreational sex *God brought me this person*	Non-use of contraceptives or condoms substance use/abuse with partners

values regarding the awareness of the body, and relative comfort with sexual behaviors and relationships may have their origins in attitudes and responses to childhood sexual abuse and as a result decrease the likelihood a woman will be able to utilize HIV protective behaviors.

When HIV-related risk behaviors are identified there is often confusion about the etiology of the behaviors for African American women. While it has been well established that a history of CSA increases risks for HIV infection, the specific effects of cultural and religious values are not well described. The ways in which sexual abuse and cultural or religious values may influence very similar effects on HIV-related risk behaviors can be sorted into three dimensions. These aspects of CSA are often understudied in HIV/AIDS behavioral research:

1. *Poor personal boundaries.* Incidents of sexual abuse where the perpetrator used psychological manipulation (e.g., "No one loves us, so we have to love each other;"), threats (e.g., "If you tell, I will kill your pet,"), financial or emotional incentives, or physical force often affect the survivor's ability to establish personal limits on their own behavior. This is especially the case when the sexual abuse occurs over long periods of time and involves vaginal or anal penetration. The survivor of abuse may struggle to learn how to identify their own sexual needs, criteria for establishing intimate relationships and their own patterns of sexual arousal or pleasure. Given that the process of intimate and trusting relationship formation is often controlled by a more powerful perpetrator, survivors tend to gravitate to controlling and powerful partners who assume control over sex-related decisions. If those partners choose to ignore HIV/STD prevention and engage in unprotected sex or have a history of multiple partners or drug use/abuse, the risks of HIV transmission can become more likely.

2. *Externalized control of the body.* Cultural values regarding body touching and conversations about sex for women endorse more passive, receptive roles (Wyatt, 1994a). The role of a male partner is perceived to be instinctive, authoritative and knowledgeable. The assumption is that the woman's role is to follow the lead of her partner. Both the abusive and cultural rationales for HIV related outcomes could increase risks of selecting controlling, authoritarian partners to limit sexual negotiations about HIV testing, contraceptive and condom use. For many individuals with conservative beliefs, passivity in women's roles are endorsed and rewarded with social, community and family recognition that a woman knows "how to keep a man." Alternatively, a man might know "how to handle a woman." The issue of disease transmission risks is not fully considered as a possible outcome of these role dichotomies.

3. *Lack of trust.* African American sexual behavior has been characterized as "risky, dangerous" and a 'threat' to public health long before HIV/AIDS (Wyatt, 1997). Some of the earliest descriptions of African women and men before slavery described them as sexually promiscuous (Wyatt, 1997). While stereotypes about African sexuality may, in part, contribute to assumptions that African Americans have high rates of HIV/AIDS, the fact that research has reported differences between racial and ethnic groups, but has not offered adequate explanations for these differences or these stereotypes.

In an attempt to understand both the range of sexual experiences and the behaviors that occur willfully and with consent as well as those where coercion, force or violence is involved, our research team has developed a system for asking about sexual experiences that occurred before and since the age of 18, where consent to participate in sexual practices with another is legal. This approach is consistent with sexuality research since the Kinsey studies beginning in the 1940s.

Research has documented the relationship between histories of early sexual abuse and an increase in HIV/AIDS risk behaviors, specifically higher numbers of partners, non-condom use, and a likelihood of engaging in a variety of sexual behaviors including vaginal, anal and oral sex (Wyatt et al., 2004). However, it is just as important to avoid assumptions about the etiology of high-risk sexual practices as it is to include other factors that may also mimic the after-effects of sexual abuse and that may have also been viewed as unimportant to our understanding of how to effectively reduce HIV related risk behaviors among African Americans. Table 1 below describes the how cultural and religious messages mimic the effects of CSA.

Gender and Race

Complicating the study of childhood sexual abuse and HIV risk behaviors among African American women are not only the cultural norms of sexual behavior within the African American community but gender stereotypes and gender expectations. Such norms often influence the manner in which African American women respond and cope with CSA. For instance, due to distrust with the legal and medical system, African American families are less likely to report CSA (Cargill et al., 2004; Wyatt, 1997). Being a part of a collectivistic culture that values family and protection of family members may also influence how African American families and victims cope with childhood sexual abuse. Moreover, as a result of the much publicized unavailability of African American males, African American women may feel less empowered to demand condom use out of fear of losing their mate and as well as beliefs about the procreational role of sex (Wyatt & Riederle, 1994a). It is therefore critical that childhood sexual abuse and HIV risk among African American women are examined through a historical and cultural frame of reference. As such, investigators have recently begun to urge researchers to utilize theoretical frameworks that integrate theories of power, specifically, as it relates to culture, gender, race, and class, in HIV behavioral studies and interventions (Amaro, 1995; Amaro & Raj, 2000).

Challenges in Intervention Implementation: Conflicting Messages from the Community and Funding Agencies

An accumulation of data underscores the need to address issues that contribute to engaging in risky behaviors, such as childhood sexual abuse (Wyatt et al., 2004). Several approaches for encouraging community-based agencies to utilize evidence-based HIV interventions that have been shown to be efficacious in reducing risk behavior. Whether referred to as dissemination, community-based partnership research, translational research or capacity building, there are standard processes of informing the community and service providers about HIV prevention interventions to reduce sexual risk and including them in the development of interventions (Kegeles, Rebchook, & Tebbetts, 2005; Kelly et al., 2000; Minkler, 2005; Rebchook et al., 2006).

Kerner, Rimer, & Emmons (2005 suggest that the National Institute of Health and other funding organizations, both governmental and non-governmental, expand their funding for dissemination research. That is, not only should projects that are assessing the process involve clinics and agencies as partners and research, they should also address the gaps in training and services provided as the intervention is implemented by their staff. The problem arises when funding dissemination research, publishing its results, and ultimately including these studies in systematic reviews of research evidence is a challenge across the board (Kerner et al., 2005). Essentially, agreements among peer reviewers about the relative advantages and disadvantages of different study designs for conducting, disseminating, and implementing research should be standardized among reviewers and funders.

Bridging the Gap: Collaborating with Community Based Organizations

The double risk of sexual trauma for HIV positive women with sexual abuse histories is of growing concern, given that most women, especially African Americans, do not disclose their abuse, receive the appropriate treatment and ancillary support and often are not included in HIV related programs that offer them an opportunity to discuss all of their sexual experiences. Indeed, sexuality includes those experiences that are engaged in willfully and those that are forced or involved coercion. Whether or not a person consents to a sexual act should not be criteria for excluding them from HIV prevention efforts. And yet, most evidenced based interventions do not specifically address some of the psycho-social issues that increase HIV risk among African American women who continue to engage in unprotected sex and drug related practices (Wyatt, 2009).

The multifaceted issues that are raised when sexual abuse among vulnerable populations occurs can increase the pressure and responsibility of communities to offer trauma-related services for African American women along with other ethnic groups. There is also a need to ensure that the focus includes gender and cultural factors that complicate trauma but yet are often overlooked in HIV prevention efforts (Wyatt, 1994b). The Sexual Health program at UCLA has been at the forefront of examining the breadth of sexual experiences of African American women and has developed an intervention for HIV positive African American women with sexual abuse histories (Wyatt et al., 2004). In order to move the intervention to the dissemination phase of HIV prevention, we conducted a needs assessment in Los Angeles County, with support from the UCLA AIDS Institute and in collaboration with the California State Office on AIDS in 2003. The one-day conference included 32 community based organizations (CBOs) who provided HIV-related services to women. In the discussion, the need for a program that focused on sexual abuse and trauma for HIV positive and at risk populations was highlighted.

Community-based stakeholders and case managers described the gaps in services that addressed the behavioral and psychological needs of HIV positive women when they had histories of sexual abuse, particularly, African American women, whose rates of AIDS continued to rise. Further, staff skills were limited to discussions about condom use and reduction of high risk behaviors without the inclusion of information that would help staff to discuss their sexual abuse experiences and to link them to later sexual and drug related practices. Indeed, the standard case management guidelines for Ryan White funded HIV clinics did not include mention of sexual abuse, how to identify sexual trauma or the similarities between cultural beliefs about women's roles as sexual partners and gender and religious socialization that endorsed unprotected sex and deference's to partners regarding the use of contraceptives including condoms (Amaro et al., 2007; Center for Disease Control and Prevention, 1997; Zlotnick, Mattia, & Zimmerman, 2001). Current efforts by the Center for Disease Control to disseminate evidence based interventions to CBOs and health facilities need to consider the following issues when considering the addition of services that include sexual abuse and trauma-related approaches:

1. The motivation of organizations to receive new training to address the aftermath of sexual abuse and trauma and increased HIV related risk taking practices.
2. The readiness of organizations to receive new training should include an assessment of
   (a) The number and clinical background of staff available to be trained.
   (b) The number and expertise of supervisors to meet weekly with group facilitators of an intervention.
3. Staff availability to call women regularly to monitor their well-being.
4. The willingness of the agency director and or administrative staff of the agency to receive an orientation about secondary interventions that focus on psychological outcomes of HIV positive women.
5. The willingness of staff to maintain ongoing collaborations with those who train the trainers to conduct monthly evaluations of the services offered to women in order to maximize the benefits of new programs that are offered.
6. The interest in and commitment to cultural and gender competence training for staff and The Community Advisory Board can help to ensure that any programs for African American women with sexual abuse will continue to address the cultural context of women's lives.

Summary

The purpose of this chapter was to provide an overview of the data on the impact of childhood sexual abuse and how it contributes to increased risk for acquiring HIV/AIDS. It is clear that significant variability exists in the psychobiological trajectory among victims, yet future studies should examine the factors that moderate and mediate such differences. This will provide a fuller understanding of the secondary problems associated with the abuse. Although not covered in this chapter, additional factors known to influence the psychosocial sequelae should be incorporated into the study of early sexual abuse and HIV risk (e.g., relationship of the perpetrator to victim, abuse severity, disclosure of abuse, and duration). Additionally, the next steps in trauma and HIV research is to develop realistic expectations about how to best support efforts to integrate trauma-related services into standard care for HIV infected women. An integrative biopsychosocial model of childhood sexual abuse that incorporates cultural and gender-related factors is needed. As such, these components should be integrated into HIV prevention and intervention programs, especially those that target ethnic minorities.

Acknowledgments Preparation of this chapter was supported by the National Institute of Mental Health (H059496-0451 and MH073453-01A1), the UCLA AIDS Institute (A128697), National Institute on Drug Abuse, (DA 01070-31), and National Institute on Drug Abuse (DA 01070-34). The first author was supported by a UCLA Psychobiology Fellowship (NIMH grant T32 MH17140) and The Pittsburgh Mind-Body Center (PMBC; NIH grant HL076852/076858). The authors acknowledge Micha Dalton and Tanishia Wright for their assistance in the preparation of this manuscript.

References

Amaro, H. (1995). Love, sex, and power: considering women's realities in HIV prevention. *The American Psychologist, 50*(6), 437–447.

Amaro, H., Jianyu, D., Arevalo, S., Acevedo, A., Matsumoto, A., Nieves, R., et al. (2007). Effects of integrated trauma treatment on outcomes in a racially/ethnically diverse sample of women in urban community-based substance abuse treatment. *Journal of Urban Health: Bulletin of the New York Academy of Medicine, 84*(4), 508–522.

Amaro, H., & Raj, A. (2000). On the margin: power and women's HIV risk reduction strategies. *Sex Roles, 42*(7–8), 723–749.

Axelrod, J., Myers, H. F., Durvasula, R. S., Wyatt, G. E., & Cheng, M. (1999). The impact of relationship violence, HIV, and ethnicity on adjustment in women [Special issue: HIV/AIDS and ethnic minority women, families, and communities]. *Cultural Diversity and Ethnic Minority Psychology, 3*, 263–275.

Baker, S. A., Beadnell, B., Stoner, S., Morrison, D. M., Gordon, J., Collier, C., et al. (2003). Skills training versus health education to prevent STDs/HIV in heterosexual women: a randomized controlled trial utilizing biological outcomes. *AIDS Education and Prevention, 15*(1), 1–14.

Bensley, L. S., Eenwyk, J. V., & Simmons, K. W. (2000). Self-reported childhood sexual and physical abuse and adult HIV-risk behaviors and heavy drinking. *American Journal of Preventive Medicine, 18*(2), 151–158.

Blankertz, L., Cnann, R., & Freedman, E. (1993). Childhood Risk Factors in Dually Diagnosed Homeless Adults. *Social Work, 38*(5), 587–596.

Boudewyn, A. C., & Liem, J. H. (1995). Childhood sexual abuse as a precursor to depression and self-destructive behavior in adulthood. *Journal of Traumatic Stress, 8*(3), 445–459.

Briere, J. (2004). Integrating HIV/AIDS prevention activities into psychotherapy for child sexual abuse survivors. In L. J. Koenig & L. S. Doll (Eds.), *From child sexual abuse to adult sexual risk: Trauma, revictimization, and intervention* (pp. 219–232). Washington, DC: American Psychological Association.

Briere, J., & Elliott, D. M. (1993). Sexual abuse, family environment, and psychological symptoms: On the validity of statistical control. *Journal of Consulting and Clinical Psychology, 61*(2), 284–288.

Briere, J., Runtz, M. (1988). Post sexual abuse trauma. In G. E. Wyatt, & G. J. Powell (Eds.), *Lasting effects of child sexual abuse (Sage focus editions)*, Vol. 100 (pp. 85-99). Thousand Oaks: Sage.

Cargill, V. A., Stone, V. E., & Robinson, M. R. (2004). HIV treatment in African Americans: Challenges and opportunities. *Journal of Black Psychology, 30*(1), 24–39.

Carrion, V. G., Weems, C. F., Garret, A., Mennon, V., & Reiss, A. L. (2007). Posttraumatic stress symptoms and brain function during a response-inhibition task: an fMRI study in youth. *Depression and Anxiety, 25*(6), 514–526.

Center for Disease Control and Prevention. (1997). *HIV prevention case management – guidance.* http://www.cdc.gov/hiv/pubs/pcmg/pcmg-doc.htm. Retrieved 26.06.2006.

Center for Disease Control and Prevention. (2005). HIV prevalence, unrecognized infection, and HIV testing among men who have sex with men – five U.S. cities, June 2004–April 2005. *MMWR. Morbidity and Mortality Weekly Report, 54*(24), 597–601.

Centers for Disease Control and Prevention. (2007). *HIV surveillance report: AIDS cases by race and ethnicity.* http://www.cdc.gov/hiv/stats.htm.

Chin, D., & Kroesen, K. W. (1999). Disclosure of HIV infection among Asian/Pacific Islander American women: cultural stigma and support [Special issue: HIV/AIDS and ethnic minority women, families, and communities]. *Cultural Diversity and Ethnic Minority Psychology, 5*(3), 222–235.

Chin, D., Wyatt, G. E., Carmona, J. V., Loeb, T. B., & Myers, H. F. (2004). Child sexual abuse and HIV: An integrative risk-reduction approach. In L. J. Koenig & L. S. Doll (Eds.), *From child sexual abuse to adult sexual risk: Trauma, revictimization, and intervention* (pp. 233–250). Washington, DC: American Psychological Association.

Cloitre, M., Scarvalone, P., & Difede, J. (1997). Posttraumatic stress disorder, self- and interpersonal dysfunction among sexually retraumatized women. *Journal of Traumatic Stress, 10*(3), 437–452.

Coe, C. L., & Laudenslager, M. L. (2007). Psychosocial influence on immunity, effects on immune maturation and senescence. *Brain Behavaviour and Immunity, 21*(8), 1000–1008.

Cohen, M., Deamant, C., Barkan, S., Richardson, J., Young, M., Holman, S., et al. (2000). Domestic violence and childhood sexual abuse in HIV-infected women and women at risk for HIV. *American Journal of Public Health, 90*(4), 560–565.

Crosby, R. A., Wingood, G. M., DiClemente, R. J., & Rose, E. S. (2002). Family-related correlates of sexually transmitted disease and barriers to care: a pilot study of pregnant African American adolescents. *Family and Community Health, 25*(2), 16–27.

Downs, W. R. (1993). Developmental considerations for the effects of childhood sexual abuse [Special issue: Research on treatment of adults sexually abused in childhood]. *Journal of Interpersonal Violence, 8*(3), 331–345.

Draucker, C. B. (1997). Early family life and victimization in the lives of women. *Research in Nursing &amp. Health, 20*(5), 399–412.

Fleming, D., & Wasserheit, J. (1999). From epidemiology synergy to public health policy and practice: the contribution of other sexually transmitted diseases to sexual transmission of HIV infection. *Sexually Transmitted Infections, 75*(1), 3–17.

Freshwater, K., Leach, C., & Aldridge, J. (2001). Personal constructs, childhood sexual abuse, and revictimization. *The British Journal of Medical Psychology, 74*, 379–397.

Friedman, M. J., Charney, D. S., & Deutch, A. Y. (1995). *Neurobiological and clinical consequences of stress: from normal adaptation to post-traumatic stress disorder* (p. 551). Philadelphia: Lippincott Williams & Wilkins.

Gibson, R. L., & Hartshorne, T. S. (1996). Childhood sexual abuse and adult loneliness and network orientation. *Child Abuse and Neglect, 20*(11), 1087–1093.

Gorcey, M., Santiago, J. M., & McCall-Perez, F. (1986). Psychological consequences for women sexually abused in childhood. *Social Psychiatry, 21*(3), 129–133.

Harlow, L. L., Rose, J. S., Morokoff, P. J., Quina, K., Mayer, K., Mitchell, K., et al. (1998). Women HIV sexual risk takers: related behaviors, issues and attitudes. *Women's Health: Research on Gender, Behavior, and Policy, 4,* 407–439.

Hays, R. B., McKusick, L., Pollack, L., Hilliard, R., Hoff, C., & Coates, T. J. (1993). Disclosing HIV seropositivity to significant others. *AIDS, 7*(3), 425–431.

Heim, C., Newport, D. J., Heit, S., Graham, Y. P., Wilcox, M., Bonsall, R., et al. (2000). Pituitary-adrenal and autonomic responses to stress in women after sexual and physical abuse in child-hood. *JAMA: Journal of the American Medical Association, 284*(18), 2321–2322.

Heise, L., Moore, K., & Toubia, N. (1995). *Sexual coercion and reproductive health: A focus on research.* New York: Ebert Program in Reproductive Health of the Population Council and the Health and Development Policy Project.

Johnsen, L. W., & Harlow, L. L. (1996). Childhood sexual abuse linked with adult substance use, victimization, and AIDS risk. *AIDS Education and Prevention, 8*(1), 44–57.

Kegeles, S. M., Rebchook, G. M., & Tebbetts, S. (2005). Challenges and facilitators to building program evaluation capacity among community-based organizations. *AIDS Education and Prevention, 17*(4), 284–299.

Kelly, B., Raphael, B., Burrows, G., Judd, F., Kernutt, G., Burnett, P., et al. (2000). Measuring psychological adjustment to HIV infection. *International Journal of Psychiatry in Medicine, 30*(1), 41–59.

Kerner, J., Rimer, B., & Emmons, K. (2005). Dissemination research and research dissemination: How can we close the gap? *Health Psychology, 24*(5), 443–446.

Kiecolt-Glaser, J. K., & Glaser, R. (1992). Stress and the immune system: Human studies. *American Psychiatric Press Review of Psychiatry, 11,* 169–180.

Koopman, C., Gore-Felton, C., Classen, C., Kim, P., & Spiegel, D. (2001). Acute stress reactions to everyday stressful life events among sexual abuse survivors with PTSD. *Journal of Child Sexual Abuse, 10*(2), 83–99.

Kopnisky, K. L., Stoff, D. M., & Rausch, D. M. (2004). Workshop report: the effects of psychological variables on the progression of HIV-1 disease. *Brain, Behavior, and Immunity, 18*(3), 246–261.

Kumar, M., Kumar, A. M., Walididrop, D., Antoni, M. H., & Eisdorfer, C. (2003). HIV-1 infection and its impact on the HPA axis, cytokins, and cognition. *Stress, 6*(3), 167–172.

Laumann, E. O., Paik, A., & Rosen, R. C. (1999). Sexual dysfunction in the United States: Prevalence and predictors. *JAMA: Journal of the American Medical Association, 281*(6), 537–544.

Loeb, T., Williams, J. K., Carmona, J. V., Rivkin, I. D., Wyatt, G., Chin, D., et al. (2002a). Child sexual abuse associations with the sexual functioning of adolescents and adults. *Annual Review of Sex Research, 13,* 307–345.

McCauley, J., Kern, D. E., Kolodner, K., Derogatis, L. R., & Bass, E. B. (1998). Relation of low-severity violence to women's health. *Journal of General Internal Medicine, 13*(10), 687–691.

Minkler, M. (2005). Community-based research partnerships: Challenges and opportunities. *Journal of Urban Health: Bulletin of the New York Academy of Medicine, 82*(Suppl. 2), ii3–ii12.

Molnar, B. E., Buka, S. L., & Kessler, R. C. (2001). Child sexual abuse and subsequent psycho-pathology: results from the National Comorbidity Survey. *American Journal of Public Health, 91*(5), 753–760.

Mullen, P. E., Martin, J. L., Anderson, J. C., Romans, S. E., & Herbison, G. P. (1994). The effect of child sexual abuse on social, interpersonal and sexual function in adult life. *The British Journal of Psychiatry, 165*(1), 35–47.

Myers, H. F., Sumner, L. A., Ullman, B. J., Loeb, T. B., Carmona, J. V., & Wyatt, G. E. (2009). Trauma and psychosocial predictors of substance abuse in women impacted by HIV/AIDS. *The Journal of Behavioral Health Services and Research, 36*(2), 233–246.

Polusny, M. A., & Follette, V. M. (1995). Long-term correlates of child sexual abuse: theory and review of the empirical literature. *Applied and Preventive Psychology, 4*(3), 143–166.

Rasmusson, A. M., Vythilingam, M., & Morgan, C. A, III (2003). The neuroendocrinology of posttraumatic stress disorder: new directions. *CNS Spectr, 8*(9), 651-656, 665-657.

Rebchook, G. M., Kegels, S. M., Huebner, D., & the TRIP Team. (2006). Transplanting research into practice: The dissemination and initial implementation of an evidence-based HIV prevention program. *AIDS Education and Prevention, 18*(Suppl. A), 119–136.

Schiffer, F., Teicher, M. H., Anderson, C., Tomoda, A., Polcari, A., Navalta, C. P., et al. (2007). Determination of hemispheric emotional valence in individual subjects: a new approach with research and therapeutic implications. *Behavioral and brain functions: BBF, 3*, 13.

Simoni, J. M., Mason, H. R. C., Marks, G., & Ruiz, M. S. (1995a). Women's self-disclosure of HIV infection: Rates, reasons, and reactions. *Journal of Consulting and Clinical Psychology, 63*(3), 474–478.

Simoni, J. M., Mason, H. R. C., Marks, G., & Ruiz, M. S. (1995b). Women living with HIV: Sexual behaviors and counseling experiences. *Women and Health, 23*(4), 17–26.

Simpson, T. L. (2002). Women's treatment utilization and its relationship to childhood sexual abuse history and lifetime PTSD. *Substance Abuse, 23*(1), 17–30.

Smith, G. (1992). The unbearable traumatogenic past: child sexual abuse. In V. P. Varma (Ed.), *The secret life of vulnerable children* (pp. 130–156). Florence: Taylor & Frances.

Smith, D. W., Letourneau, E. J., Saunders, B. E., Kilpatrick, D. G., Resnick, H. S., & Best, C. L. (2000). Delay in disclosure of childhood rape: results from a national survey. *Child Abuse and Neglect, 24*(2), 273–287.

Stein, M. B., Koverola, C., Hanna, C., Torchia, M. G., & McClarty, B. (1997). Hippocampal volume in women victimized by childhood sexual abuse. *Psychological Medicine, 27*(4), 951–959.

Thompson, N. J., Potter, J. S., Sanderson, C. A., & Maibach, E. W. (1997). The relationship of sexual abuse and HIV risk behaviors among heterosexual adult female STD patients. *Child Abuse and Neglect, 21*(2), 149–156.

Urquiza, A. J., & Goodlin-Jones, B. L. (1994). Child sexual abuse and adult revictimization with women of color [Special issue: Violence against women of color]. *Violence and Victims, 9*(3), 223–232.

Vogeltanz, N. D., Wilsnack, S. C., Harris, T. R., Wilsnack, R. W., Wonderlich, S. A., & Kristjanson, A. F. (1999). Prevalence and risk factors for childhood sexual abuse in women: national survey findings. *Child Abuse and Neglect, 23*(6), 579–592.

West, C. M., Williams, L. M., & Siegel, J. A. (2000). Adult sexual victimization among Black women sexually abused in childhood: a prospective examination of serious consequences of abuse [Special focus section: Repeat victimization]. *Child Maltreatment: Journal of the American Professional Society on the Abuse of Children, 5*(1), 49–57.

Wingood, G. M., & DiClemente, R. (1997a). Child sexual abuse, HIV sexual risk, and gender relations of African-American women. *American Journal of Preventive Medicine, 13*(5), 380–384.

Wingood, G., & DiClemente, R. (1997b). The effects of an abusive primary partner on the condom use and sexual negotiation practices of African-American women. *American Journal of Public Health, 87*(6), 1016–1018.

World Health Organization. (2002). *World report on violence and health.* http://www.who.int/violence_injury_prevention/violence/world_report/

Wyatt, G. E. (1985). The sexual abuse of Afro-American and White-American women in childhood. *Child Abuse and Neglect, 9*(4), 507–519.

Wyatt, G. E. (1992). The sociocultural context of African American and White American women's rape. *Journal of Social Issues, 48*(1), 77–91.

Wyatt, G. E. (1994a). *The sociocultural relevance of sex research: challenges for the 1990s and beyond.* Paper presented at the 101st Annual Convention of the American Psychological Association, Toronto, Canada.

Wyatt, G. E. (1994b). The sociocultural relevance of sex research: Challenges for the 1990s and beyond. *The American Psychologist, 49*(8), 748–754.

Wyatt, G. E. (1997). *Stolen women: reclaiming our sexuality, taking back our lives.* New York: Wiley.

Wyatt, G. E. (2009). Enhancing cultural and contextual intervention strategies to reduce HIV/AIDS among African Americans. *American Journal of Public Health, 99*(11), 1941–1945.

Wyatt, G. E., & Riederle, M. (1994a). Sexual harassment and prior sexual trauma among African-American and White American women [Special issue: Violence against women of color]. *Violence and Victims, 9*(3), 233–247.

Wyatt, G. E., & Riederle, M. H. (1994b). Reconceptualizing issues that affect women's sexual decision-making and sexual functioning [Special issue: Transformations: reconceptualizing theory and research with women]. *Psychology of Women Quarterly, 18*(4), 611–625.

Wyatt, G. E., Axelrod, J., Chin, D., Carmona, J. V., & Loeb, T. B. (2000). *Examining Patterns of Vulnerability to Domestic Violence Among African American Women*. Paper presented at the African American Institute on Domestic Violence in the Community, St Paul, MN, US.

Wyatt, G. E., Carmona, J. V., Loeb, T. B., Ayala, A., & Chin, D. (2002). Sexual abuse. In G. M. Wingood & R. J. DiClemente (Eds.), *Handbook of women's sexual and reproductive health. Issues in women health* (pp. 195–216). New York: Kluwer Academic.

Wyatt, G. E., Carmona, J. V., Loeb, T. B., & Williams, J. K. (2005). HIV-positive black women with histories of childhood sexual abuse: patterns of substance use and barriers to health care. *Journal of Health Care for the Poor and Underserved, 16*(4 Suppl. B), 9–23.

Wyatt, G. E., Guthrie, D., & Notgrass, C. M. (1992). Differential effects of women's child sexual abuse and subsequent sexual revictimization. *Journal of Consulting and Clinical Psychology, 60*(2), 167–173.

Wyatt, G. E., Longshore, D., Chin, D., Carmona, J. V., Loeb, T. B., Myers, H. F., et al. (2004). The efficacy of an integrated risk reduction intervention for HIV-positive women with child sexual abuse histories. *AIDS and Behavior, 8*(4), 453–462.

Wyatt, G. E., Myers, H. F., Williams, J. K., Kitchen, C. R., Loeb, T., Carmona, J. V., et al. (2002). Does a history of trauma contribute to HIV risk for women of color? Implications for prevention and policy. *American Journal of Public Health, 92*(4), 660–665.

Wyatt, G. E., Newcomb, M. D., & Riederle, M. H. (1993). *Sexual abuse and consensual sex: women's developmental patterns and outcomes*. Thousand Oaks: Sage.

Wyatt, G., Notgrass, C. M., & Gordon, G. (1995). The effects of African American women's sexual revictimization: Strategies for prevention. In C. Swift (Ed.), *Sexual assault and abuse: sociocultural context of prevention* (pp. 111–134). New York: Haworth.

Wyatt, G., Tucker, B., Romero, G. J., Vargas-Carmona, J., Newcomb, M. D., Wayment, H. A., et al. (1997). Adapting a comprehensive approach to African-American women's sexual risk taking. *Journal of Health Education, 28*(Suppl. 6), S52–S60.

Zlotnick, C., Mattia, J., & Zimmerman, M. (2001). Clinical features of survivors of sexual abuse with major depression. *Child Abuse and Neglect, 25*(3), 357–367.

Part III
Interventions

Chapter 9
A Systematic Review of Evidence-Based Behavioral Interventions for African American Youth at Risk for HIV/STI Infection, 1988–2007

Khiya Marshall, Nicole Crepaz, and Ann O'Leary

In the United States, African American youth are disproportionally affected by human immunodeficiency virus (HIV) and sexually transmitted infections (STIs). An estimated 1.2 million people are living with HIV/AIDS (Glynn & Rhodes, 2005). Data from 33 states in the United States with confidential name-based reporting show that in 2006 African Americans of all ages represented 49% of HIV/AIDS diagnosis, although African Americans accounted for only 13% of the U.S. population (Centers for Disease Control and Prevention (CDC), 2008b). During this same period, although adolescents aged 13–19 represented 16% of the U.S. population, African American youth accounted for 69% of reported AIDS cases. The primary mode of transmission of HIV/AIDS among African American adolescents aged 13–19 is male-to-male sexual contact for males (60%) and high-risk heterosexual contact for females (59%; CDC, 2008c). Also, in 2006, a larger proportion of STIs (e.g., gonorrhea, Chlamydia, and syphilis) were transmitted among African Americans than among other racial/ethnic groups (CDC, 2008b).

Given the high rates of sexually transmitted HIV infections and other STIs among African American youth, it is important to better understand sex behaviors within this group. African American adolescents report a higher rate of sex behaviors than other racial/ethnic groups. Data from the 2007 Youth Risk Behavior Survey (YRBS) indicated that almost half (47.8%) of U.S. students, grades 9–12th had previously engaged in sexual intercourse (CDC, 2008d). African Americans had the highest prevalence rate of students who had previously had sexual intercourse (66.5% compared to 43.7% of white and 52.0% of Hispanic students), had sex with ≥4 persons (27.6% compared to 11.5% of white and 17.3% of Hispanic students), had sex before the age of 13 (16.3% compared to 4.4% of white and 8.2% of Hispanic students), or were sexually active within the past 3 months (46.0% compared to 32.9% of white and 37.4% of Hispanic students; CDC, 2008d).

K. Marshall (✉)
Division of HIV/AIDS Prevention, Centers for Disease Control and Prevention,
Atlanta, GA 30333, USA
e-mail: kmarshall@cdc.gov

D.H. McCree et al. (eds.), *African Americans and HIV/AIDS*,
DOI 10.1007/978-0-387-78321-5_9,

Although the prevalence rate of sex behaviors was higher for African American adolescents, they were more likely to have used a condom during last sexual intercourse (67.3% compared to 59.7% of white and 61.4% of Hispanic students) and to have ever been tested for HIV (22.4% compared to 10.7% of white and 12.7% of Hispanic students; CDC, 2008d). Among all adolescents, trends from 1991 to 2007 showed a decrease in the number who had previously engaged in sexual intercourse, had ≥4 sex partners, or were currently sexually active (CDC, 2008d). Trends among African American adolescents showed a decrease in the number that had ≥4 sex partners (from 1991 to 2007), but there was no change in the number that had ever had sex (from 2001 to 2007) or used a condom during last sexual intercourse (from 1999 to 2007; CDC, 2008d).

Additionally, sex behaviors differ by gender. The YRBS showed that African American male adolescents were more likely than African American female adolescents to have ever had sexual intercourse (72.6 vs. 60.9%), had sex with ≥4 persons (37.6 vs. 18.1%), had sex before the age of 13 (26.2 vs. 6.9%), to be sexually active within the past 3 months (48.7 vs. 43.5%) or used condoms during last sex (74.0 vs. 60.1%). However, females were more likely than males to have ever been tested for HIV (27.2 vs. 17.3%; CDC, 2008d).

The levels of HIV and STI risk associated with sex behaviors are reflected in African American youth's knowledge and attitudes toward HIV and STIs. More African Americans than any other racial/ethnic group considered sexual health issues such as HIV, STIs, and pregnancy as personally important in a national survey of adolescents and young adults (Hoff, Greene, & Davis, 2003). African Americans were more knowledgeable about STI and HIV/AIDS information; but, of particular concern, African American youth were more likely to believe that STIs can only be spread when symptoms are present. Additionally, they were more likely to have been tested for HIV or other STIs, to have been asked to be tested, and to be "very likely" or "somewhat likely" to get tested for HIV in the next year compared to other racial/ethnic groups. They reported having an STI more than other racial/ethnic groups, possibly because they were more likely to have been tested and to know their HIV status (Hoff et al., 2003).

Taken as a whole, comparing to other racial/ethnic groups, African American youth are, in general, more sexually active and experienced, generally more knowledgeable of basic sexual health, and more likely to be tested for HIV and STIs. It is important to better understand potential protective and risk factors associated with risky sex behaviors that put them at risk for HIV and STI infection.

Adolescent Risk and Protective Factors

Multiple protective and risk factors influence adolescent sex behavior, including individual, interpersonal, environmental, societal, and cultural. It would be informative to have a better understanding of these factors and their associations with HIV and STI risk behaviors. A better understanding would allow for the development of interventions that are likely to achieve successful changes in behavior among African American youth.

Individual Factors

Evidence suggests that African American youth who have high self-esteem (Belgrave, Van Oss Marin, & Chambers, 2000; Salazartet et al., 2005; Wills et al., 2007) and self-control (Wills et al., 2007), and who are afraid of acquiring an STI (Brown & Waite, 2005), are less likely to engage in HIV/STI risk behaviors. On the other hand, older youth (Black et al., 1997), youth with negative body image (Wingood, DiClemente, Harrington, & Davies, 2002), and youth using substances (Bachanas etal., 2002; Cooper & Guthrie, 2007) are susceptible to sex risk behaviors.

Interpersonal and Environmental Factors

Family, peers, religion, and the school environment play important roles in African American youth's risk of HIV and STI infections. Protective interpersonal factors include parental supervision and monitoring (Black et al., 1997; Mandara, Murray, & Bangi, 2003), family interactions and support (Black et al., 1997; Cooper & Guthrie, 2007; Crosby et al., 2001; Perrino, Gonzalez-Soldevilla, Pantin, & Szapocznik, 2000), parental connectedness (Perrino et al., 2000), positive peer behaviors (Black et al., 1997; Cooper & Guthrie, 2007), religiosity (McCree, Wingood, DiClemente, Davies, & Harrington, 2003), spiritual interconnectedness (Holder et al., 2000), involvement in black organizations (Crosby et al., 2002a, b), and ethnic pride and identity (Belgrave et al., 2000; Salazar et al., 2005; Wills et al., 2007). Living in a two-parent household (Cooper & Guthrie, 2007; Felton & Bartoces, 2002) has also been shown to be a protective factor. One study conducted with rural African American youth and their parents found that after-school activities and parental monitoring are perceived HIV-related resiliency factors mentioned by both adolescents and their parents (Brown & Waite, 2005). Other protective factors stated exclusively by adolescents included wanting to be a role model, having friends who are not sexually active, not wanting to lose self-image or become ashamed, family, attending church, and having pastor's encouragement (Brown & Waite, 2005).

Several environmental factors are also found to be associated with youth's risk for HIV/STI. Perceptions and feelings regarding neighborhood toughness (Cooper & Guthrie, 2007) and living in rural areas (Milhausen et al., 2003) are associated with engaging in risky sexual behaviors. On the other hand, availability of condoms in schools has been shown to increase the use of condoms during last sex and condom use for pregnancy prevention (Blake et al., 2003).

Societal and Cultural Factors

Societal factors that may affect African American youth's risk for contracting HIV and STIs include poverty, social capital, and mass media messages. Poverty is an important risk factor in adolescents' sex-risk behavior (Aral, 2001; Sionéan et al., 2001). In 2006, more African Americans were living in poverty – more specifically, 24.3% of African Americans were living below poverty and had the lowest median income compared to other racial/ethnic groups (DeNavas-Walt, Proctor, & Smith, 2007). Communities with high rates of poverty have been shown to be at increased risk for STIs. Research has shown that African American adolescent females who have a low socioeconomic status (i.e., lived in a single-parent household and had parental unemployment) were more likely to self-report a history of gonorrhea than African American females who lived in two-parent households and whose parents were employed (Sionéan et al., 2001).

On the other hand, *social capital* may play a more important role in protective and risk behavior than income and poverty (Crosby, Holtgrave, DiClemente, Wingood, & Gayle, 2003). Social capital is recognized as "a population-level attribute that measures social relations and connections among people and social organization of communities," (Bourdieu, 1985; Putnam, 2002). Emerging evidence shows that risky sexual behavior among adolescents (Crosby et al., 2003), teenage pregnancy (Crosby & Holtgrave, 2006), and rates of AIDS cases (Holtgrave & Crosby, 2003) are inversely correlated with social capital measured by Putnam's 14-item Social Capital Index (2000, 2001). Among African American adolescent females, being members of social organizations has been shown to be a protective factor for engaging in risky sexual behaviors (Crosby et al., 2002a, b).

Societal factors also include mass media and the impact it has on adolescents' risk and protective factors. Media influences, including TV, magazines, and music have been linked to both sexual intentions and behaviors (L'Engle, Brown, & Kenneavy, 2006), and they play a significant role in adolescent development. For African American adolescents, of whom 81% listen to hip-hop music (Hoff, Greene, & Davis, 2003), the hip-hop culture (including fashion, music, television, and movies) strongly influences how they dress, what they listen to, and how they behave.

In general, adolescents listen to music approximately 1.5–2.5 h a day (Martino et al., 2006; Roberts, Foehr, & Rideout, 2005). There is a direct correlation between the length of time adolescents watch hip-hop music videos and listen to hip-hop music and their views toward sex and gender roles (Ward, Hansbrough, & Walker, 2005). A recent study (Martino et al., 2006) examined adolescent's sexual behavior and exposure to degrading and non-degrading music lyrics over time and across a range of musical genres (hard rock, alternative rock, rap-rock, rap, rap-metal R&B, country, and teen pop). Overall, rap music included the highest percentage of songs with degrading sexual content. Adolescent boys and girls were similarly affected by degrading lyrics. A more important finding is that listening to more degrading lyrics was related to earlier initiation of sexual intercourse and non-coital sexual activity, regardless of race or gender (Martino et al., 2006).

Additional evidence from Wingood et al. (2003) showed a significant connection between exposure to rap music videos and sexual health among adolescent African American females. Female youth who had more exposure to rap music were more likely to have multiple sex partners, acquire an STI, get arrested, and use drugs and alcohol 12 months after being exposed to rap music videos. A similar study showed that African American adolescent females who perceived more portrayals of sexual stereotypes (African American women touched or fondled, treated disrespectfully, controlled, or portrayed as sex objects by African American men) in rap music videos were more likely to report multiple sex partners, a negative body image, binge drinking, and to test positive for marijuana (Peterson, Wingood, DiClemente, Harrington, & Davies, 2007). Although the direction of causality between listening to rap music and engaging in HIV risk behavior cannot be determined based on those data (Wingood et al., 2003), the results suggest the potential importance of developing interventions that address a sense of ethnic and gender pride with an attempt to counter balance the negative and damaging images that are portrayed in some of today's hip-hop music, especially music videos.

HIV/STI Prevention Interventions

Identifying, packaging, and disseminating culturally sensitive evidence-based behavioral interventions (EBIs) for African American youth are important strategies for HIV and STI prevention. EBIs are interventions that have been tested using a methodologically rigorous design and have demonstrated evidence of efficacy in reducing HIV incidence or HIV risk indirectly by reducing STI incidence or sex- or injection drug-related risk behaviors (Lyles, Crepaz, Herbst, & Kay, 2006). Increased use of such interventions can expand the overall success of HIV prevention efforts in the affected communities (Collins, Harshbarger, Sawyer, & Hamdallah, 2006).

The evidence-based prevention approach is made using relevant and rigorous scientific evidence, most appropriately identified through a systematic research synthesis process as a basis for prevention efforts in the field. The CDC, 2007b initiated the HIV/AIDS Prevention Research Synthesis (PRS) project in 1996 (Lyles et al., 2006; Sogolow, Peersman, Semaan, Strouse, & Lyles, 2002) to translate scientific evidence from the research literature into practical information that can be used by prevention providers and state and local health departments throughout the United States. The PRS project has been conducting systematic reviews to identify EBIs for various at-risk populations. Below, we describe the method used to identify evidence-based interventions, summarize the best evidence and promising evidence individual-level and group-level behavioral interventions that target African American adolescents, and address the research gaps for interventions with this population at risk for HIV/STI infection. Best evidence-based interventions have been comprehensively evaluated and they demonstrate the "strongest evidence of efficacy." Promising evidence-based interventions have not met the same standards as best evidence-based interventions, but they are sound and have "sufficient evidence of efficacy" (CDC, 2008a).

Methods

Search Strategy

Multiple search strategies were conducted to build a cumulative PRS database. The systematic search strategy includes automated and manual search components. The automated search is conducted annually in four electronic databases (EMBASE, MEDLINE, PsycINFO, and SocioFile, including AIDSLINE before December 2000). Manual searches of 35 key journals have been conducted biannually to identify articles that have not yet been indexed. More information about the PRS systematic search strategy can be found elsewhere (Deluca et al., 2008).

Eligibility of Citations

Interventions were considered to be eligible for this review if they met all of the following criteria:

- Were conducted in the United States.
- Prevention focus was on HIV/AIDS/STI.
- Had controlled trials (i.e., with a comparison group).
- They targeted youth regardless of school status (currently attending or not attending school).
- They targeted African Americans or included a population that was at least 50% African American per study arm.
- Studies had an outcome evaluation.
- Were delivered to individuals or small groups of youth.
- Included behavioral outcome data (abstinence, condom use, number of sexual partners, refusal to have unsafe sex) or biologic outcome (incident STI).

Qualitative Data Coding

After the relevant reports were identified, the process of identifying the linking reports in a single study was conducted. Then, all citations, including linked citations, were coded on the basis of efficacy criteria (described below) and all discrepancies were reconciled. All the procedures were carried out by pairs of trained content analysts.

Efficacy Criteria for Best and Promising Evidence-Based Interventions

Each eligible intervention evaluation study was evaluated based on the execution of the study, the quality of design, implementation and analysis, and the strength of the evidence. "Best-evidence" interventions are required to meet all the following criteria: significant and positive intervention effects on relevant outcomes, no significant and negative intervention effects on relevant outcomes measured in the study, a comparison group, unbiased assignment, ≥3 months follow-up in both groups, ≥70% retention in both groups, analyses adjusted for baseline differences in outcome measures (if non-RCT), at least 50 participants in the analytic sample in each group, and no evidence that any additional limitation was a fatal flaw. "Promising-evidence" interventions are required to meet the following criteria: significant and positive intervention effects on relevant outcomes, no significant and negative intervention effects on relevant outcomes measured in the study, a comparison group, unbiased or moderately biased assignment, ≥1 month follow-up in both groups, ≥60% retention in both groups, analyses adjusted for baseline differences in outcome measures (if non-RCT), at least 40 participants in the analytic sample in each group, and no evidence that any additional limitation was a fatal flaw (CDC, 2008a). A more thorough description of the criteria can be found elsewhere (CDC, 2008a; Lyles et al., 2006).

Results

The systematic review of the HIV behavioral intervention literature published between 1988 and 2007 yielded 11 evidence-based interventions for high-risk African American youth.[1] The seven best EBIs include: *Be Proud! Be Responsible!* (Jemmott, Jemmott, & Fong, 1992), *Becoming a Responsible Teen (BART*; St. Lawrence et al., 1995), *Making Proud Choices* (Jemmott, Jemmott, & Fong, 1998), *Focus on Kids plus Informed Parents and Children Together (FOK+ ImPACT[2]*; Wu et al., 2003), *Sistering, Informing, Healing, Living, and Empowering*

---

[1] The scope of this chapter is broader than CDC's Compendium Update (CDC, 2008a). In this book chapter, we also evaluated interventions for youth in schools as well as interventions delivered in school settings. As a result, we identified two evidence-based interventions, *Making Proud Choices* and *Project AIM* that are not part of the Updated Compendium as of September 2008.

[2] *Focus on Kids (FOK)* and *Focus on Kids plus Informed Parents and Children Together (FOK+ ImPACT)* were used by the authors in the original publications. The names on the intervention packages available on the Diffusion of Effective Behavioral Interventions (DEBI, n.d.) website were changed to *Focus on Youth (FOY)* and *Focus on Youth plus Informed Parents and Children Together (FOY + ImPACT)*.

(SiHLE; DiClemente et al., 2004), *Project AIM (Adult Identity Mentoring*; Clark et al., 2005), and *Sisters Saving Sisters* (Jemmott, Jemmott, Braverman, & Fong, 2005). The four promising EBIs include: *Intensive AIDS Education* (Magura, Kang, & Shapiro, 1994), *Focus on Kids (FOK*; Stanton et al., 1996), *Street Smart* (Rotheram-Borus et al., 2003), and *Responsible, Empowered, Aware, Living (REAL) Men* (Dilorio, McCarty, Resnicow, Lehr, & Denzmore, 2007).

Concerning study design for these 11 interventions, nine were randomized controlled trials (Clark et al., 2005; DiClemente et al., 2004; Dilorio et al., 2007; Jemmott et al., 1992, 1998; Jemmott et al., 2005; Stanton et al., 1996; St. Lawrence et al., 1995; Wu et al., 2003) and two were non-randomized controlled trials (Magura et al., 1994; Rotheram-Borus et al., 2003). The population and intervention characteristics are presented in Tables 9.1 and 9.2.

Population Characteristics

The interventions all included an HIV/AIDS prevention focus. However, in addition to HIV/AIDS prevention, four programs focused on STI prevention (Clark et al., 2005; DiClemente et al., 2004; Dilorio et al., 2007; Jemmott et al., 2005), one also focused on pregnancy prevention (DiClemente et al., 2004), and one had an additional focus on sexual education and sexual health promotion (Clark et al., 2005).

Of the 11 interventions, eight targeted African American adolescents (Clark et al., 2005; DiClemente et al., 2004; Jemmott et al., 1992, 1998, 2005;

Stanton et al., 1996; St. Lawrence et al., 1995; Wu et al., 2003) while one intervention targeted male adolescents and their fathers (or father figures), but the study participants were predominately African American (Dilorio et al, 2007), one intervention specifically targeted incarcerated male adolescent drug users (Magura et al., 1994) and one targeted runaway adolescents (Rotheram-Borus et al., 2003). Two of 11 interventions involved the adolescent's parent or guardian (Dilorio et al., 2007; Wu et al., 2003). Among the 11 interventions, three focused exclusively on males (Dilorio et al., 2007; Jemmott et al., 1992; Magura et al., 1994) and two included only females (DiClemente et al., 2004; Jemmott et al., 2005). The sample size of all studies ranged from 157 to 817 participants; while the mean age of all participants was 14.5 years old (range 9–19).

Intervention Characteristics

A theoretical framework or model was exclusively stated in all except one intervention (Magura et al., 1994). The Social Cognitive Theory/Social Learning Theory ($n = 7$) was used by the most interventions; followed by the Theory of Reasoned Action ($n = 3$); and the Theory of Planned Behavior ($n = 3$; not mutually exclusive). Three interventions used three theories (Jemmott et al., 1992, 1998, 2005),

Table 9.1 Population characteristics of best and promising evidence-based interventions for African American youth at risk for HIV/STI Infection ($n=11$)

Best/ Promising	Intervention Name	Author	Target Population	No.	Gender % M/F	% African American	Mean age (range)
Best	BART	St. Lawrence et al. (1995)	African American adolescents	246	28/72	100	15 (14–18)
Best	Be proud! be responsible!	Jemmott et al. (1992)	Inner-city African American male adolescents	157	100/0	100	15
Best	FOK + ImPACT	Wu et al. (2003)	High-risk African American youth living in low-income urban community sites	817	42/58	100	14 (13–16)
Best	Making Proud Choices	Jemmott et al. (1998)	Inner-city African American adolescents	659	47/53	100	12
Best	Project AIM	Clark et al. (2005)	Low-income African American youth	211	55/45	100	13 (12–14)
Best	SiHLE	DiClemente et al. (2004)	Sexually experienced African American adolescent girls	522	0/100	100	16 (14–18)
Best	Sisters Saving Sisters	Jemmott et al. (2005)	Sexually-active African American and Latina adolescent female patients at family planning clinics	682	0/100	68	16 (12–19)
Promising	FOK	Stanton et al. (1996)	Low-income, urban African American youth	383	56/44	100	11 (9–15)
Promising	Intensive AIDS education	Magura et al. (1994)	Incarcerated, male adolescent drug users	157	100/0	66	18 (16–19)
Promising	REAL men	Dilorio et al. (2004)	Adolescent boys and their fathers	273	100/0	96	13 (11–14)
Promising	Street smart	Rotheram-Borus et al. (2003)	Runaway youth	187	51/49	53	16 (11–18)

Table 9.2 Intervention characteristics of best and promising-evidence based interventions for African-American youth at risk for HIV/STI infection ($n = 11$)

Intervention Name	Theories/ Model*	Culturally Sensitive and Developmentally Appropriate	Intervention Components	Delivery Method	Intervention Setting(s)
BART	IMB, SLT	culturally sensitive and developmentally appropriate	• Cognition (self-efficacy, empowerment) • Knowledge (information on HIV/AIDS and methods of preventing HIV infection) • Skills building (condom use, assertiveness, communication)	group discussion, role plays, exercises/ games, video, lectures, practice, demonstration	A public health clinic serving low-income families
Be Proud! Be Responsible!	SCT, TRA, TPB	culturally sensitive and developmentally appropriate	• Cognition (pride in making safer sexual choices, sexual responsibility and accountability, focus on family/ community as well as self, weaken problematic attitudes towards risky sexual behaviors) • Knowledge (increase knowledge of AIDS and STIs, increase information about risks with IV drug use) • Skills building (implement safer sex practices including abstinence; condom use)	group discussion, role plays, exercises/ games, video, lectures, practice	Local community building

Unit of Delivery (Range)	Deliverer	Intervention Duration	Relevant Outcomes Measured and Follow-up Time	Intervention Effects
Group (5-15)	Two co-facilitators (one male and one female); a small group of local youth who were HIV-positive led a discussion in one session	Eight 90-120 minute sessions delivered over 8 weeks	• Sexual risk behaviors during past two months (including frequency of unprotected and condom-protected vaginal, oral, and anal sex; and number of sex partners) measured immediately after the intervention and at 6- and 12-months post-intervention.	• A significantly lower percentage of intervention youth reported being sexually active compared to comparison youth at the 12 month follow-up (p < .05). • For the subgroup of youths who were not sexually active at baseline, there was a significantly smaller percentage of intervention youth who reported initiating sexual activity compared to the comparison youth by 12 months (p <.01). • Sexually active intervention youth reported a significantly greater percentage of sexual intercourse occasions that were condom-protected than comparison youth at the 6-month (p < .01) and 12-month (p < .05) follow-ups.
Group (5-6)	African-American men and women facilitators	One 5-hour session	• Sexual risk behaviors during past 3 months (including number of days respondent had sex, number of sex partners, number of sex partners involved with other men, and occurrence of anal sex) were measured at the 3-months post-intervention. • Condom use during past 3 months (including frequency of condom use scale and number of days of not using a condom during coitus) were measured at the 3-months post-intervention.	• Intervention youth reported significantly less risky sexual behavior (using the combined scale, p < .01) and fewer number of female sex partners (p < .003) than the comparison youth at the 3-month follow-up.

(continued)

Table 9.2 (continued)

Intervention Name	Theories/ Model*	Culturally Sensitive and Developmentally Appropriate	Intervention Components	Delivery Method	Intervention Setting(s)
FOK + ImPACT	PMT	culturally sensitive and developmentally appropriate	• Cognition (decision-making, goal-setting) • Knowledge (abstinence and safe sex, drugs, alcohol, and drug selling, AIDS and STIs, contraception, and human development) • Skills building (communication, decision-making, negotiation) • Emotional well-being (ethnic and gender pride)	group discussion, role plays, exercises/ games, video, lectures, risk-reduction supplies (condoms)	Housing developments and community sites
Making Proud Choices	SCT, TRA, TPB	developmentally appropriate	• Cognition (ethnic and gender pride, self-efficacy, strengthen abstinence beliefs) • Knowledge (increase HIV/AIDS knowledge) • Skills building (condom use, negotiation)	group discussion, exercises/ games, video	Middle schools
Project AIM	TPS	culturally sensitive and developmentally appropriate	• Cognition (sexual intentions, future possible self) • Knowledge • Skills building (skills necessary to reach personal goals)	group discussion, exercises, role plays	Middle schools

Unit of Delivery (Range)	Deliverer	Intervention Duration	Relevant Outcomes Measured and Follow-up Time	Intervention Effects
Group (5-12)	Interventionist and assistant group leader (for FOK); interventionist (for ImPACT)	Nine intervention sessions (8 for FOK and 1 for ImPACT) last approximately 1.5 hours each, and are generally delivered one session per week.	• Sexual risk behaviors during the previous 6 months (including sexual intercourse and unprotected sex at last sexual encounter) were measured at 6-, 12-, and 24-months post-intervention.	• Intervention youth who were sexually active at baseline reported significantly lower rates of sexual intercourse (p = .05) and unprotected sex (p = .005) than youth in the FOK only comparison at the 6-month follow-up.
Group (6-8)	Peer co-facilitator and adult facilitator	Eight 1-hour sessions delivered over two consecutive Saturdays	• Condom use, frequency of sex, and unprotected sex measured at 0, 3, 6, and 12-months after the intervention.	• Intervention youth reported significantly higher frequency of condom use than the comparison youth at the 3-month follow-up (p = .05), 6-month follow-up (p = .03), and 12-month follow-up (p = .04). – A significant larger proportion of intervention youth than the comparison youth reported consistent condom use at the 3-month follow-up (p = .02). – A significantly smaller proportion of intervention youth than the comparison youth reported unprotected sexual intercourse at the 3-month follow-up (p = .04).
Group (entire health education class)	One male and one female African-American graduate students	Ten 50-minute sessions once or twice a week over a 6-week period	• Abstinence was measured 19 weeks post-baseline and 12-months post-intervention.	• Intervention youth were significantly less likely to report nonabstience (any sexual intercourse) than the comparison youth at the 3-month follow-up.

(continued)

Table 9.2 (continued)

Intervention Name	Theories/ Model*	Culturally Sensitive and Developmentally Appropriate	Intervention Components	Delivery Method	Intervention Setting(s)
SiHLE	SCT, TGP	culturally sensitive and developmentally appropriate	• Cognition (risk perception, confidence, gender pride, ethnic pride, cognitive rehearsal, enhanced awareness) • Knowledge (HIV risk reduction strategies) • Skills building (condom use, safer sex conversations) • Emotional well-being (ethnic pride, gender pride, confidence, support, joys and challenges of being an African American female) • Normative influence (group norms supportive of HIV prevention)	group discussion, role plays, lectures, demonstration	Family medicine clinic
Sisters Saving Sisters	SCT, TRA, TPB	culturally sensitive and developmentally appropriate	• Cognition (personal risk)• Knowledge (HIV/STI risk reduction) • Skills building (condom use demonstration, negotiation)	group discussion, role plays, exercises/games, video, practice, demonstration	Adolescent medicine clinic

Unit of Delivery (Range)	Deliverer	Intervention Duration	Relevant Outcomes Measured and Follow-up Time	Intervention Effects
Group (10-12)	African-American female health educator and peer educators	Four 4-hour sessions delivered weekly on consecutive Saturdays	• Sexual risk behaviors in the past 30 days and past 6 months (including consistent condom use, condom use at last sex, percent condom protected vaginal sex acts, number of unprotected vaginal sex acts, new vaginal sex partner, and frequency of applying condom on sex partner) were measured 6- and 12-months post-intervention. • Incident STIs (including Chlamydia, gonorrhea, or trichomonas infection) were measured during the 12 month follow-up.	• Intervention youth reported significantly greater increases in consistent condom use, percentage of condom-protected vaginal sex acts, frequency of applying condoms on a sex partner, and condom use during last sex than the comparison youth over the 6- and 12-month follow-up periods. - Intervention youth reported significantly fewer new vaginal sex partners and episodes of unprotected vaginal sex during the 6- and 12-month follow-up periods than the comparison youth. - Intervention youth were also significantly less likely to acquire a new Chlamydia infection over 12 months of follow-up than the comparison youth.
Group (2-10)	African-American women facilitators	One 250-minute session	• Sex risk behaviors during past 3 months (including unprotected sex, unprotected sex with drugs or alcohol, and number of sex partners) were measured at 3-, 6-, and 12-month follow-ups. • New STI infections (including gonorrhea, Chlamydia, or trichomonas) were measured at 6- and 12-month follow-ups.	• Skills-based intervention youth, compared to Health Promotion comparison youth, - reported significantly fewer days of sex without condom use ($p = .002$) and significantly fewer days of unprotected sex while high on drugs or alcohol ($p = .02$) at the 12-month follow-up. - reported fewer sexual partners ($p = .04$) at the 12-month follow-up. - were significantly less likely to report having multiple sex partners ($p = .002$) at the 12-month follow-up. - were significantly less likely to test positive for a new STI during the 12-month follow-up period ($p = 0.05$).

(continued)

Table 9.2 (continued)

Intervention Name	Theories/ Model*	Culturally Sensitive and Developmentally Appropriate	Intervention Components	Delivery Method	Intervention Setting(s)
FOK	PMT	culturally sensitive and developmentally appropriate	• Cognition (goal setting; decision making; values clarification) • Knowledge (facts about AIDS/STI; contraception; human development) • Skills building (decision-making, communication) • Emotional well-being (friendship groups) • Access (condoms)	group discussion, role plays, exercises/ games, video, lectures, risk-reduction supplies (condoms), arts and crafts, social event, storytelling	Recreation center meeting room; a rural campsite
Intensive AIDS Education	NR	developmentally appropriate	• Cognition (high-risk attitudes and behaviors) • Knowledge (general HIV education information, general health knowledge, drug use initiation/ continuation; information on health care services, social services, an drug treatment) • Skills building (decision-making, problem solving)	group discussion, role plays, exercises, problem solving therapy	New Adolescent Reception and Detention Center
REAL Men	SCT	developmentally appropriate	• Cognition (intentions to have sexual intercourse) • Knowledge (transmission and prevention of HIV and AIDS, sex education) • Skills building (father-son communication) • Emotional well-being (encouragement, support from others)	group discussion, role plays, games, video, lectures	Boys & Girls Clubs

Unit of Delivery (Range)	Deliverer	Intervention Duration	Relevant Outcomes Measured and Follow-up Time	Intervention Effects
Group (3-10)	Two trained adult interventionists, typically African American community members, at least one of whom is gender matched to the group	Eight weekly meetings: seven 90-minute sessions and one day-long session. Monthly and annual 90-minute booster sessions	• Sexual risk behaviors in the past 6 months (including having sex, condom use at last sex, and unprotected sex) were measured at 6-, 12-, 18-, 24-, and 36-month follow-ups.	• Sexually active FOK intervention youth were significantly less likely to report unprotected sex compared to the comparison youth at the 18-month follow-up ($p < .05$).
Group (8)	Male counselor	Four 1-hour sessions delivered twice a week over a 2-week period	• Sexual risk behaviors measured during time in the community since release from jail were: having multiple sex partners, having any high-risk sex partners, having any anal sex, and frequency of condom use during vaginal, oral, and anal sex; outcomes were measured at a median of 10 months after baseline, which was a median of 5 months after release from jail, indicating a follow-up of at least 5 months (but less than 10 months).	• Intervention youth reported a significantly greater frequency of condom use during vaginal sex than the control participants ($p = .02$, one-tailed test) at the 5-month or greater follow-up.
Group (groups of fathers in first 6 sessions; groups of father and son dyads in last session)	Facilitator	Seven 2-hour sessions (6 sessions for fathers; 1 joint session) delivered over a 7-week period	• Increased condom use and increased abstinence rate measured 1, 4, and 10-months post-intervention.	• Intervention youth reported a significantly higher rates of abstinence than the comparison youth at the 4-month follow-up ($p = 0.05$, one-tailed test). • Among sexually active, a significantly smaller proportion of intervention youth than the comparison youth reported sexual intercourse without a condom at 4-month follow-up ($p = .02$, one-tailed test) and 10-month follow-ups ($p = .03$, one-tailed test).

(continued)

Table 9.2 (continued)

Intervention Name	Theories/ Model*	Culturally Sensitive and Developmentally Appropriate	Intervention Components	Delivery Method	Intervention Setting(s)
Street Smart	SLT	developmentally appropriate	• Cognition (self-efficacy, personal risk, intentions, attitudes) • Knowledge (general HIV/STI risk information) • Skills building (communication, coping skills, safer sex negotiation, assertiveness) • Emotional well-being (self-esteem, social support networks, emotional state-anxiety, depression, anger) • Access (condoms and health care services)	group discussion, role plays, exercises/ games, video, practice, risk-reduction supplies (condoms), counseling, developing video and art media, goal setting, homework	Four runaway youth shelters

NR not reported; *IMB* information motivation behavior model; *PMT* protective motivation theory; theory of planned behavior; *TRA* theory of reasoned action; *TPS* theory of possible selves

two interventions used two theories (DiClemente et al., 2004; St. Lawrence et al., 1995), and five interventions used only one theory (Clark et al., 2005; Dilorio et al., 2007; Rotheram-Borus et al., 2003; Stanton et al., 1996; Wu et al., 2003).

All of the interventions incorporated cognition (e.g., self-efficacy, attitudes, intentions, perceptions of risk), knowledge (e.g., increase HIV/AIDS knowledge and risk reduction), and skills building (e.g., condom use, communication, negotiation) as part of the study content. Several interventions also addressed ethnic and gender pride (e.g., incorporating videos that included an African American or multiethnic cast or highlighted the accomplishments of African American women) and/ or social support (DiClemente et al., 2004; Dilorio et al., 2007; Jemmott et al., 1998; Rotheram-Borus et al., 2003), three explicitly stated that condoms were provided (Rotheram-Borus et al., 2003; Stanton et al., 1996; Wu et al., 2003), and one addressed normative influence (peer influences; DiClemente et al., 2004). The most common methods used to deliver the interventions were group discussion ($n=11$), role plays ($n=10$), exercises and games ($n=7$), videos ($n=8$), lectures ($n=6$), practice ($n=4$), and demonstration ($n=3$), which are not mutually exclusive.

Various methods of delivery were used to implement the specific content (e.g., cognition, knowledge, and skills building) of each intervention. Several interventions relied on demonstration and practice for condom skills, role plays for negotiation and communication skills, and practicing how to be assertive for negotiation and communication. Additionally, a video depicting parent and child communication (with role play) was used, along with games, exercises, and group

Unit of Delivery (Range)	Deliverer	Intervention Duration	Relevant Outcomes Measured and Follow-up Time	Intervention Effects
Individual and group (6-10)	Co-led by a trained researcher (the same gender and typically the same ethnicity) and a shelter staff	10 sessions (9 small-group and 1 individual) delivered over a 3 week period	• Sexual risk behaviors in the past 3 months (the number of sex partners, number of insertive or receptive vaginal, anal, or oral sex acts, number of unprotected sex acts of each type, and abstinent from vaginal or anal sexual acts) measured at 0, 3, 9, 15, and 21 months after the intervention.	• Among female youth, intervention youth reported significantly fewer unprotected sex acts than comparison youth at 21 months after the intervention (p = .018).

SCT social cognitive theory; *SLT* social learning theory; *TGP* theory of gender and power; *TPB*
[a]Theories/model

discussions regarding the risk of HIV/AIDS (Wu et al., 2003). Videos depicting African American youth and correct condom use and condom negotiation were also incorporated into the interventions.

With regard to deliverers, most interventions used gender- and ethnicity-matched deliverers. Eight interventions stated that they were gender matched (Clark et al., 2005; DiClemente et al., 2004; Jemmott et al., 1992; 2005; Magura et al., 1994; Rotheram-Borus et al., 2003; Stanton et al., 1996; St. Lawrence et al., 1995). For the interventions that included a population that was 100% female or 100% male, all deliverers were matched by race and gender. The evaluation of the *Making Proud Choices* intervention specifically tested gender and age matching and found that neither altered the results of the study (Jemmott et al., 1998). For the three interventions that reported educational attainment of deliverers, all had at least a college degree (Clark et al., 2005; Jemmott et al., 1992; 2005). Three studies provided information on the background of the deliverers, which included training in human sexuality, education, nursing, social work, and small group facilitation (Jemmott et al., 1992), experience with inner-city youth (Jemmott et al., 2005), and involvement with community-based organizations (Stanton et al., 1996). Among the three studies that reported the number of hours the deliverers were trained, training was conducted for 6 (Jemmott et al., 1992), 8 (Jemmott et al., 2005) and 24 h (Stanton et al., 1996). Two interventions were delivered by a peer in addition to adult facilitators or adult health educators (DiClemente et al., 2004; Jemmott et al., 1998).

Interventions were conducted in community-based establishments or public venues, such as Boys & Girls Clubs, YMCA, recreation centers, and shelters (Dilorio et al., 2007; Jemmott et al., 1992; Rotheram-Borus et al., 2003; Stanton et al., 1996; Wu et al., 2003), health care settings, including family planning and STI clinics (DiClemente et al., 2004; Jemmott et al., 2005; St. Lawrence et al., 1995), educational settings, including high schools and middle schools (Clark et al., 2005; Jemmott et al., 1998), and at a detention center (Magura et al., 1994).

All of the interventions were delivered in group settings, with two interventions also involving a parent or guardian (Dilorio et al., 2007; Wu et al., 2003). Each intervention consisted of 1 to 10 sessions and ranged from 2 to 20 total hours. Six interventions were conducted in 6 to 10 sessions (Dilorio et al., 2007; Jemmott et al., 1998; Rotheram-Borus et al., 2003; Stanton et al., 1996; St. Lawrence et al., 1995; Wu et al., 2003) and five interventions were conducted in 1 to 5 sessions (Clark et al., 2005; DiClemente et al., 2004; Jemmott et al., 1992; 2005; Magura et al., 1994). Additionally, five interventions lasted less than 10 h (Clark et al., 2005; Jemmott et al., 1992; Jemmott et al., 1998; 2005; Magura et al., 1994), five interventions lasted 10 or more hours (DiClemente et al., 2004; Dilorio et al., 2007; Stanton et al., 1996; St. Lawrence et al., 1995; Wu et al., 2003), and one intervention did not report the total time (Rotheram-Borus et al., 2003). The follow-up time ranged from 1 to 36 months after the completion of the intervention, with all studies reporting at least a 1-month follow-up (promising-evidence interventions) or a 3 month follow-up (best-evidence interventions).

Intervention Effects

Compared to the youth in the comparison group, youth receiving an intervention reported the following: reduced unprotected sex (DiClemente et al., 2004; Dilorio et al, 2007; Jemmott et al., 1992, 1998; 2005; Rotheram-Borus et al., 2003; Stanton et al., 1996; St. Lawrence et al., 1995; Wu et al., 2003); increased condom use/consistent condom use (DiClemente et al., 2004; Jemmott et al., 1998; Magura et al., 1994; St. Lawrence et al., 1995); reduced number of sex partners, including new sex partners (DiClemente et al., 2004; Jemmott et al., 1992, 2005); reduced sexual activity (Clark et al., 2005; Jemmott et al., 1998; St. Lawrence et al., 1995; Wu et al., 2003); reduced new STI (DiClemente et al., 2004; Jemmott et al., 2005); increased abstinence (Clark et al., 2005; Dilorio et al., 2007); and reduced unprotected sex while under the influence of drugs or alcohol (Jemmott et al., 2005).

Several of the best evidence-based intervention effects remained significant throughout the follow-up period, although none of the promising evidence-based interventions remained significant. Three interventions (DiClemente et al., 2004; Jemmott et al., 1998; St. Lawrence et al., 1995) were sustained 6 and 12 months after the intervention. They remained significant for increasing condom use

(DiClemente et al., 2004; Jemmott et al., 1998; St. Lawrence et al., 1995) and reducing new STIs and new vaginal sex partners (DiClemente et al., 2004).

Discussion

Despite differences in population and intervention characteristics, the 11 EBIs we identified in this review showed several similarities: incorporating a behavioral theory to guide intervention development; addressing cognition, knowledge, and skills building; delivering intervention content with multiple methods, such as group discussion, role plays, videos (many of them culturally sensitive), and exercises and games. Most of these interventions were conducted in health care or community settings, were culturally sensitive and developmentally appropriate, and included ethnic and gender matched deliverers. The outcomes included a decrease in unprotected sex, number of sex partners, as well as an increase in condom use and abstinence.

The characteristics of the deliverers may be critical in the overall efficacy of the intervention. Although most of the EBIs had deliverers matched by gender and ethnicity to the target group, one study (Jemmott et al., 1998) specifically tested the matching issue and found that gender or age (peer or adult) of the deliverers did not have a significant effect on the intervention findings. This is consistent with previous findings in the literature (Jemmott & Jemmott, 2002; Jemmott, Jemmott, Fong, & McCaffree, 1999). It is plausible that whether the deliverer is culturally or gender competent is more important than the deliverers being of the same race/ethnicity or gender as the participants (Jemmott et al., 1999). It is important that the deliverers are properly trained and have a good understanding of the culture and subject matter they are trying to convey to the adolescents. This will not only be beneficial to the deliverer, but also to the adolescents participating in the intervention. Many of the EBIs did not mention the specific training (time or content) of the deliverers or their respective backgrounds (e.g., adolescents, the African American community, human sexuality). This information should be reported for better understanding of the intervention effect.

Similarly, several EBIs stated that they were culturally sensitive and developmentally appropriate; however, few actually described these components. Cultural sensitivity (e.g., respecting and understanding the African American community) is essential for some African Americans to fully participate in interventions designed specifically for them (Stevenson & Davis, 1994; Stevenson, Gay, & Josar, 1995), and developmental appropriateness is important for adolescents to comprehend and understand the content being delivered. Clearly, a description of the operationalization of these important elements would be very informative for intervention providers to understand what actually works. Research has shown the importance of including developmentally appropriate material for interventions that target adolescents (Pedlow & Carey, 2004).

Research Gaps and Recommendations

The best and most promising evidence-based interventions described in this chapter demonstrate how behavioral interventions can help African American adolescents reduce their risk for HIV and STIs. Many of those EBIs addressed the risk and protective factors associated with African American youth's risk behaviors as we described earlier in this chapter. However, several research gaps remain. Below, we discuss what has been addressed in those EBIs, what the research gap is, and research recommendations derived from this review. They are divided into three categories: individual, interpersonal and environmental, and societal and cultural factors.

Individual Factors

The age of the participants in the EBIs included in this chapter ranged from 9 to 19 years old, which represents a wide age range. An intervention that is effective for a 9-year-old may not work for a 19-year-old. It is critical that interventions narrow the age of the participants or have different content depending on the ages of the participants. Additionally, we only identified one EBI specifically for African American males (Jemmott et al., 1992). Including more interventions that specifically target African American male adolescents, especially because they are at high risk for acquiring an STI, including HIV (Jemmott & Jemmott 1996), is extremely important.

The primary mode of HIV transmission among African American males is male-to-male sexual contact (CDC, 2008c); therefore, interventions targeting this population are greatly needed. None were identified in this chapter. Stigma and discrimination in the African American community and society in general, makes this population hard to reach and incorporate appropriately tailored interventions. Young African American men who have sex with men (MSM) might be unsure of their sexuality or might not be gay-identified, making it difficult to tailor needed interventions for this population. Limited research has been published on prevention interventions for gay, lesbian, and bisexual (GLB) adolescents (Blake et al., 2001; Malow, Kershaw, Sipsma, Rosenberg, & Dévieux, 2007). Of the interventions that have focused on GLB adolescents, most included a broad age range and viewed sexual risk behaviors only, not including identity or developmental issues. Moreover, most of the studies had a population that was less than 50% African American. Examining the relevant literature, studies showed that GLB adolescents were more likely to have used alcohol and drugs, to have used alcohol/drugs before sex, ever had sexual intercourse, were younger at first sexual intercourse, had more sexual partners, were currently sexually active (past 3 months), and had ever been or gotten someone pregnant compared to heterosexual adolescents (Blake et al., 2001; Garofalo, Wolf, Kessel, Palfrey, & DuRant, 1998). Some interventions based on one-group pre- and post-intervention data showed a decrease in unprotected same-sex sexual behavior (anal and oral sex) and number of sex partners among gay and bisexual adolescent males (Remafedi, 1994; Rotheram-Borus, Reid, & Rosario, 1994; Rotheram-Borus, Rosario, Reid, & Koopman, 1995). Although those interventions show potential, more rigorous evaluation should be conducted to determine the efficacy of those interventions.

Substance use is another factor that interventions need to address, because it has been shown to be directly related to adolescents engaging in risky sex behaviors (Bachanas et al., 2002; Brook et al., 2004; Cooper, Peirce, & Huselid, 1994; Fullilove et al., 1993; Kingree & Betz, 2003; Stanton, Li, Cottrell, & Kaljee, 2001). Of the EBIs included in this chapter, only one, *Intensive AIDS Education* (Magura et al., 1994), targeted drug users (who were also male and incarcerated). Several of the other interventions, *Street Smart* (Rotheram-Borus et al., 2003), *Be Proud! Be Responsible!* (Jemmott et al., 1992), *FOK+ ImPACT* (Wu et al., 2003), and *Sisters Saving Sisters* (Jemmott et al., 2005) included a component of substance use in their interventions (e.g., drug and alcohol use, drug selling, drug delivery, intravenous drug use). They discussed how substance use can affect sexual control and judgment; as well as risks associated with engaging in drugs and alcohol before sex and the fact that drugs and alcohol are barriers to using condoms. In one study (Bachanas et al., 2002), minority adolescent females who used more drugs or alcohol were more likely to report STIs, pregnancies, sexual partners, and engage in unprotected sex compared to minority adolescent females who did not use these substances.

Self-esteem and skills for making the right decisions are important protective factors associated with youth's risk behavior. They are also a component that both adolescents and parents identified as needing to be incorporated into interventions (Brown & Waite, 2005). Learning how to resist peer pressure and choosing the right peers, and knowing how to say no are critical to youth staying safe. Additionally, developing lifelong skills was important. Lifelong skills include empowering adolescents with basic knowledge skills (beyond drug and sex education), teaching work ethics, professional and technical skills, incorporating academics and athletics, black history, and teaching respect. These ideas are similar to *Project AIM*, in which adolescents created a positive self image in order to eliminate risky sexual behaviors, by achieving their personal goals (Clark et al., 2005).

Interpersonal and Environmental Factors

Parental monitoring, supervision, closeness, and increased support have shown to be both protective and risk factors of adolescent's sexual behavior and intentions (Buhi & Goodson, 2007). A systematic review of the literature related to the aforementioned concerns is needed to better understand the role, positive or negative, that parents play in their adolescents decision-making and risk behaviors (Buhi & Goodson, 2007). *FOK+ ImPACT* (Wu et al., 2003), which involved a parent or guardian to promote safe sex behaviors among youth showed significant results in reducing sexual risk behaviors among adolescents. Parental monitoring and communication was an essential component of this intervention. Compared to the comparison group (*FOK*), the adolescents who received the intervention with a parent or guardian (*FOK* + *ImPACT*) had significantly lower rates of sexual intercourse and unprotected sex 6 months after the intervention. Another intervention, *REAL Men* (Dilorio et al., 2007), that is intended to increase father and son communication about safe sex showed positive results in practicing safer sex behaviors among boys. It is vital to increase communication between African American adolescents and parents.

In addition to parents and guardians, other people in the community who interact with African American youth could also play an important role in influencing adolescents' behavior. In one study (Brown & Waite, 2005), African American youth wanted to include after-school and church activities, as well as promote self-esteem, condom use, and HIV and drug education in the creation of HIV prevention messages. African American youth wanted to include not only their parents, but their church pastors and police officers in the staffing of the prevention program (Brown & Waite, 2005). The church is the main focal point in many African American communities and should be included in any intervention that is created, especially since religion (McCree et al., 2003) and spiritual interconnectedness (Holder et al., 2000) have been shown to be protective factors.

It has been noted that the community needs to be involved in various aspects of the intervention, from creation to evaluation (Hatch, Moss, Saran, Presley-Cantrell, & Mallory, 1993). Community involvement in the direction and focus of the research is especially important for underserved minority populations. Community members can also be used to give advice, serve as gatekeepers, or actively participate in the delivery of the intervention (Hatch et al., 1993). HIV/AIDS is not only a personal risk factor but a growing problem among families and communities. Interventions should also incorporate a sense of family and community (Jemmott & Jemmott, 2002). *Be Proud! Be Responsible!* not only viewed the adolescent's risk but also included the need to protect the family and community (Jemmott et al., 1992). *SiHLE* included the theme of protecting the community as well as the adolescent as part of the intervention (DiClemente et al., 2004).

Making condoms available in schools has been shown to increase condom use (Blake et al., 2003). This is especially important for African American adolescents, who have higher rates of STIs (CDC, 2007a), including HIV/AIDS (CDC, 2008c). Condom acquisition by students was greatest when students did not have to directly ask for them (e.g., in bowls or baskets) and when a clinic was available at the school (Kirby & Brown, 1996). Making condoms available to youth and allowing students to obtain condoms could be an effective way to encourage safer behaviors (Kirby & Brown, 1996).

The environment in which an adolescent lives helps to determine the specific needs of that individual. An intervention targeted to a specific residency (urban, suburban, and rural) of adolescents may need different components, since each environment presents its own set of challenges. Research has shown that rural adolescents are more likely to have ever had sex and to have had unprotected sex compared to non-rural adolescents (Milhausen et al., 2003). This may be due in part to the lack of extracurricular activities in many rural communities, especially in the evening (Brown & Waite, 2005). Adolescents who are home alone (without a parent) have been shown to engage in sex earlier (Dilorio et al., 2004) and to have increased sexual activity (Perkins, Luster, Villarruel, & Small, 1998). After-school programs and activities should be considered as a structural-level intervention.

Societal and Cultural Factors

The media has a great influence on adolescent development. It has been previously noted how the media, including the hip-hop culture, can have a potentially negative effect on adolescents engaging in risk sex behaviors. Over the past 25 years, media campaigns have expanded to incorporate every segment of the population, and they have included print, radio, and television. The hip-hop culture has included some public service announcements (PSAs) that have incorporated many of today's artists. The Kaiser Family Foundation has been working with MTV's *Fight For Your Rights: Protect Yourself* campaign along with Black Entertainment Television's (BET) *Rap it Up* campaign to promote HIV/AIDS knowledge through various PSAs, special programming, as well as print and Web information free of charge (Davis, 2006).

A range of media outlets can be used for positive change for HIV/AIDS prevention among adolescents (Delgado & Austin, 2007). Several international studies using the media have been conducted (Bertrand, O'Reilly, Denison, Anhang, & Sweat, 2006; Underwood, Hachonda, Serlemitsos, & Bharath-Kumar, 2006), but research in the United States is scarce (Delgado & Austin, 2007). Future interventions should incorporate the media, especially the hip-hop culture to assert a positive influence on adolescent's behavior.

Adolescence is recognized as a period of risk-taking behavior, including experimentation with smoking, drugs and alcohol, as well as sexual activity. At this stage in life, these behaviors may be impulsive, exploratory, and excitable. However, the idea of engaging in risky sexual behaviors may have consequences that could result in unwanted pregnancy or STIs, including HIV/AIDS. Therefore, it is necessary to create culturally sensitive and developmentally appropriate evidenced-based behavioral interventions to combat the spread of STIs and HIV/AIDS among today's adolescent population. Our review showed that behavioral interventions are efficacious in increasing abstinence and consistent condom use as well as reducing sexual intercourse, unprotected sex, number of sex partners, and number of new STI infections. In order to move research targeting African American youth to the next phase, individual, interpersonal and environmental, and societal and cultural factors we discussed in this chapter should be considered and incorporated.

Furthermore, translating and disseminating evidence-based research into the field is vital in having an effect on the HIV/AIDS epidemic. Some progress has been made in translating scientific-based knowledge into user friendly intervention packages for dissemination through two CDC projects: Replicating Effective Programs (REP) Plus (2008)) and diffusion of effective behavioral interventions

(DEBI, n.d.). Several EBIs for youth have been packaged or are in the process of packaging by CDC and commercial venues (CDC, 2007b). For EBIs specifically for African American youth identified in this review (*FOK + ImPACT, Project AIM, SiHLE, and Street Smart*) are available or soon to be available through the DEBI dissemination (DEBI, n.d.). With a wide dissemination of EBIs to the community in need, we expect to see a substantial reduction in HIV/STI risk behaviors and infections among African American youth in the near future.

References

Aral, S. O. (2001). Sexually transmitted diseases: magnitude, determinants and consequences. *International Journal of STD and AIDS, 12*(4), 211–215.

Bachanas, P. J., Morris, M. K., Lewis-Gess, J. K., Sarett-Cuasay, E. J., Flores, A. L., Sirl, K. S., et al. (2002). Psychological adjustment, substance use, HIV knowledge, and risky sexual behavior in at-risk minority females: developmental differences during adolescence. *Journal of Pediatric Psychology, 27*(4), 373–384.

Belgrave, F. Z., Van Oss Marin, B., & Chambers, D. B. (2000). Cultural, contextual, and intrapersonal predictors of risky sexual attitudes among urban African American girls in early adolescence. *Cultural Diversity and Ethnic Minority Psychology, 6*(3), 309–322.

Bertrand, J. T., O'Reilly, K., Denison, J., Anhang, R., & Sweat, M. (2006). Systematic review of the effectiveness of mass communication programs to change HIV/AIDS-related behaviors in developing countries. *Health Education Research, 21*(4), 567–597.

Blake, S. M., Ledsky, R., Goodenow, C., Sawyer, R., Lohrmann, D., & Windsor, R. (2003). Condom availability programs in Massachusetts high schools: relationships with condom use and sexual behavior. *American Journal of Public Health, 93*(6), 955–962.

Blake, S. M., Ledsky, R., Lehman, T., Goodenow, C., Sawyer, R., & Hack, T. (2001). Preventing sexual risk behaviors among gay, lesbian, and bisexual adolescents: the benefits of gay-sensitive HIV instruction in schools. *American Journal of Public Health, 91*(6), 940–946.

Black, M. M., Ricardo, I. B., & Stanton, B. (1997). Social and psychological factors associated with AIDS risk behaviors among low-income, urban, African American adolescents. *Journal of Research on Adolescence, 7*(2), 173–195.

Bourdieu, P. (1985). The forms of social capital. In J. G. Richardson (Ed.), *Handbook of theory and research for the sociology of education* (pp. 241–258). New York: Greenwood.

Brook, J. S., Adams, R. E., Balka, E. B., Whiteman, M., Zhang, C., & Sugerman, R. (2004). Illicit drug use and risky sexual behavior among African American and Puerto Rican urban adolescents: the longitudinal links. *The Journal of Genetic Psychology, 165*(2), 203–220.

Brown, E. J., & Waite, C. D. (2005). Perceptions of risk and resiliency factors associated with rural African American adolescents' substance abuse and HIV behaviors. *Journal of the American Psychiatric Nurses Association, 11*(2), 88–100.

Buhi, E. R., & Goodson, P. (2007). Predictors of adolescent sexual behavior and intention: a theory-guided systematic review. *The Journal of Adolescent Health, 40*(1), 4–21.

Centers for Disease Control and Prevention. (2007a). *Sexually transmitted disease surveillance, 2006*. Atlanta, GA: U.S. Department of Health and Human Services

Centers for Disease Control and Prevention. (2007b). *HIV/AIDS prevention research synthesis project*. Retrieved September 3, 2008, from http://www.cdc.gov/hiv/topics/ research/prs/index. htm.

Centers for Disease Control and Prevention. (2008a). *Efficacy review: efficacy criteria*. Retrieved October 1, 2008, from http://www.cdc.gov/hiv/topics/research/prs/efficacy_criteria.htm.

Centers for Disease Control and Prevention. (2008b). *HIV/AIDS in the United States. CDC HIV/ AIDS facts.* Retrieved June 4, 2008, from http://www.cdc.gov/hiv/resources/factsheets/PDF/ us.pdf.

Centers for Disease Control and Prevention. (2008c). *HIV/AIDS surveillance in adolescents and young adults (through 2006).* Retrieved June 5, 2008, from http://www.cdc.gov/hiv/topics/ surveillance/resources/slides/adolescents/index.htm.

Centers for Disease Control and Prevention. (2008d). Youth risk behavior surveillance-United States. *Surveillance Summaries, MMWR, 57*(4), 1–131.

Clark, L. F. Miller, K. S., Nagy, S. S., Avery, J., Roth, D. L., Liddon, N., et al. (2005). Adult identity mentoring: Reducing sexual risk for African-American seventh grade students. *Journal of Adolescent Health, 37*(4), 337.e1-337.e10.

Collins, C., Harshbarger, C., Sawyer, R., & Hamdallah, M. (2006). The diffusion of effective behavioral interventions project: development, implementation, and lessons learned. *AIDS Education and Prevention, 18*(Suppl. A), 5–20.

Cooper, S. M., & Guthrie, B. (2007). Ecological influences on health-promoting and health-compromising behaviors: a socially embedded approach to urban African American girls' health. *Family and Community Health, 30*(1), 29–41.

Cooper, M. L., Peirce, R. S., & Huselid, R. F. (1994). Substance use and sexual risk taking among black adolescents and white adolescents. *Health Psychology, 13*(3), 251–262.

Crosby, R. A., DiClemente, R. J., Wingood, G. M., Cobb, B. K., Harrington, K., Davies, S. L., et al. (2001). HIV/STD-protective benefits of living with mothers in perceived supportive families: a study of high-risk African American female teens. *Preventive Medicine, 33*(3), 175–178.

Crosby, R. A., DiClemente, R. J., Wingood, G. M., Harrington, K., Davies, S., & Malow, R. (2002a). Participation by African-American adolescent females in social organizations: associations with HIV-protective behaviors. *Ethnicity and Disease, 12*(2), 186–192.

Crosby, R. A., DiClemente, R. J., Wingood, G. M., Harrington, K., Davies, S., & Oh, M. K. (2002b). Activity of African-American female teenagers in black organisations is associated with STD/HIV protective behaviours: A prospective analysis. *Journal of Epidemiology and Community Health, 56*(7), 549–550.

Crosby, R. A., & Holtgrave, D. R. (2006). The protective value of social capital against teen pregnancy: a state-level analysis. *The Journal of Adolescent Health, 38*(5), 556–559.

Crosby, R. A., Holtgrave, D. R., DiClemente, R. J., Wingood, G. M., & Gayle, J. A. (2003). Social capital as a predictor of adolescents' sexual risk behavior: a state-level exploratory study. *AIDS and Behavior, 7*(3), 245–252.

Davis, J. (2006). *Evolution of an epidemic: 25 years of HIV/AIDS media campaigns in the U.S.* Menlo Park, CA: Henry Kaiser Family Foundation. Retrieved February 22, 2008, from http:// www.kff.org/entpartnerships/upload/7515.pdf.

Delgado, H. M., & Austin, S. B. (2007). Can media promote responsible sexual behaviors among adolescents and young adults? *Current Opinion in Pediatrics, 19*(4), 405–410.

DeLuca, J. B., Mullins, M. M., Lyles, C. M., Crepaz, N., Kay, L., & Thadiparthi, S. (2008). Developing a comprehensive search strategy for evidence-based systematic review. *Evidence Based Library and Information Practice, 3*(1), 3–32.

DeNavas-Walt, C., Proctor, B. D., & Smith, J. (2007). U.S. Census Bureau, Current Population Reports, P60–233. *Income, poverty, and health insurance coverage in the United States: 2006.* Washington, DC.: U.S. Government Printing Office.

DiClemente, R. J., Wingood, G. M., Harrington, K. F., Lang, D. L., Davies, S. L., Hook, E. W., III, et al. (2004). Efficacy of an HIV prevention intervention for African American adolescent girls: a randomized controlled trial. *Journal of the American Medical Association, 292*(2), 171–179.

Diffusion of effective behavioral interventions. (DEBI). (n.d.). Retrieved February 22, 2008, from http://www.kff.org/entpartnerships/upload/7515.pdf.

Dilorio, C., Dudley, W. N., Soet, J. E., & McCarthy, F. (2004). Sexual possibility situations and sexual behaviors among young adolescents: the moderating role of protective factors. *Journal of Adolescent Health, 35*(6), 528.e11–528.e20.

Dilorio, C., McCarty, F., Resnicow, K., Lehr, S., & Denzmore, P. (2007). REAL men: a group-randomized trial of an HIV prevention intervention for adolescent boys. *American Journal of Public Health, 97*(6), 1084–1089.

Felton, G. M., & Bartoces, M. (2002). Predictors of initiation of early sex in black and white adolescent females. *Public Health Nursing, 19*(1), 59–67.

Fullilove, M. T., Golden, E., Fullilove, R. E., III, Lennon, R., Porterfield, D., Schwarcz, S., et al. (1993). Crack cocaine use and high-risk behaviors among sexually active black adolescents. *The Journal of Adolescent Health, 14*(4), 295–300.

Garofalo, R., Wolf, R. C., Kessel, S., Palfrey, J., & DuRant, R. H. (1998). The Association between health risk behaviors and sexual orientation among a school-based sample of adolescents. *Pediatrics, 101*(5), 895–902.

Glynn, M., & Rhodes, P. (2005, June). Estimated HIV prevalence in the United States at the end of 2003. National HIV Prevention Conference. Atlanta. Abstract T1-B1101. Retrieved December 14, 2007, from, http://www.aegis.com/conferences/NHIVPC/2005/ T1-B1101.html.

Hatch, J., Moss, N., Saran, A., Presley-Cantrell, L., & Mallory, C. (1993). Community research: partnership in black communities. *American Journal of Preventive Medicine, 9*(6 Suppl.), 27-31; 32-34.

Hoff, T., Greene, L., & Davis, J. (2003). *National survey of adolescents and young adults: sexual health knowledge, attitudes and experiences.* Menlo Park, CA: Henry Kaiser Family Foundation. Retrieved December 14, 2007, from http://www.kff.org/youthhivstds/ upload/National-Survey-of-Adolescents-and-Young-Adults.pdf.

Holder, D. W., DuRant, R. H., Harris, T. L., Daniel, J. H., Obeidallah, D., & Goodman, E. (2000). The association between adolescent spirituality and voluntary sexual activity. *The Journal of Adolescent Health, 26*(4), 295–302.

Holtgrave, D. R., & Crosby, R. A. (2003). Social capital, poverty, and income inequality as predictors of gonorrhoea, syphilis, Chlamydia and AIDS case rates in the United States. *Sexually Transmitted Infections, 79*(1), 62–64.

Jemmott, J. B., III, & Jemmott, L. S. (1996). Strategies to reduce the risk of HIV infection, sexually transmitted diseases, and pregnancy among African American adolescents. In R. J. Resnick & R. H. Rozensky (Eds.), *Health psychology through the life span: practice and research opportunities* (pp. 395–422). Washington, D.C.: American Psychological Association.

Jemmott, J. B., III, & Jemmott, L. S. (2002). Empowering African American adolescents at risk: community-based strategies for reducing risk through enhancing self-efficacy. In M. A. Chesney & M. H. Antoni (Eds.), *Innovative approaches to health psychology: prevention and treatment lessons from AIDS* (pp. 45–70). Washington, D.C.: American Psychological Association.

Jemmott, J. B., III, Jemmott, L. S., Braverman, P. K., & Fong, G. T. (2005). HIV/STD risk reduction interventions for African American and Latino adolescent girls at an adolescent medicine clinic: a randomized controlled trial. *Archives of Pediatrics and Adolescent Medicine, 159*(5), 440–449.

Jemmott, J. B., III, Jemmott, L. S., & Fong, G. T. (1992). Reductions in HIV risk-associated sexual behaviors among black male adolescents: Effects of an AIDS prevention intervention. *American Journal of Public Health, 82*(3), 372–377.

Jemmott, J. B., III, Jemmott, L. S., & Fong, G. T. (1998). Abstinence and safer sex HIV risk-reduction interventions for African American adolescents: a randomized controlled trial. *Journal of the American Medical Association, 279*(19), 1529–1536.

Jemmott, J. B., III, Jemmott, L. S., Fong, G. T., & McCaffree, K. (1999). Reducing HIV risk-associated sexual behavior among African American adolescents: testing the generality of intervention effects. *American Journal of Community Psychology, 27*(2), 161–187.

Kingree, J. B., & Betz, H. (2003). Risky sexual behavior in relation to marijuana and alcohol use among African-American, male adolescent detainees and their female partners. *Drug and Alcohol Dependence, 72*(2), 197–203.

Kirby, D. B., & Brown, N. L. (1996). Condom availability programs in U.S. schools. *Family Planning Perspectives, 28*(5), 196–202.

L'Engle, K. L., Brown, J. D., & Kenneavy, K. (2006). The mass media are an important context for adolescents' sexual behavior. *The Journal of Adolescent Health, 38*(3), 186–192.

Lyles, C. M., Crepaz, N., Herbst, J. H., Kay, L. S., & for the HIV/AIDS Prevention Research Synthesis Team. (2006). Evidence-based HIV behavioral prevention from the perspective of the CDC's HIV/AIDS Prevention Research Synthesis Team. *AIDS Education and Prevention, 18*(Suppl. A), 21–31.

Magura, S., Kang, S. Y., & Shapiro, J. L. (1994). Outcomes of intensive AIDS education for male adolescent drug users in jail. *The Journal of Adolescent Health, 15*(6), 457–463.

Malow, R. M., Kershaw, T., Sipsma, H., Rosenberg, R., & Dévieux, J. G. (2007). HIV preventive interventions for adolescents: a look back and ahead. *Current HIV/AIDS Reports, 4*(4), 173–180.

Mandara, J., Murray, C. B., & Bangi, A. K. (2003). Predictors of African American adolescent sexual activity: an ecological framework. *Journal of Black Psychology, 29*(3), 337–356.

Martino, S. C., Collins, R. L., Elliott, M. N., Strachman, A., Kanouse, D. E., & Berry, S. H. (2006). Exposure to degrading versus nondegrading music lyrics and sexual behavior among youth. *Pediatrics, 118*(2), e430–e41.

McCree, D. H., Wingood, G. M., DiClemente, R., Davies, S., & Harrington, K. F. (2003). Religiosity and risky sexual behavior in African-American adolescent females. *The Journal of Adolescent Health, 33*(1), 2–8.

Milhausen, R. R., Crosby, R., Yarber, W. L., DiClemente, R. J., Wingood, G. M., & Ding, K. (2003). Rural and nonrural African American high school students and STD/HIV sexual-risk behaviors. *American Journal of Health Behavior, 27*(4), 373–379.

Pedlow, C. T., & Carey, M. P. (2004). Developmentally appropriate sexual risk reduction interventions for adolescents: Rationale, review of interventions, and recommendations for research and practice. *Annals of Behavioral Medicine, 27*(3), 172–184.

Perkins, D. F., Luster, T., Villarruel, F., & Small, S. A. (1998). An ecological, risk-factor examination of adolescents' sexual activity in three ethnic groups. *Journal of Marriage and the Family, 60*(3), 660–673.

Perrino, T., González-Soldevilla, A., Pantin, H., & Szapocznik, J. (2000). The role of families in adolescent HIV prevention: A review. *Clinical Child and Family Psychology Review, 3*(2), 81–96.

Peterson, S. H., Wingood, G. M., DiClemente, R. J., Harrington, K., & Davies, S. (2007). Images of sexual stereotypes in rap videos and the health of African American female adolescents. *Journal of Women's Health, 16*(8), 1157–1164.

Putnam, R. D. (2000). *Bowling alone: the collapse and revival of American community*. New York: Touchstone.

Putnam, R. D. (2001). *Comprehensive Social Capital Index*. Retrieved December 20, 2007, from http://www.bowlingalone.com.

Putnam, R. D. (2002). *Bowling alone: the collapse and revival of American community*. New York: Simon and Schuster.

Remafedi, G. (1994). Cognitive and behavioral adaptations to HIV/AIDS among gay and bisexual adolescents. *The Journal of Adolescent Health, 15*(2), 142–148.

Replicating Effective Programs (REP) Plus. (2008). Centers for Disease Control and Prevention. Retrieved June 4, 2008, from http://www.cdc.gov/hiv/topics/prev_prog/rep/index.htm.

Roberts, D. F., Foehr, U. G., & Rideout, V. (2005). *Generation M: media in the lives of 8–18 year-olds*. Washington, DC: Kaiser Family Foundation Study.

Rotheram-Borus, M. J., Reid, H., & Rosario, M. (1994). Factors mediating changes in sexual HIV risk behaviors among gay and bisexual male adolescents. *American Journal of Public Health, 84*(12), 1938–1946.

Rotheram-Borus, M. J., Rosario, M., Reid, H., & Koopman, C. (1995). Predicting patterns of sexual acts among homosexual and bisexual youths. *The American Journal of Psychiatry, 152*(4), 588–595.

Rotheram-Borus, M., Song, J., Gwadz, M., Lee, M., Van Rossem, R., & Koopman, C. (2003). Reductions in HIV risk among runaway youth. *Prevention Science, 4*(3), 173–187.

Salazar, L. F., Crosby, R. A., DiClemente, R. J., Wingood, G. M., Lescano, C. M., Brown, L. K., et al. (2005). Self-esteem and theoretical mediators of safer sex among African American female adolescents: Implications for sexual risk reduction interventions. *Health Education and Behavior, 32*(3), 413–427.

Sionéan, C., DiClemente, R. J., Wingood, G. M., Crosby, R., Cobb, B. K., Harrington, K., et al. (2001). Socioeconomic status and self-reported gonorrhea among African American female adolescents. *Sexually Transmitted Diseases, 28*(4), 236–239.

Sogolow, E., Peersman, G., Semaan, S., Strouse, D., Lyles, C. M., & the HIV/AIDS Prevention Research Synthesis Project Team. (2002). The HIV/AIDS prevention research synthesis project: scope, methods, and study classification results. *Journal of Acquired Immune Deficiency Syndromes, 30*(Suppl. 1), S15–S29.

St. Lawrence, J. S., Brasfield, T. L., Jefferson, K. W., Alleyne, E., O'Bannon, R. E., & Shirley, A. (1995). Cognitive-behavioral intervention to reduce African American adolescents' risk for HIV infection. *Journal of Consulting and Clinical Psychology, 63*(2), 221–237.

Stanton, B., Li, X., Cottrell, L., & Kaljee, L. (2001). Early initiation of sex, drug-related risk behaviors, and sensation-seeking among urban, low-income African-American adolescents. *Journal of the National Medical Association, 93*(4), 129–138.

Stanton, B. F., Li, X., Ricardo, I., Galbraith, J., Feigelman, S., & Kaljee, L. (1996). A randomized, controlled effectiveness trial of an AIDS prevention program for low-income African-American youths. *Archives of Pediatrics and Adolescent Medicine, 150*(4), 363–372.

Stevenson, H. C., & Davis, G. (1994). Impact of culturally sensitive AIDS video education on the AIDS risk knowledge of African-American adolescents. *AIDS Education and Prevention, 6*(1), 40–52.

Stevenson, H. C., Gay, K. M., & Josar, L. (1995). Culturally sensitive AIDS education and perceived AIDS risk knowledge: reaching the "know-it-all" teenager. *AIDS Education and Prevention, 7*(2), 134–144.

Underwood, C., Hachonda, H., Serlemitsos, E., & Bharath-Kumar, U. (2006). Reducing the risk of HIV transmission among adolescents in Zambia: Psychosocial and behavioral correlates of viewing a risk-reduction media campaign. *Journal of Adolescent Health, 38*(1), 55. e1–55.e13.

Ward, L. M., Hansbrough, E., & Walker, E. (2005). Contributions of music video exposure to black adolescents' gender and sexual schemas. *Journal of Adolescent Research, 20*(2), 143–166.

Wills, T. A., Murry, V. M., Brody, G. H., Gibbons, F. X., Gerrard, M., Walker, C., et al. (2007). Ethnic pride and self-control related to protective and risk factors: test of the theoretical model for the strong African American families program. *Health Psychology, 26*(1), 50–59.

Wingood, G. M., DiClemente, R. J., Bernhardt, J. M., Harrington, K., Davies, S. L., Robillard, A., et al. (2003). A prospective study of exposure to rap music videos and African American female adolescents' health. *American Journal of Public Health, 93*(3), 437–439.

Wingood, G. M., DiClemente, R. J., Harrington, K., & Davies, S. L. (2002). Body Image and African American Females' Sexual Health. *Journal of Women's Health and Gender-Based Medicine, 11*(5), 433–439.

Wu, Y., Stanton, B. F., Galbraith, J., Kaljee, L., Cottrell, L., Li, X., et al. (2003). Sustaining and broadening intervention impact: a longitudinal randomized trial of 3 adolescent risk reduction approaches. *Pediatrics, 111*(1), e32–e38.

Chapter 10
HIV Behavioral Interventions for Heterosexual African American Men: A Critical Review of Cultural Competence

Kirk D. Henny, Kim M. Williams, and Jocelyn Patterson

In the United States, the rate of HIV infection transmitted through high-risk heterosexual contact is disproportionately higher among African American than among persons of other races or ethnicities (Centers for Disease Control and Prevention [CDC], 2009). Therefore, African American men who have sex[1] with women represent a critical target for behavioral interventions designed to reduce HIV incidence in this community. Among men in the United States, African Americans account for most of the HIV infections transmitted through high-risk heterosexual contact: African Americans, 63%; Hispanics, 21%; whites, 13% (CDC, 2009). In addition, nearly half (44%) of the recent HIV/AIDS cases among African American women, were acquired through high-risk heterosexual contact (CDC, 2009). Because most sexual-partner networks are intraracial (Laumann, Ellingson, Mahay, Paik, & Youm, 2004), interventions that reduce high-risk sexual behaviors among heterosexual AA men are likely to reduce HIV infection in the African American community.

In recent years, several HIV behavioral interventions have been developed specifically for heterosexual African American (AA) men or have been evaluated on the basis of samples composed primarily of these men. These interventions have focused on various subsets of heterosexual AA men, including adolescents and substance users. After a rigorous evaluation of the study implementation, design, analysis, and strength of the findings, some of these interventions have been designated by the Centers for Disease Control and Prevention (CDC) as evidence-based interventions (EBIs; i.e., interventions having strong evidence of efficacy in reducing

---

[1] We will use the term "heterosexual African American men" to refer to African American men who have sex with woman (MSW). The authors are aware of the differences between sexual identity (i.e., heterosexual) and sexual behavior (men who have sex with women). However, we will use heterosexual to refer to MSW in this chapter.

K.D. Henny (✉)
Division of HIV/AIDS Prevention, Centers for Disease Control and Prevention,
1600 Clifton Road NE, MS E-37, Atlanta, GA 30333, USA
e-mail: KHenny@cdc.gov

D.H. McCree et al. (eds.), *African Americans and HIV/AIDS*,
DOI 10.1007/978-0-387-78321-5_10,

HIV risk behaviors and the incidence of HIV/sexually transmitted infections (STIs)) (CDC, 2007b). EBIs are making inroads in the HIV epidemic among African Americans. The efficacy of both CDC EBIs and other studies depend on designing key components to yield desired outcomes (e.g., reducing risky behaviors and the incidence of STIs, including HIV). One intervention component that may enhance the efficacy of HIV behavioral interventions designed for African Americans is cultural competence (Beatty, Wheeler, & Gaiter, 2004; Scott, Gilliam, & Braxton, 2005; Torre & Estrada, 2001; Williams, 2003). Cultural competence refers to the ability of designers and facilitators to implement intervention components that are based on the cultural constructs of the target population (Torre & Estrada, 2001). This includes attending to both the intervention presentation, strategies designed to appeal to a particular cultural group, and the intervention content which intertwines culturally relevant messages into an intervention's activities (Wilson & Miller, 2003). Furthermore, cultural competency should carefully consider the cultural context associated with sex (Beatty et al., 2004; Scott et al., 2005) and sexual identity as distinct influences that uniquely interact with race and ethnic identity (Wilson & Miller, 2003). There is evidence that suggests such interventions may increase the likelihood of acceptance and efficacy for various target populations who may be resistant to HIV-related activities (Nobles, Goddard, & Gilbert, 2009). However, the literature includes only few analyses of the cultural competence of HIV behavioral interventions for heterosexual AA men.

The purpose of this chapter is to provide a critical review of HIV behavioral prevention interventions for heterosexual AA men (EBIs and other interventions) and the extent to which these interventions include elements of culturally competence. Specifically, we

1. Describe the criteria used to select interventions for this review and the measures used to analyze cultural competence.
2. Critically review the extent to which cultural competence was reflected in the evaluation reports of HIV behavioral interventions for heterosexual AA men.
3. Identify gaps and future directions regarding the use of cultural competence in HIV behavioral prevention interventions targeting heterosexual AA men.

Background

African Americans and HIV

The literature suggests that HIV-related disparities among African Americans are the byproduct of contextual factors that contribute to an increased risk for HIV acquisition and transmission (Adimora et al., 2008; Friedman, Cooper, & Osburne, 2009). These contextual factors include general health-related issues that negatively affect African American men. For example, African American men, compared with white men, have less access to health care services because many of them are underinsured or are not insured (DeNavas-Walt, Proctor, & Smith, 2007). In addition, it has been suggested that African American patients, compared with white patients, are more likely to receive health care from physicians with less training (Bach, Pham, Schrag, Tate, & Hargraves, 2004). Further, African American men who do access health care services are more likely to seek primary care at an emergency department than through ambulatory health services (e.g., a primary care clinic), which results in less favorable health outcomes (Shenolikar & Balkrishnan, 2007). Finally, compounding these structural factors is the fact that many African Americans are reluctant to seek medical care because of a commonly shared distrust of the government and public health entities (Bogart & Thorburn, 2005).

Given these barriers to health care, African Americans, compared with Whites, are less likely to receive a diagnosis of HIV in the early stages of infection and less likely to adhere to antiretroviral medication regimens (Milberg et al., 2001; Reif, Whetten, & Thielman, 2007; Schwarcz et al., 2007). Late HIV diagnosis and lack of adherence to treatment regimens contribute to higher viral loads and increased risk of transmitting HIV to sexual partners (Quinn et al., 2000).

Another contextual factor that contributes to the HIV risk factors of African American men is the higher prevalence of other STIs in the community. The rate of STIs is higher among African Americans than among Whites (CDC, 2007a) – a fact that is important because the presence of STIs increases the risk of acquiring and transmitting HIV (Fleming & Wasserheit, 1999). Therefore, because of the higher STI prevalence in the sexual partner pool, all African Americans (including heterosexual AA men) are at increased risk of HIV even when risky sexual behaviors such as sex with multiple partners are taken into account (Adimora & Schoenbach, 2002; Adimora et al., 2008).

Additional contextual factors associated with increased HIV risk among heterosexual AA men are high rates of incarceration (Raj et al., 2008) and poverty (Adimora & Schoenbach, 2002), which has been associated with risky sexual behaviors (Nattrass, 2009). The high rates of incarceration among African American men are exacerbated by disproportionately intensive policing patterns in African American neighborhoods. Incarceration further reduces opportunities to earn income, adds to a higher level of poverty, and disrupts social and sexual networks within the community (Abiona, Adefuye, Balogun, & Sloan, 2009; Friedman et al., 2009). All of these factors have the potential to increase HIV acquisition and transmission within the community.

Heterosexual AA Men and HIV. In addition to health-related challenges facing African American men in general, King and Williams (1995) suggested that the context of HIV risk among heterosexual AA men is significantly affected by cultural norms. Culture has been shown to play a significant role in the epidemiology of chronic diseases, including HIV (King & Williams, 1995; Larkey, Hecht, Miller, & Alatorre, 2004). For example, many heterosexual AA men adhere to the masculine ideology, black machismo, which is associated with a perspective that emphasizes male dominance over females (Pleck, Sonenstein, & Ku, 1993). Adherence to this ideology may result in overemphasis on financial wealth, sexual prowess, and physical dominance (Bowleg, 2004). Because the socioeconomic status of heterosexual AA men is disproportionately lower than that of men of other races/ethnicities, adherents of this ideology may attempt to compensate for the lack of material wealth by overemphasizing sexual prowess (Whitehead, 1997). This pattern may result in negative attitudes about condom use, inconsistent condom use, greater and multiple sexual partners (Pleck et al., 1993). Therefore, adherence to Black machismo may contribute to increased HIV transmission risk (e.g., through unprotected sex) particularly among African American men of lower socioeconomic status (Whitehead, 1997).

The emphasis on heterosexuality that is associated with black machismo includes the public rejection of activities associated with gay men or bisexuality (Diaz, 1998; Harris, 1995). Adherence to this ideology may lead to cultural norms that reduce the motivation to engage in HIV risk-reduction behaviors. On the other hand, understanding cultural norms can lead to the development of theory-based components of risk-reduction interventions that are specific to heterosexual AA men.

Cultural Competence. Cultural competence has emerged as an increasingly important component in the development and implementation of behavioral interventions (Cross, Bazron, Dennis, & Isaacs, 1989; Williams, 2003; Wilson & Miller, 2003; Wyatt & Williams, 2008). The US Department of Health and Human Services published the national standards for culturally and linguistically appropriate services (CLAS) (Office of Minority Health, 2001). CLAS established an overarching definition of cultural competence based on the work of Cross et al. (1989), and we used this work to guide our review. The definition of cultural competence is as follows:

> Cultural and linguistic competence is a set of congruent behaviors, attitudes, and policies that come together in a system, agency, or among professionals that enables effective work in cross-cultural situations. "Culture" refers to integrated patterns of human behavior that include the language, thoughts, communications, actions, customs, beliefs, values, and institutions of racial, ethnic, religious, or social groups. "Competence" implies having the capacity to function effectively as an individual and an organization within the context of the cultural beliefs, behaviors, and needs presented by consumers and their communities (adapted from Cross et al., 1989).

It is important to distinguish cultural sensitivity and cultural competence in the context of intervention development and implementation. Cultural sensitivity is a subset of cultural competence and refers to the tangible aspects of intervention development and implementation (Torre & Estrada, 2001). Examples of these tangible aspects are culturally sensitive materials and having a staff trained to be culturally competent (Torre & Estrada, 2001). Further, cultural competence includes a focus on building the intervention on cultural constructs and the normative beliefs of the target population (Torre & Estrada, 2001). Designing a culturally competent intervention requires tailoring theoretically sound risk-reduction interventions to the proper context of the populations targeted.

The following are specifics of the domains of cultural competence that are relevant to health-related services and interventions

- *Cultural sensitivity*: The regard for a participant's beliefs, values, and practices within a cultural context and the awareness that a service provider's background may influence professional practice, most notably communication (Lister, 1999).
- *Policies and procedures*: Includes the recruitment and retention of culturally competent staff that represent the races and ethnicities being served (Office of Minority Health, 2001).
- *Intervention and treatment models*: Models that include culturally and linguistically competent evaluation, treatment, and services; traditional beliefs;

and inclusive decision making (Substance Abuse and Mental Health Services Administration, 1998).

- *Monitoring, evaluation, and research*: Critical to cultural competence because these tasks highlight areas of progress and areas where improvement is needed. These tasks include organizational assessment and an evaluation of consumer satisfaction. Preparing and disseminating information about cultural competence is another arena for issues related to cultural competence. Before conducting an organizational assessment, the organization should conduct a community needs assessment to become more knowledgeable about the community it serves (Substance Abuse and Mental Health Services Administration, 1998).

These domains served as the foundation for our review of cultural competence. The operationalization of the concepts and the methods used to conduct the review are described later in this chapter.

Methods

Selection of Heterosexual AA Men Interventions

The criteria for selecting studies for review was that the interventions were evaluated with samples that were ≥50% male and ≥50% African American. There were two categories of interventions that were selected for this review. Studies that met these criteria were categorized into one of two groups: (a) CDC EBIs that targeted high-risk heterosexuals and (b) other relevant studies identified through a literature search.

A multi-phased search method was used to identify published reports (January 1998–May 2008) of interventions designed to reduce HIV risk behaviors among heterosexual AA men in the United States. This strategy was based on a search model created by CDC's Prevention Research Synthesis Project (Lyles, Crepaz, Herbst, & Kay, 2006). Both automated and manual search methods were used to find relevant studies. A comprehensive search of electronic bibliographic databases was performed on the following: AIDSLINE (1988 to discontinuation in December 2000), CINHAL, PsychINFO, EMBASE, SocioFile, and Science Citation and Social Sciences Citation indexes (January 1998 through December 2005). Standardized search terms were cross-referenced in three areas: (a) HIV, AIDS, or STD (sexually transmitted disease); (b) intervention evaluation; and (c) behavior or biologic outcomes (either HIV or STI infection). A manual search of over 30 key journals that regularly publish HIV or STD prevention research was conducted to locate additional intervention reports for the period January 2004 through May 2008.

After the initial search, interventions were selected if they explicitly targeted heterosexual AA men or if at least 50% of the sample were heterosexual AA men. For the articles that did not report exact percentages, we used marginal estimates to calculate the proportion of African American men in the sample. Marginal estimates were calculated by multiplying the percentages of men and African Americans in a study sample. If the product was 50% or larger, the intervention was included in the review. We acknowledge that these estimates can vary significantly; thus, the actual percentage of African American men in a sample may be below the 50% threshold. However, this approach allowed us to maximize the number of studies in the review and remain focused on the goal of providing an extensive review of the cultural competence of HIV behavioral interventions targeting heterosexual AA men.

Inclusion/Exclusion Criteria

Prevention intervention studies were included in this review if they met the following criteria: (a) were individual-, group-, community-, or structural-level interventions specifically designed to decrease sexual risk behaviors; (b) used a quasi-experimental or experimental design; (c) reported at least one post-intervention outcome that measured sexual risk behaviors or biologic outcomes; and (d) were delivered to a sample population that was at least 50% African American men. Sexual risk behavior variables were (a) unprotected vaginal intercourse or anal intercourse, (b) condom use; and the biologic variable was (c) incident HIV/STI.

Studies were excluded if the intervention was intended for youth (persons aged ≤18 years) or more than 50% of the sample were youth (differences in intervention activities for adults and those for adolescents would have made aggregate analysis inappropriate). Additionally, we excluded studies that explicitly targeted illicit drug users, men who have sex with men, or bisexual men because these populations are addressed in other chapters. A total of 20 HIV/STI behavioral prevention intervention studies met the study criteria and were included in the review (Table 10.1).

Critical Review of Included Studies

We reviewed each article to determine whether the descriptions of the following intervention elements included mention of cultural competence domains: (1) sample composition, (2) recruitment setting, (3) intervention materials, and (4) staffing.

Sample composition refers to the distribution of participants by specified demographic characteristics (e.g., race, gender) and is directly related to the cultural competence domain called monitoring, evaluation, and research (Office of Minority Health, 2001). This domain emphasizes the importance of assessing the needs of the community before delivering an intervention. The more homogenous the composition of the target population, the more the intervention should reflect the cultural norms of the population. The more heterogeneous the group, the larger the extent to which the intervention components should reflect the shared norms of subgroups while minimizing bias toward any specific subgroup. Although this concept may be

Table 10.1 Summary of Eligible HIV Behavioral Interventions studies for Heterosexual African American Men

Author (date), intervention	Recruitment/intervention setting/sample description	Study groups and assignment method	Intervention components/cultural and gender relevancy (materials, facilitator/participant matching)	Assessments period(s) and outcomes
Cohen et al. (1992), Doing Something Right	*Recruitment* STD clinic	One comparison group: (Standard care), one intervention group: (Group counseling)	*Comparison group* Routine care	*Assessment* Baseline and follow-up at 7–9 months
	Intervention STD Clinic	Assignment: Non-random (time of day)	*Intervention group* Group counseling	Source: Medical records
	Sample N=426, 65% AA male	Unit of delivery: Group	*Components* HIV knowledge, safer-sex negotiation skills, condom-use skills)	*Outcomes* New incidence of STIs lower among interv group compared with comparison group among men.
			Cultural and gender relevancy Ethnic and gender matching of facilitator (females only)	No differences were found among women.
El-Bassel et al. (2003), Project Connect	*Recruitment* Clinic (hospital-based)	One comparison group: (Education), two intervention groups: (Couples, women only)	*Comparison group:* HIV/STD education (video)	*Assessments* Baseline and 3-month follow-up
	Intervention Clinic (hospital-based)	Assignment: Random	*Intervention components (couples and women only)*	*Outcomes* Protected Sex Acts higher among interv groups compared to comparison groups
	Sample N=434 (217 couples), 55% AA, 50% male	Unit of delivery: Group)	Communication skills, safer-sex negotiation skills, problem-solving skills	UPS lower among interv groups compared to comparison groups
			Cultural and gender relevancy Gender matched facilitators for orientation sessions. Female facilitators for comparison group and women-only intervention group	No differences found between two intervention groups

(continued)

Table 10.1 (continued)

Author (date), intervention	Recruitment/intervention setting/sample description	Study groups and assignment method	Intervention components/cultural and gender relevancy (materials, facilitator/participant matching)	Assessments period(s) and outcomes
Kalichman et al. (1999), Project Nia	*Recruitment* STD Clinic *Intervention* STD Clinic *Sample* N=117, 100% AA male	One comparison group, one intervention group: (Motivational skills building) Assignment: Random Unit of delivery: Group	*Comparison group:* HIV prevention information, HIV Counseling and Testing, condom discussion *Intervention group components* Personal risk reduction plan, HIV knowledge, motivation to protect oneself and others,, self-esteem, condom use skills, assertiveness skills, problem-solving skills, safer sex negotiation skills *Cultural and gender relevancy* Culturally and gender specific materials. Gender matched facilitators	*Assessment* Baseline. 3 and 6 months *Outcomes* UPS lower among interv group compared with comparison group, condom use higher among interv group compared with comparison group, # sex ptrs lower among comparison group compared with interv group
Kamb (1998), Project RESPECT	*Recruitment* STD Clinics *Intervention* STD Clinic *Sample* N=5,758, 59% AA. 57% male, Assignment: Block randomization (computer-generated)	One comparison group: Routine HIV/STD information, two intervention groups: (Enhanced counseling, Brief counseling) Unit of delivery: Group	*Comparison groups* Typical STD clinic didactic messages promoting consistent condom use with all partners *Intervention group components* Same as above and adding…	*Assessments* Baseline and 3, 6, 9, 12-month follow-up *Outcomes* Increased condom use Shown between comparison and intervention groups at 3-month, less pronounced at 6-month; no differences at 9, 12-month

	Enhanced counseling: Information to encourage changes in self-efficacy, attitude, perceived norms about condom use. Goals for reducing risk were developed for each participant Intervention based on theory of reason action and social cognitive theory. Brief counseling: Information to assess actual and self-perceived HIV/STD risk and develop risk reduction plan (modeled after CDC plan) *Cultural and gender relevancy* None reported	Decreased reporting of new STIs between comparison and intervention groups – no differences between two intervention groups
NIMH (1998), Project "LIGHT"	*Recruitment* STD Clinic	One comparison group (Education), one intervention group (Small group sessions focusing on risk reduction skills-building)	*Comparison group* Education session	*Assessments* Baseline and 3, 6, 12-month follow-ups
	Intervention STD Clinic		*Intervention group components* Condom use skills, problem-solving skills, HIV knowledge, safer sex negotiation	*Outcomes* Reduced UPS, increased condom use, reduced STI incidence
	Sample $N=3{,}706$, *74% AA male*	Unit of delivery: Group	*Cultural and gender relevancy* None reported	

(continued)

Table 10.1 (continued)

Author (date), intervention	Recruitment/intervention setting/sample description	Study groups and assignment method	Intervention components/cultural and gender relevancy (materials, facilitator/participant matching)	Assessments period(s) and outcomes
Wenger et al. (1991), HIV Education and Testing	*Recruitment* STD clinic *Intervention* STD Clinic *Sample* N=256, Approximately 55% AA male	One comparison group: (AIDS education alone), one intervention group: (AIDS education and HIV test with results) Assignment: Random Unit of delivery: Individual	*Comparison group:* AIDS Education *Intervention group components* HIV knowledge and personal risk, condom use skills, and HIV C&T *Cultural and gender relevancy* None reported	*Assessments* Baseline and 2-month follow-up (via mail questionnaire) *Outcomes* Condom use with last partner increased for intervention group compared to comparison group
Wolitski et al. (2006), Project START	*Recruitment* Correctional *Intervention* Correctional *Sample* N=522, 52% AA male	One comparison group: (Standard Education), one intervention group: (Enhanced Intervention) Assignment: Random Unit of delivery: Individual	*Comparison group:* HIV knowledge, personalized risk reduction plans, referrals, skills training *Intervention group components* Personalized risk reduction plan, HIV knowledge, motivation to protect oneself and others, prevention case mgmt., harm reduction, problem solving skills *Cultural and gender relevancy* None reported	*Assessments* Baseline and 24-week follow-up *Outcomes* UPS lower among interv group compared with comparison

				Assessments
Berkman et al. (2006)	*Recruitment* Community-based establishment	One comparison group: (HIV education group), one intervention group (SexG-Brief group)	*Comparison group:* HIV education and condom use skills	Baseline and 6-month follow-up
	Intervention Community	Assignment: Random	*Intervention group components* HIV/STD knowledge and information, motivation and intention, condom use skills, decision-making and problem solving, safer sex negotiation skills	*Outcomes* Unprotected sex lower among intervention group compared with comparison group
	Sample N=92, 65% AA male	Unit of delivery: Group	*Cultural and gender relevancy* None reported	
Berkman et al. (2007)	*Recruitment* Psychiatric Outpatient Clinic	One comparison group: (Attention control), one Intervention Group (Enhanced SexG+booster group)	*Comparison group:* Money management, social skills	*Assessments* Baseline, 3M, 6M, 9M, 12M follow-ups (plus boosters)
	Intervention Psychiatric Outpatient Clinic	Assignment: Random	*Intervention group components* HIV&STD knowledge and information, motivation and intention, normative influence, condom use skills, decision-making/problem solving skills, social support, evaluation of personal goals	*Outcomes* Unprotected sex lower among intervention group compared with comparison group
	Sample N=149, 54% AA male	Unit of delivery: Individual	*Cultural and gender relevancy* Gender matched facilitators	Condom use higher among intervention group compared with comparison group

(continued)

Table 10.1 (continued)

Author (date), intervention	Recruitment/intervention setting/sample description	Study groups and assignment method	Intervention components/cultural and gender relevancy (materials, facilitator/participant matching)	Assessments period(s) and outcomes
Branson et al. (1998)	*Recruitment* STD Clinic	One comparison group: (Standard care), one intervention group: (Multisession group counseling)	*Comparison Group:* Standard HIV prevention counseling	*Assessments* Baseline and 12-month follow-up
		Assignment: Random	*Intervention group components* Addresses HIV knowledge, motivation to protect oneself and others, empowerment, personal responsibility, self-esteem, decision-making skills, condom use skills, needle-cleaning skills	*Outcomes* Condom use increased similarly in both interv and comparison group
	Intervention STD Clinic			Incident of new STIs lowered similarly in both interv and comparison group
	Sample N=964, 50% AA male	Unit of delivery: Group	*Cultural and gender relevancy* None reported	# of partners lowered similarly in both interv and comparison group

Crosby et al. (2009)	**Recruitment** STD Clinic	One comparison group: (Standard care), one intervention group (Lay Health Advisor)	*Comparison group:* Nurse-delivered messages regarding condom use knowledge, access to condoms	*Assessments* Baseline and 3-month follow-up
	Intervention STD Clinic	Assignment: Random Unit of delivery: Individual	*Intervention group components* Addresses knowledge/information; motivation/intention; self-efficacy for condom use, correct condom use skills, lubrication use, access to condoms and lubrication	*Outcomes* New incidence of STIs lower among interv group compared with comparison group among men
				Condom use at last sex higher among intervention group compared with comparison group
	Sample N = 266, 100% AA male		*Cultural and gender relevancy* Ethnic-matched facilitator. Culturally-competent facilitator (facilitator raised in catchment area). Gender-matched facilitator.	Fewer sex partners among intervention group compared with comparison group
				No significant differences in number of unprotected sex during last 3 months
Grinstead et al. (1999)	**Recruitment** Correctional	One comparison group: (Standard care), one intervention group (Pre-release HIV Prevention Interv.)	*Comparison group:* Access to HIV educational materials, informal access to peer educators	*Assessments* Baseline and 2–4 week follow-up
	Intervention Correctional	Assignment: Random	*Intervention group components* Addresses personal risk, personalized risk reduction plan, and HIV knowledge, HIV testing referrals, needle exchange	*Outcomes* Condom use during first sex encounter post-release higher among interv group than comparison group
	Sample N = 414, 51% AA male	Unit of delivery: Individual	*Cultural and gender relevancy* Gender matched facilitator (male)	

(continued)

Table 10.1 (continued)

Author (date), intervention	Recruitment/intervention setting/sample description	Study groups and assignment method	Intervention components/cultural and gender relevancy (materials, facilitator/participant matching)	Assessments period(s) and outcomes
Kalichman et al. (2005)	*Recruitment* STD Clinic	One comparison group, three intervention groups: (Motivational enhancement, Behavioral self-management and sexual communication, Full IMB model)	*Comparison group:* HIV education about transmission, risk factors, and disease processes	*Assessments* Baseline and 3, 6, 9-month follow-ups
			Intervention groups components (four groups)	*Outcomes* New STIs (decreased): Greatest reduction among men receiving full IMB model
	Intervention STD Clinic		*Motivational Enhancement:* Emphasizes personal behavioral change based on personal responsibility	Unprotected sex (decreased): Greatest reduction among men receiving IMB model
	Sample N=612, Approximately 59% AA male	Unit of delivery: Group	*Behavioral self-management and sexual communication:* Emphasize strategies to reduce high risk behavior and communicating safe sex practices with partner	Note: Motivational enhancement associated with more positive outcomes for women
			Full IMB model: Includes all components listed above	
			Video: used as part of intervention delivery	
			Cultural and gender relevancy Culturally and gender specific materials. Gender-matched facilitators	

	Recruitment / Intervention / Sample	Design	Intervention/Comparison components	Assessments / Outcomes
Lurigio et al. (1992)	*Recruitment* Adult Probation Depart. *Intervention* Adult Probation Dept. *Sample* N=99, Approximately 77% AA male	*One comparison group* Education: (Heart Disease), one intervention group: (HIV education) Assignment: Random Unit of delivery: Individual and group	*Comparison groups:* Heart disease prevention strategies *Intervention group components* HIV/STD knowledge and information, motivation and intention, condom use skills, skills using lubricants, cleaning needles; using dental dams *Cultural and gender relevancy* None reported	*Assessments* Baseline and (approximately) 1 month follow-up *Outcomes* Condom use
McMahon et al. (2001)	*Recruitment* Drug Treatment Program (VA Hospital) *Intervention* Drug Treatment Program (VA Hospital) *Sample* N = 149, 59% AA male	*One comparison group:* (Standard care), one intervention group (Cognitive-behavioral HIV risk reduction group) Assignment: Random Unit of delivery: Group	*Comparison group:* Basic information about HIV, HIV risk behaviors, and risk reduction practices *Intervention group components* HIV knowledge/information, condom use skills, safer sex negotiation skills, other sex-related communication skills, needle use skills, personal risk/vulnerability assessment *Cultural and gender relevancy* Cultural and gender specific materials	*Assessments* Baseline and 12-month follow-up *Outcomes* Increases in # of unprotected sex acts

(continued)

Table 10.1 (continued)

Author (date), intervention	Recruitment/intervention setting/sample description	Study groups and assignment method	Intervention components/cultural and gender relevancy (materials, facilitator/participant matching)	Assessments period(s) and outcomes
Maher et al. (2003)	*Recruitment* STD Clinic	One comparison group: (Routine counseling), one intervention group (Intensive counseling) Assignment: Random	*Comparison group* Standard of care (STD clinic):	*Assessments* Baseline and 12 months
	Intervention Community location convenient to participant		*Intervention group components* Personal risk assessment, HIV knowledge, motivation to protect oneself and others, attitude and beliefs about STDs, changing social norms, condom use skills, safer sex negotiation skills, alternatives to intercourse, future education and job plans	*Outcomes* STD incidence lower for interv group compared to comparison group
	Sample N=581, 100% AA male	Unit of delivery: Individual	*Cultural and gender relevancy* Intervention materials culturally specific. Counselors familiar and sensitive to cultural norms, values, and traditions	

O'Donnell et al. (1998)	*Recruitment* STD Clinic	One comparison group: (Standard care), two intervention groups: (Video viewing only, Video viewing followed by interactive group discussion)	*Comparison group:* Standard of care	*Assessments* Baseline and follow-up (average. 17 months) via clinical records
	Intervention STD Clinic *Sample* $N=2,004$, 62% AA male	Assignment: Proportionate random sampling plan (reflective of clinic patient population) Unit of delivery: Group	*Intervention groups components (two groups)* Video viewing only: Provided education about STDs and prevention, positive attitudes about condom use, and modeled strategies for condom use in various sexual relationships Video viewing/discussion: Addresses HIV knowledge, motivation to protect oneself and others, and attitudes toward condom use, safer sex negotiation skills, overcoming barriers to condom use *Cultural and gender relevancy* AA and gender specific materials (videos). Gender matched facilitator (men)	*Outcomes* New STIs lower among interv (video/discussion) group compared to comparison group

(continued)

Author (date), intervention	Recruitment/intervention setting/sample description	Study groups and assignment method	Intervention components/cultural and gender relevancy (materials, facilitator/participant matching)	Assessments period(s) and outcomes
O'Leary et al. (1998)	*Recruitment* STD Clinic	One comparison group: (Standard Care), one intervention group (Intensive HIV Risk Reduction)	*Comparison group:* Standard care	*Assessments* Baseline and 3 months
	Intervention STD Clinic	Assignment: Random	*Intervention group components* Addresses personal risk, HIV/STD knowledge, and condom use self-efficacy, correct condom use skills, negotiating safer sex skills	*Outcomes* # of sex ptrs lower among interv group # of unprotected sex acts lower overall between BL and 3M assessments in both groups
	Sample N=659.Approximately 54% AA male	Unit of delivery: Group	*Cultural and gender relevancy* None reported	
Ross et al. (2004)	*Recruitment* Community (by zip codes via street intercepts)	One comparison group, one intervention group	*Comparison group:* Provision of condoms at selected business venues	*Assessments* Baseline and 24 month follow-up
	Intervention Community	Assignment: two community samples defined by zip codes	*Intervention group components* Exposure to media campaign with messages encouraging syphilis testing, treatment, and condom use	*Outcomes* Condom use with last partner increased for interv group compared to comparison group
	Sample N=808, Approximately 50% AA male	Unit of delivery: Community	*Cultural and gender relevancy* Culturally specific materials (messages tailored to community based on formative work)	Note – Significant cross contamination of media campaign

| Susser et al. (1998) | *Recruitment*
Community Based Establishment

Intervention
Community

Sample
N=59, 58% AA male | One comparison group (Education), one intervention group (Sex, Games, and Videotape)

Assignment: Random

Unit of delivery: Group | *Comparison group:*
HIV/STD knowledge, condom use instructions

Intervention group components
HIV knowledge/information, condom use skills, safer sex negotiation skills, sex risk reduction self-efficacy, personal risk/vulnerability assessment

Cultural and gender relevancy
Ethnic-matched facilitators | *Assessments*
Baseline, 6, and 12-month follow-ups

Outcomes
Unprotected sex episodes lower in intervention group compared to comparison group |

straightforward in theory, practical implementation can be challenging and complex. It can be difficult to make an intervention culturally appropriate to various groups while maintaining fidelity to the intervention (Office of Minority Health, 2001).

The cultural competence domain called cultural sensitivity should be reflected in the settings chosen for recruitment (Office of Minority Health, 2001). That is, the recruitment settings should represent the target population's behavioral patterns in terms of geospatial movement (Office of Minority Health, 2001). The geospatial patterns of participants partly reflect their cultural norms and behavior (Lee, Moudon, & Courbois, 2006) (e.g., young African American men on college campuses vs. young African American men in correctional facilities). Therefore, recruitment should facilitate access to a subpopulation that has shared cultural experiences beyond demographic characteristics, and the intervention contents should reflect the cultural norms of the participants recruited at those locations. In our review, we examined the diversity of recruitment settings to determine whether they reflected an effort to include various subpopulations of heterosexual AA men.

The cultural sensitivity domain should also be reflected in intervention materials. This domain emphasizes regard for a participant's beliefs, values, and practices within a cultural context and awareness of how a provider's background may influence professional practice, most notably communication (Lister, 1999; Puebla-Fortier & Shaw-Taylor, 1999; Substance Abuse and Mental Health Services Administration, 1998). The definitions of *culturally appropriate materials* varied widely: some of the articles provided no definition; some provided an author-specific definition.

Culturally competent staffing reflects the domain emphasizing cultural competence in policies and procedures. This domain emphasizes the importance of recruiting and retaining culturally competent staff that represents the races/ethnicities of the populations served (Office of Minority Health, 2001). However, the interpretations of *culturally competent staff* range from simply matching the demographic backgrounds of participant and provider (e.g., by race or gender) to the completion of "sensitivity" courses by the intervention staff (Substance Abuse and Mental Health Services Administration, 1998). For this review, the measures of culturally competent staff included any mention of participant-facilitator matching (e.g., by race, gender, socioeconomic status) or reports that staff were specifically trained in cultural sensitivity. Our focus was the extent to which the articles included mention of culturally competent staff.

Results

Sample Composition

A total of 20 studies were eligible for this review: the samples of 3 were 100% African American men (presumably heterosexual AA men) (Crosby, DiClemente, Charnigo, Snow, Troutman, 2009; Kalichman, Cherry, & Browne-Sperling, 1999; Maher, Peterman, Osewe, Odusanya, & Scerba, 2003). The remaining studies reported separate proportions for race and gender but did not provide specific data on heterosexual AA men. Therefore, heterosexual AA men sample proportions were estimated from the reported univariate measures of race and gender (e.g., Kalichman et al., 2005; Lurigio, Petraitis, & Johnson, 1992). For some studies, identifying heterosexual AA men as the majority of the sample was straightforward, given that the samples were either all African American or all male (e.g., Berkman, Cerwonka, Sohler, & Susser, 2006; Branson, Peterman, Cannon, Ransom, & Zaidi, 1998). The fact that very few of the samples were 100% African American men (assumed to be heterosexual AA men) is consistent with the findings of other reviews (Neumann et al., 2002).

Recruitment Venues

Of the 20 interventions, 11 recruited participants from STD clinics. Other venues were correctional venues (e.g., jails, prisons, probation departments) (Grinstead, Zack, Faigeles, Grossman, & Blea, 1999; Lurigio et al., 1992; Wolitski & Project START Writing Group, 2006); community-based establishments (Berkman et al., 2006; Susser et al., 1998); hospital-based clinics (El-Bassel et al., 2003); outpatient psychiatric clinics (Berkman et al., 2007); drug treatment centers (McMahon, Malow, Jennings, & Gomez, 2001); and street intercepts (Ross, Chatterjee, & Leonard, 2004).

Culture- and Gender-Specific Materials

Our review includes any reported use of culture- or gender-specific materials reflective of heterosexual AA men. The concept "gender-specific materials" was operationalized as any report of the use of intervention materials that were tailored to, or developed specifically for, male populations.

Six studies reported use of culture-specific materials (Kalichman et al., 1999, 2005; Maher et al., 2003; McMahon et al., 2001; O'Donnell, O'Donnell, San Doval, Duran, & Labes, 1998; Ross et al., 2004). Of these six interventions, two were delivered to sample populations composed entirely of heterosexual AA men (Kalichman et al., 1999; Maher et al., 2003), and four reported the use of electronic or mass media campaigns (Kalichman et al., 1999, 2005; O'Donnell et al., 1998; Ross et al., 2004). In addition to reporting culturally specific materials, four studies reported the use of gender-specific materials (Kalichman et al., 1999, 2005; McMahon et al., 2001; O'Donnell et al., 1998).

Culturally Competent Facilitators

Of the 20 interventions reviewed, 3 reported facilitator-participant matching by race or ethnicity (Cohen, MacKinnon, Dent, Mason, & Sullivan, 1992; Crosby et al., 2009; Susser et al., 1998), and six studies reported matching by gender (Berkman et al., 2007;

Crosby et al., 2009; Grinstead et al., 1999; Kalichman et al., 1999, 2005; O'Donnell et al., 1998). The Cohen et al. (1992) study was not included among studies with facilitators matched by gender because the authors reported only a female facilitator (i.e., gender-matched only for female participants). None of the studies reported training in cultural competence.

Limitations of Review

Our review had several limitations. A major limitation was the lack of reporting of all cultural competence domains in the interventions reviewed. This finding is particularly applicable to the review of culturally specific materials and participant-facilitator matching by race or gender. The lack of consistency in the reporting of sociodemographic and sexual behavior data further limited our review. Although many of the studies targeted heterosexual participants, some of male participants who identified themselves as heterosexual may also have had sex with other men (i.e., bisexual). Therefore, some of the studies may have included studies in which some of the men were bisexual because not all the studies explicitly reported the gender of sex partners in addition to, or in lieu of, sexual orientation.

Discussion

In spite of the limitations, our review yielded information that can provide some direction for future research. The efficacy of behavioral prevention interventions is dependent on many factors related to the intervention design and implementation (Lyles et al., 2006). Because evidence suggests that cultural competence may one of the key factors (Office of Minority Health, 2001), this review assessed the extent to which cultural competence domains were addressed in the selected studies.

Although cultural competence is not the sole determining factor in developing efficacious interventions for heterosexual AA men, cultural competence may be a particularly important facet of interventions targeting heterosexual AA men (Office of Minority Health, 2001).

Sample Composition

A sizable void was the lack of explicit reporting of race/sex proportions of the samples. This information would markedly enhance the feasibility of performing either primary (e.g., evaluation studies) or secondary review (e.g., meta-analyses) of cultural competence for heterosexual AA men interventions. The reporting of race/sex proportions could include various cross-tabulations of the demographic characteristics that are associated with HIV risk (e.g., homosexual or bisexual behavior, injection drug use). The reporting of these cross-tabulations could increase the number of cultural competence review of interventions targeting heterosexual AA men and thus lead to the development of more efficacious risk-reduction interventions for this population

Notwithstanding the limited information about sample composition, most of the selected studies included populations that were heterogeneous in terms of race or gender. An intervention delivered to a heterogeneous group can certainly be culturally competent (e.g., Cohen et al., 1992; El-Bassel et al., 2003). The caveat, however, is that to design intervention components that reflect all the groups, one must first have adequate information about each group. Developing interventions for heterogeneous populations without proper formative work to ensure cultural competence may decrease the potential efficacy of the intervention. If little is known about any distinct group, then extensive formative work or developing interventions targeting a more homogenous group could be the best initial course of action.

Recruitment Venues

Of 20 studies, 11 recruited participants from STD clinics. Accessibility to persons engaging in high-risk sexual behaviors is an important reason for recruiting in STD clinics. Furthermore, STD clinics have educational materials and personnel that can complement and simplify the development and implementation of interventions. However, HIV behavioral interventions targeting heterosexual AA men should not limit recruitment to STD clinics. Expanding recruitment venues will allow access to at-risk heterosexual AA men who are not accessible through traditional recruitment settings such as STD clinics. Additionally, heterosexual AA men participants recruited from STD clinics may represent a subgroup whose health-care–seeking behavior differs from that of other African American men (Agho & Lewis, 2001; Farkas, Marcella, & Rhoads, 2000). Further, the literature suggests that higher-income persons are more likely to seek STI treatment from private physicians (Brackbill, Sternberg, & Fishbein, 1999). Therefore, risk-reduction interventions designed for STD clinic populations may not be culturally relevant or efficacious for higher-income heterosexual AA men who may be at risk for HIV. Developing HIV behavioral interventions for higher-income heterosexual AA men may be an important strategy for reducing HIV incidence among African Americans in general. Although low income is associated with increased HIV risk (Adler, 2006), racial disparities in HIV incidence exist even when analysis is adjusted for income (Kraut-Becher et al., 2008).

Culture- and Gender-Specific Materials

The use of cultural-specific materials reflects the core domain called cultural sensitivity (Lister, 1999). For interventions targeting heterosexual AA men, cultural-specific materials should relate to this population both as African Americans (i.e., cultural background) and men (i.e., gender). As stated earlier, cultural-specific materials may include text or images that are tailored to the cultural background of participants.

The use of gender-specific materials is particularly important for HIV prevention targeting heterosexual AA men, given the influence of masculine ideology in this population (Bowleg, 2004; Whitehead, 1997). Only 4 out of 20 studies reported use of gender-specific materials.

Culturally Competent Facilitators

Only three studies reported participant-facilitator matching by race, six reported matching by gender, and none reported staff training in cultural competence. The inclusion of culturally competent facilitators and support staff is a major emphasis in the CLAS report. Cultural competence could be achieved through training. The goal of cultural competence training is to ensure that facilitators are knowledgeable and respectful of the participants' cultural norms (as defined partly by their race/ ethnicity and gender) so that facilitator-participant interactions can be based on common understanding and respect. Respect from facilitators and intervention staff may be particularly relevant in interventions targeting heterosexual AA men because many African Americans distrust public health entities (Bogart & Thorburn, 2005). The training of culturally competent facilitators could symbolize an effort by researchers to change that distrust felt by many African Americans (King & Williams, 1995).

The assessments of participant-facilitator matching by race/ethnicity and gender are mixed (Huddy et al., 1997; Jemmott, Jemmott, Fong, & McCaffree, 1999; Pollner, 1998; Prewett-Livingston, Field, Veres, & Lewis, 1996; Rhodes, 1994). But the guiding principle of cultural competence is to develop and implement interventions that add the cultural constructs (i.e., measures of cultural-specific behaviors) of the target population (Torre & Estrada, 2001). Participant-facilitator matching (as well as cultural competence training) may help facilitate that process. Heterosexual AA men participating in HIV prevention interventions can benefit from the presence of heterosexual AA men professional facilitators who can combine their technical expertise and their cultural background to enhance the intervention delivery and in some instances, serve as role models.

Recommendations

This critical review has led to several recommendations for researchers and practitioners to consider in developing HIV behavioral interventions targeting heterosexual African American men. Authors are recommended to report elements related to cultural competence. Overall, it is difficult to determine the cultural competence level of interventions without the reporting of key measures related to the major domains aforementioned in the chapter. It is also recommended that HIV prevention efforts targeting heterosexual AA men include men who are at *elevated risk* of HIV, not simply those who are at high risk of HIV. *Elevated risk* may be defined in various ways. Analyses of social networks indicate that the degrees of separations pertaining to sexual contacts between persons at high risk and persons at low risk are relatively small (Friedman et al., 1997; Yuom & Laumann, 2002). For example, a person who is considered at low risk at the time of an intervention may have been at high risk a year earlier or may be at high risk a year later (depending on the operational definitions used by evaluators). Given the disproportionate prevalence of HIV/STIs within many African American sexual networks, a broader scope for heterosexual AA men at-risk groups is needed to compensate for disease prevalence. One strategy that could assist in this effort is to increase formative research activities that include recruitment from nontraditional settings. Such formative activities could be conducted at relatively low cost and could also help to develop innovative strategies for more efficiently recruiting hard-to-access at-risk heterosexual AA men.

We further recommend expanding the types of heterosexual AA men included in HIV behavioral intervention trials to encourage the creation of interventions that are more specifically tailored to the cultural norms of various subgroups. These subgroups may be defined in terms of the many differences that have implications for HIV risk (e.g., education, religious beliefs, socioeconomic status).

In addition, we recommend cultural competence training for facilitators. According to the principles reported in the CLAS report, this component has the potential to increase the efficacy of interventions designed for heterosexual AA men.

Finally, developing culturally competent interventions for heterosexual AA men will require the inclusion of culturally relevant materials. For heterosexual AA men, this can be facilitated by the use of intervention materials that reflect both race and gender. One possible approach is the use of social marketing campaigns that incorporate culturally specific images. Social marketing campaigns, which are community-level interventions, can directly or indirectly influence the knowledge, attitudes, and behaviors of an entire community (Wolitski et al., 2006). Studies have shown that African Americans do stigmatize persons living with HIV/AIDS (Herck & Capitanio, 1993). Perhaps more passive approaches delivered to large numbers of persons, such as social marketing campaigns, may simultaneously help reduce stigma and raise HIV/AIDS awareness without singling out participants in a group setting.

Application of the principles regarding cultural competence as outlined in the CLAS report could represent a step forward in improving and increasing the number of efficacious interventions available to heterosexual AA men. The HIV/AIDS epidemic among African Americans is in a state of crisis. In lieu of a vaccine or cure, all strategies and approaches must be considered to reduce the incidence of the disease. In pursuit of this public health effort, prevention strategies and activities should be imbedded in the reality of African American lives, particularly the lives of heterosexual AA men. If strategies and approaches are applied without regard for the cultural context, the acceptance and sustainability of prevention activities will be attenuated. Emphasizing cultural competence provides an opportunity to integrate larger segments of heterosexual AA men as partners instead of vectors and victims in fighting HIV.

References

Abiona, T. C., Adefuye, A. S., Balogun, J. A., & Sloan, P. E. (2009). Relationship between incarceration frequency and human immunodeficiency virus risk behaviors of African American inmates. *Journal of the National Medical Association, 101*, 308–315.

Adimora, A. A., & Schoenbach, V. (2002). Contextual factors and the black-white disparity in heterosexual HIV transmission. *Epidemiology, 13*, 707–712.

Adimora, A., Schoenbach, V., Martinson, F., Coyne-Beasley, T., Doherty, I., Stancil, T., et al. (2008). Heterosexually transmitted HIV infection among African Americans in North Carolina. *Journal of Acquired Immune Deficiency Syndromes, 41*, 616–623.

Adler, N. E. (2006). Overview of health disparities. In G. E. Thompson, F. Mitchell, & M. Williams (Eds.), *Examining the health disparities research plan of the National Institutes of Health: Unfinished business* (pp. 129–188). Washington, DC: National Academic Press.

Agho, A. O., & Lewis, M. A. (2001). Correlates of actual and perceived knowledge of prostate cancer among African Americans. *Cancer Nursing, 24*, 165–171.

Bach, P. B., Pham, H. H., Schrag, D., Tate, R. C., & Hargraves, J. L. (2004). Primary care physicians who treat blacks and whites. *New England Journal of Medicine, 351*, 575–584.

Beatty, L., Wheeler, D., & Gaiter, J. (2004). HIV prevention research for African Americans: Current and future directions. *Journal of Black Psychology, 31*, 40–58.

Berkman, A., Cerwonka, E., Sohler, N., & Susser, E. (2006). A randomized trial of a brief HIV risk reduction intervention for men with severe mental illness. *Psychiatric Services, 57*, 407–409.

Berkman, A., Pilowsky, D. J., Zybert, P. A., Herman, D. B., Conover, S., Lemelle, S., et al. (2007). HIV prevention with severely mentally ill men: A randomised controlled trial. *AIDS Care, 19*, 579–588.

Bogart, L., & Thorburn, S. (2005). Are HIV/AIDS conspiracy beliefs a barrier to HIV prevention among African Americans? *Journal of Acquired Immune Deficiency Syndromes, 38*, 213–218.

Bowleg, L. (2004). Love, sex, and masculinity in sociocultural context: HIV concerns and condom use among African American men in heterosexual relationships. *Men and Masculinities, 7*(2), 166–186.

Brackbill, R. M., Sternberg, M. R., & Fishbein, M. (1999). Where do people go for treatment of sexually transmitted diseases? *Family Planning Perspectives, 31*(1), 10–15.

Branson, B. M., Peterman, T., Cannon, R., Ransom, R., & Zaidi, A. (1998). Group counseling to prevent sexually transmitted disease and HIV: A randomized controlled trial. *Sexually Transmitted Diseases, 25*, 553–560.

Centers for Disease Control and Prevention. (2007a). *Sexually transmitted disease surveillance, 2006.* Washington, DC: US Department of Health and Human Services, Centers for Disease Control and Prevention.

Centers for Disease Control and Prevention. (2007b). *Updated compendium of evidence-based interventions.* Retrieved January 14, 2008, from http://www.cdc.gov/hiv/topics/research/prs/evidence-based-interventions.htm

Centers for Disease Control and Prevention. (2009). *HIV/AIDS surveillance report, 2007* (Vol. 19, pp. 17–22). Atlanta, GA: U.S. Department of Health and Human Services, Centers for Disease Control and Prevention.

Cohen, D., MacKinnon, D., Dent, C., Mason, H., & Sullivan, E. (1992). Group counseling at STD clinics to promote use of condoms. *Public Health Reports, 107*(6), 727–731.

Crosby, R., DiClemente, R., Charnigo, R., Snow, G., & Troutman, A. (2009). Evaluation of a lay health advisor model risk reduction intervention for promoting safer sex among heterosexual African American men newly diagnosed with an STD: A randomized controlled trial. *American Journal of Public Health, 99*, S96–S103.

Cross, T., Bazron, B., Dennis, K., & Isaacs, M. (1989). *Towards a culturally competent system of care* (Vol. 1). Washington, DC: Georgetown University Child Development Center.

DeNavas-Walt, C., Proctor, B., & Smith, J. (2007). *Income, poverty, and health insurance coverage in the United States: 2006.* Washington, DC: U.S. Government Printing Office.

Diaz, R. (1998). *Latino gay men and HIV: Culture, sexuality and risk behavior.* New York: Routledge.

El-Bassel, N., Witte, S., Gilbert, L., Wu, E., Chang, M., Hill, J., et al. (2003). The efficacy of a relationship-based HIV/STD prevention program for heterosexual couples. *American Journal of Public Health, 93*(6), 963–969.

Farkas, A., Marcella, S., & Rhoads, G. G. (2000). Ethnic and racial differences in prostate cancer incidence and mortality. *Ethnicity and Disease, 10*(1), 69–75.

Fleming, D., & Wasserheit, J. (1999). From epidemiological synergy to public health policy and practice: The contribution of other sexually transmitted diseases to sexual transmission of HIV infection. *Sexually Transmitted Infections, 75*, 3–17.

Fortier, J. P. and shaw, T. (1999). Cutural and linguistic competence students and Research Ayerdu Project Part One: Reconerdutirs for National Standards. Resewies for cross Cultural Health Care and the Center for the Advancement of Health.

Friedman, S. R., Cooper, H. L. F., & Osburne, A. H. (2009). Structural and social contexts of HIV risk among African Americans. *American Journal of Public Health, 99*(6), 1002–1008.

Friedman, S. R., Neaigus, A., Jose, B., Curtis, R., Goldstein, M., Ildefonso, G., et al. (1997). Sociometric risk networks and risk for HIV infection. *American Journal of Public Health, 87*(8), 1289–1296.

Grinstead, O. A., Zack, B., Faigeles, B., Grossman, N., & Blea, L. (1999). Reducing postrealease HIV risk among male prison inmates: A peer-led intervention. *Criminal Justice and Behavior, 26*, 453–465.

Harris, S. (1995). Psychosocial development and Black male masculinity: Implications for counseling economically disadvantaged African American male adolescents. *Journal of Counseling and Development, 73*(3), 279–287.

Herck, G. M., & Capitanio, J. P. (1993). Public reactions to AIDS in the United States: A second decade of stigma. *American Journal of Public Health, 83*, 574–577.

Huddy, L., Billig, J., Bracciodieta, J., Hoeffler, L., Moynihan, P. J., & Pugliani, P. (1997). The effect of interviewer gender on the survey response. *Political Behavior, 19*(3), 197–220.

Jemmott, J., Jemmott, L., Fong, G., & McCaffree, K. (1999). Reducing HIV risk-associated sexual behavior among African American adolescents: Testing the generality of intervention effects. *American Journal of Community Psychology, 27*(2), 161–187.

Kalichman, S. C., Cherry, C., & Browne-Sperling, F. (1999). Effectiveness of a video-based motivational skills-building HIV risk-reduction intervention for inner-city African American men. *Journal of Counseling and Clinical Psychology, 67*, 959–966.

Kalichman, S. C., Weinhardt, L., Benotsch, E., Zweben, A., Bjodstrup, B., Cain, D., et al. (2005). Experimental components analysis of brief theory-based HIV-AIDS risk reduction counseling for sexually transmitted infection patients. *Health Psychology, 24*, 198–208.

King, G., & Williams, D. (1995). Race and health: A multidimensional approach to African American health. In B. C. Amick, S. Levine, A. R. Tarlov, & D. C. Walsh (Eds.), *Society and health* (pp. 93–130). New York: Oxford University Press.

Kraut-Becher, J., Eisenberg, M., Voytek, C., Brown, T., Metzger, D., & Aral, S. (2008). Examining racial disparities in HIV: Lessons from sexually transmitted infections research. *Journal of Acquired Immune Deficiency Syndromes, 47*(Suppl. 1), S20–S27.

Larkey, L. K., Hecht, M. L., Miller, K., & Alatorre, C. (2004). Hispanic cultural norms for health-seeking behaviors in the face of symptoms. *Health Education Behavior, 28*, 65–80.

Laumann, E. O., Ellingson, S., Mahay, J., Paik, A., & Youm, Y. (2004). *The sexual organization of the city*. Chicago, IL: Chicago University Press.

Lee, C., Moudon, A. V., & Courbois, J. Y. (2006). Built environment and behavior: Spatial sampling using parcel data. *Annals of Epidemiology, 16*(5), 387–394.

Lister, P. (1999). A taxonomy for developing cultural competence. *Nurse Education Today, 19*(4), 313–318.

Lurigio, A., Petraitis, J., & Johnson, B. R. (1992). Joining the front line against HIV: An education program for adult probationers. *AIDS Education and Prevention, 4*, 205–218.

Lyles C., Crepaz N., Herbst J., Kay L., for the HIV/AIDS Prevention Research Synthesis (PRS) Team. (2006). Evidence-based HIV behavioral prevention from the perspective of CDC's HIV/AIDS Prevention Research Synthesis Team. *AIDS Education and Prevention, 18*(Suppl. A), 21–31.

Maher, J. E., Peterman, T. A., Osewe, P. L., Odusanya, S., & Scerba, J. R. (2003). Evaluation of a community-based organization's intervention to reduce the incidence of sexually transmitted diseases: A randomized, controlled trial. *Southern Medical Journal, 96*, 248–253.

McMahon, R. C., Malow, R. M., Jennings, T. E., & Gomez, C. (2001). Effects of a cognitive-behavioral HIV prevention intervention among HIV negative male substance abusers in VA residential treatment. *AIDS Education and Prevention, 13*, 91–107.

Milberg, J., Sharma, R., Scott, F., Conviser, R., Marconi, K., & Parham, D. (2001). Factors associated with delays in accessing HIV primary care in rural Arkansas. *AIDS Patient Care and STDs, 15*(10), 527–532.

Nattrass, N. (2009). Poverty, sex, and HIV. *AIDS and Behavior, 13*(5), 833–840.

Neumann, M., Johnson, W., Semaan, S., Flores, S., Peersman, G., Hedges, L., et al. (2002). Review and meta-analysis of HIV prevention intervention research for heterosexual adult populations in the United States. *Journal of Acquired Immune Deficiency Syndromes, 30*(Suppl. 1), S106–S117.

Nobles, W., Goddard, L., & Gilbert, D. (2009). Culturecology, women, and African-centered HIV prevention. *Journal of Black Psychology, 35*, 228–246.

O'Donnell, C., O'Donnell, L., San Doval, A., Duran, R., & Labes, K. (1998). Reductions in STD infections subsequent to an STD clinic visit: Using video-based patient education to supplement provider interactions. *Sexually Transmitted Diseases, 25*, 161–168.

O'Leary, A., Ambrose, T. K., Raffaelli, M., Maibach, E., Jemmott, L. S., Jemmott, J. B., et al. (1998). Effects of an HIV risk reduction project on sexual risk behavior of low-income STD patients. *AIDS Education and Prevention, 10*, 483–492.

Office of Minority Health. (2001). *National standards for culturally and linguistically appropriate services in health care – Final report*. Retrieved March 22, 2009, from http://www.omhrc.gov/assets/pdf/checked/finalreport.pdf

Pleck, J., Sonenstein, F., & Ku, L. (1993). Masculinity ideology: Its impact on adolescent males' heterosexual relationships. *Journal of Social Issues, 49*(3), 11–29.

Pollner, M. (1998). The effects of interviewer gender in mental health interviews. *Journal of Nervous and Mental Disease, 186*, 369–373.

Prewett-Livingston, A., Field, H., Veres, J., & Lewis, P. (1996). Effects of race on interview ratings in a situational panel interview. *Journal of Applied Psychology, 81*, 178–186.

Quinn, T. C., Wawer, M. J., Sewankambo, N., Serwadda, D., Li, C., Wabwire-Mangen, F., et al. (2000). Viral load and heterosexual transmission of human immunodeficiency virus type 1. *New England Journal of Medicine, 34*, 921–929.

Raj, A., Reed, E., Santana, M., Welles, S., Horsburgh, C., Flores, S., et al. (2008). History of incarceration and gang involvement are associated with recent sexually transmitted disease/HIV diagnosis in African American men. *Journal of Acquired Immune Deficiency Syndromes, 47*, 131–134.

Reif, S., Whetten, K., & Thielman, N. (2007). Association of race and gender with use of antiretroviral therapy among HIV-infected individuals in the southeastern United States. *Southern Medical Journal, 100*(8), 775–781.

Rhodes, P. (1994). Race-of-interviewer effects: A brief comment. *Sociology, 28*, 547–558.

Ross, M., Chatterjee, N., & Leonard, L. (2004). A community level syphilis prevention programme: Outcome data from a controlled trial. *Sexually Transmitted Infections, 80*(2), 100–104.

Schwarcz, S., Weinstock, H., Louie, B., Kellogg, T., Douglas, J., LaLota, M., et al. (2007). Characteristics of persons with recently acquired HIV infection: Application of the serologic testing algorithm for recent HIV seroconversion in 10 US cities. *Journal of Acquired Immune Deficiency Syndromes, 44*(1), 112–115.

Scott, K. D., Gilliam, A., & Braxton, K. (2005). Culturally competent HIV prevention strategies for women of color in the United States. *Health Care for Women International, 26*, 17–45.

Shenolikar, R., & Balkrishnan, R. (2007). Racial differences in emergency room visits associated with medication use in Medicaid enrollees with type 2 diabetes. *Value in Health, 10*(3), A17.

Substance Abuse and Mental Health Services Administration. (1998). *Cultural competence performance measures for managed behavioral healthcare programs.* Substance Abuse and Mental Health Services Administration. Retrieved March 23, 2009, from http://mentalhealth. samhsa.gov/publications/allpubs/SMA00-3457/default.asp

Susser, E., Valencia, E., Berkman, A., Sohler, N., Conover, S., Torres, J., et al. (1998). Human immunodeficiency virus sexual risk reduction in homeless men with mental illness. *Archives of General Psychiatry, 55*, 266–272.

Torre, A., & Estrada, A. (2001). *Mexican Americans and health.* Tucson, AZ: University of Arizona Press.

Wenger, N., Linn, L., Epstein, M., & Shapiro, M. (1991). Reduction of high risk sexual behavior among heterosexuals undergoing HIV antibody testing: A randomized clinical trial. *American Journal of Public Health, 81*, 1580–1585.

Whitehead, T. (1997). Urban low-income African American men, HIV/AIDS, and gender identity. *Medical Anthropology Quarterly, 11*(4), 411–447.

Williams, P. B. (2003). HIV/AIDS case profile of African Americans. Guidelines for ethnic-specific health promotion, education, and risk reduction activities for African Americans. *Family Community Health, 26*, 289–306.

Wilson, B. D. M., & Miller, R. L. (2003). Examining strategies for culturally grounded HIV prevention: A review. *AIDS Education and Prevention, 15*, 184–202.

Wolitski, R., Henny, K., Lyles, C., Purcell, D., Carey, J., Crepaz, N., et al. (2006). Evolution of HIV/AIDS prevention programs – United States, 1982–2006. *Morbidity and Mortality Weekly Report, 55*(21), 597–603.

Wolitski, R., & Project START Writing Group. (2006). Relative efficacy of a multisession sexual risk – reduction intervention for young men released from prisons in 4 states. *American Journal of Public Health, 96*, 1854–1861.

Wyatt, G. E., & Williams, J. K. (2008). African-American sexuality and HIV/AIDS: Recommendations for future research. *Journal of the National Medical Association, 100*, 44–48.

Yuom, Y., & Laumann, E. O. (2002). Social network effects on the transmission of sexually transmitted diseases. *Sexually Transmitted Diseases, 29*(11), 689–697.

Chapter 11
HIV Prevention for Heterosexual African-American Women

Gina M. Wingood and Ralph J. DiClemente

Epidemiology of HIV/AIDS Among African-American Women

Early in the epidemic, HIV infection and AIDS were diagnosed among relatively few women and female adolescents. Currently, women account for more than 25% of all new HIV/AIDS diagnoses. Historically, African-American women have been disproportionately affected by the HIV epidemic. In 2002, the most recent year for which data are available, HIV infection was the leading cause of death for African-American women 25–34 years old; the third leading cause of death for African-American women aged 35–44 years old and the fourth leading cause of death for African-American women 45–54 years old. In this same year, HIV infection was the fifth leading cause of death among all women 35–44 years of age and the six leading cause of death among all women aged 25–34 year old. The only diseases causing more death of women were cancer and heart disease (Anderson & Smith, 2005).

As of 2004, among the 123,405 women living with HIV/AIDS 64% were African-American (Centers for Disease Control and Prevention [CDC], 2005a). While African-American women represent about 13% of all US women (CDC, 2005a, b), in 2004 they accounted for 68% of the estimated total of AIDS diagnoses. African-American women's vulnerability to AIDS is also illustrated by the fact that in 2004, the rate of AIDS diagnoses for African-American women (48.2/100,000) was approximately 23 times the rate for white women (2.1/100,000) and 4 times the rate for Hispanic women (11.1/100,000) (CDC, 2004). Unfortunately, young African-American women are also at risk of HIV. According to a 1998 CDC study of Job Corps entrants aged 16–21 years, African-American women in this study were seven times as likely as white women and eight times as likely as Hispanic women to be HIV-positive (Valleroy, MacKellar, Karon, Janssen, & Hayman, 1998).

G.M. Wingood (✉)
SCD, MPH is the Agnes Moore Endowed Faculty in HIV/AIDS Research,
Emory University, Rollins School of Public Health, 1518 Clifton Rd, Room 556,
Atlanta, GA 30322, USA
e-mail: gwingoo@sph.emory.edu

D.H. McCree et al. (eds.), *African Americans and HIV/AIDS*,
DOI 10.1007/978-0-387-78321-5_11, © Springer Science+Business Media, LLC 2010

Heterosexually acquire HIV/AID is the predominant route of transmission for African-American women. Among African-American women diagnosed with HIV/ AID during 2001–2004, 78% contracted the infection via heterosexual contact (Stephenson, 2000). Unfortunately, African-American women are being devastated by the HIV/AIDS epidemic. Greater examination of the risk factors and exposures increasing their vulnerability is warranted.

Correlates of HIV Risk among African-American Women

Nearly, one in four African-Americans live in poverty (United States Census Bureau, 2003). Socioeconomic problems associated with poverty including having a limited education (Anderson, Brackbill, & Mosher, 1996; Stephenson, 2000), having a lower income (Peterson et al., 1992), being underemployed (Wingood & DiClemente, 1998a, b, c), having limited access to high-quality health care (Diaz et al., 1994) consuming alcohol (Graves & Hines, 1997; Wingood & DiClemente, 1998a, b, c) and, using non-injection drugs (Edlin et al., 1994; Fullilove, Fullilove, Bowser, & Goss, 1990) have all been associated with increased HIV risk behaviors among African-American women. Other individual-level factors associated with African-American women's risk of HIV include having personal attitudes and belief nonsupportive of safer sex (Catania et al., 1992; Jemmott, Jemmott, Spears, Hewitt, & Cruz-Collins, 1992) and having a low perceived risk of HIV infection (Nyamathi, Bennett, Leake, Lewis, & Flaskerud, 1993). While this body of research is useful in characterizing African-American women's sexual risk, over the last few decades greater attention has been focused on examining relational factors enhancing African-American women's HIV risk.

Numerous studies have demonstrated that having poor communication skills (Catania et al., 1992; Wingood & DiClemente, 1998a, b, c), having a male partner that abuses drugs or alcohol (Sterk, 1999, 2000), having a sexually abusive (Wyatt, 1992) having a physically abusive male partner (Wingood & DiClemente, 1997; Wingood, DiClemente, McCree, Harrington, & Davies, 2001), having a male partner who disapproves of practicing safer sex (Wingood & DiClemente, 1998a, b, c) and, having an older male partner (Miller, Clark, & Moore, 1997) all significantly increase African-American women's HIV risk. Partner influences effect women's HIV risk further, by being exposed to the partner's risky sexual behaviors.

Many African-American women may be unaware of their male partner's risk for HIV. In a study of HIV-infected people (5,156 men and 3,139 women), 34% of African-American men who have sex with men (MSM); 26% of Hispanic MSM, and 13% of white MSM reported having sex with women. However, only 14% of white women, 6% of and African-American women and 6% of Hispanic women in this study acknowledged having a bisexual partner (Montgomery, Mokotoff, Gentry, & Blair, 2003). Unfortunately, many women, particularly African-American women may not know of their male partner's bisexual activity. These studies highlight that African-American women's risk of HIV is not solely a function of their behavior, but is largely attributed to the behaviors of their male sexual partners. In addition, to this body of research on interpersonal and relational influences, more recent research has examined the influence of concurrency and marriage rates.

A concurrent partnership is a sexual partnership in which one or more of the members has other sexual partners, with repeated sexual activity with at least the original partner (Adimora & Schoenbach, 2002; Gorbach, Stoner, Aral, Whittington, & Holmes, 2002). Concurrent partnerships have been associated with transmission of chlamydia, (Potterat et al., 1999) gonorrhea, (Ghani, Swinton, & Garnett, 1997) syphilis (Morris & Kretzschmar, 1997) and HIV (Koumans et al., 2001). Concurrent relationships are much more prevalent among males, particularly African-American males, than among females (Adimora & Schoenbach, 2002; Gorbach et al., 2002). Other relational factors, such as marriage rates could also affect women's HIV risk. Compared to people who are married, people who are not married are more likely to have more than one sexual partner and thus at greater risk of acquiring HIV (Laumann, Gagnon, Michael, & Michaels, 1994) According to the U.S. census data, males are significantly more likely to have never been married than women (U.S. Bureau of the Census, 1998). Moreover, the proportion of unmarried adults is marked by significant racial distinctions. Among U.S. residents older than age 15 in 1998, 46% of black men compared to 29% of white men reported having never been married; and 22% of white women compared with 41% of black women reported never having been married. African-American women's HIV risk must also be examined within the context of these social influences.

Application of the Theory of Gender and Power to Understand Women's HIV Risk

The state-of-the science of research on African-American women and HIV has progressed to address the broader array of gender-related social and contextual factors prevalent in women's lives. Recognizing the importance of this milestone there is a need to address the theoretical limitations inherent in studies of women's HIV risk. Theoretical frameworks applied to examine women's HIV risk, historically did not take into account women's social and relational lives. In an attempt to address this limitation, the Theory of Gender and Power was adapted and modified to enhance understanding of the diverse array of influences that affect women risk of HIV. The theory of Gender and Power is a *social structural model* that attempts to understand women's risk as a function of different structures (none of which can be independent of the others) (Wingood & DiClemente, 2001). According to the theory of Gender and Power, there are three major structures that characterize the gendered relationships between men and women. These three structures are: (1) the sexual division of labor (examines economic inequities favoring males), (2) the sexual division of power (examines inequities and abuses of authority and control in relationships and institutions favoring males), and (3) the structure of cathexis (examines social norms and affective attachments) (see Fig. 11.1).

Societal Level	Institutional Level	Social Mechanisms	Exposures	Risk Factors	Disease
Sexual Division of Labor	Neighborhood School Family	Manifested as unequal pay produces economic inequities for women.	Economic Exposures	Socioeconomic Risk Factors ↘	
Sexual Division of Power	Relationships Worksite	Manifested as imbalances in control power for women.	Physical Exposures	Behavioral Risk Factors ↗	→ HIV Media
Structure of Cathexis: Social Norms & Affec- tive Attachments	Relationships Family Church	Manifested as con- straints in expectations produces disparities in norms for women.	Social Exposures	Personal Risk Factors	

Fig. 11.1 Model conceptualizing the influence of the theory of gender and power on women's risk of HIV

The three structures exist at two levels, the societal and the institutional level (Connell, 1987). The societal level is the highest level in which the three social structures are embedded. The three structures are rooted in society through numerous abstract, historical and sociopolitical forces that consistently segregate power and ascribe norms on the basis of gender-determined roles. The three structures are also evident at a lower level, the institutional level. Social institutions include, but are not limited to, families, relationships, religious institutions, the medical system and the media. The social structures are maintained within institutions through social mechanisms such as unequal pay for comparable work, the imbalance of control within relationships, and the degrading images of women as portrayed in the media. The presence of these and other social mechanisms constrain women's daily life by producing gender-based inequities in women's economic potential, in their control of resources, and in gender-based expectations.

In the adaption of the theory of gender and power, it is postulated that the gen-der-based inequities and disparities in expectations that arise from each of the three structures (sexual division of labor, sexual division of power, structure of cathexis) generate different exposures and risk factors@ that influence women's risk for HIV. Exposures are variables that are external to women which may influence their sexual risk behavior. Exposures include, but are not limited to, residence in a poor neighborhood, having an abusive male partner, and having limited pool of available partners. While the term risk factor is traditionally used to denote *any influence* that enhances risk for HIV, the theory of Gender and Power reserves this term specifi-cally to denote intrapersonal variables that emanate from within women and influ-ence their risk for HIV. Risk factors include, but are not limited to, having attitudes and beliefs non-supportive of condom use and having limited self-efficacy to use or negotiate condom use. Below, each structure in the theory is defined.

The inequities resulting from the *sexual division of labor* are manifested as economic exposures and risk factors. According to the sexual division of labor, as the economic inequity between men and women increases and favors men (making women more dependent on men), women will be at greater risk for HIV. HIV-related *economic exposures* include, but are not limited to, residing in a poor neighborhood, limited social cohesion within a neighborhood and partner pay inequities. *Socioeconomic risk factors* include being younger, unemployed and having a limited education (Wingood & DiClemente, 2001).

The inequities resulting from the *sexual division of power* are manifested as physical exposures and behavioral risk factors. According to the sexual division of power, as the power inequity between men and women increases and favors men, women's sexual choices and behavior may be constrained enhancing their risk for HIV. HIV-related physical exposures include interpersonal (partner-related) and institutional (i.e., media, worksite) factors. *Physical exposures* include having a sexually abusive, physically abusive, drug-abusing sexual partner; being exposed to sexually explicit media, racial discrimination, exposure to sexual harassment at the worksite. *Behavioral risk factors* are conceptualized as women who perceived themselves as having less power to avoid unhealthy behaviors. Behavioral risk factors include using alcohol or drugs; being less efficacious in negotiating condoms (Wingood & DiClemente, 2001).

The inequities resulting from the *structure of cathexis* (i.e., social norms and affective attachments) are manifested as social exposures and as personal risk factors. According to the structure of cathexis, women who are more accepting of conventional social norms and beliefs will be at greater risk of HIV. *Social and affective exposures* including, but are not limited to, having an older partner, having a partner who desires a pregnancy and having a limited partner pool. *Personal risk factors* are conceptualized as desiring pregnancy, being in a long term relationship, and possessing conservative or traditional gender norms (Wingood & DiClemente, 2001).

Employing the theory of Gender and Power to examine gender-based exposures and risk factors influencing African-American's women's risk of HIV has a number of positive attributes. First it marshals new kinds of data and allows us to ask new and broader questions regarding African-American women's vulnerability for HIV. Further, use of such a theory creates new ways of understanding why African-American women are at greater risk of HIV.

HIV Prevention Interventions for Heterosexual African-American Women

To reduce African-American women's vulnerability to HIV, the examination of risk factors and exposures associated with women's HIV risk must be accompanied by effective behavioral prevention efforts. Since 2000 a number of HIV interventions have been designed, implemented and evaluated in which a majority of the sample are African-American women. This chapter will focus on five HIV prevention interventions that have been conducted, since 2000, in which 70% of the sample is African-American women and, that use a randomized controlled trial with at least a 6-month follow-up to evaluate the efficacy of the intervention.

In 2002, Ehrhardt et al. (2002) published a study that assessed the short- and long-term effect of a gender-specific group intervention for women on unsafe sexual encounters and strategies for protection against HIV/STD infection. Family planning clients ($N=360$) from a high HIV seroprevalence area in New York City were randomized to an eight-session, a four-session or a control condition and followed at 1, 6 and 12 months post-intervention. Using an intention-to-treat analysis, women who were assigned to the eight-session group had about twice the odds of reporting decreased or no unprotected vaginal and anal intercourse compared to controls at 1 month (OR=1.93, 95% confidence interval [CI]=1.07, 3.48, $p=0.03$) and at 12-month follow-up (OR=1.65, 95% CI=0.94, 2.90, $p=0.08$). Relative to controls, women assigned to the eight-session condition reported during the previous month approximately three-and-a-half ($p=0.09$) and five ($p<0.01$) fewer unprotected sex occasions at 1- and 12-month follow-up, respectively. Women in the eight-session group also reduced the number of sex occasions at both follow-ups, and had a greater odds of first time use of an alternative protective strategy (refusal, outercourse, mutual testing) at 1-month follow-up. Results for the four-session group were in the expected direction but overall were inconclusive. Thus, gender-specific interventions of sufficient intensity can promote short- and long-term sexual risk reduction among women in a family planning setting.

In 2003, Sterk and colleagues published a study to evaluate the effectiveness of an HIV intervention for African American women who use crack cocaine (Sterk, Theall, & Elifson, 2003). Two hundred and sixty-five women (aged 18–59 years) were randomly assigned to one of two enhanced intervention conditions or to the National Institute on Drug Abuse standard condition. A substantial proportion of women reported no past 30-day crack use at 6-month follow-up. Significant ($p<0.05$) decreases in the frequency of crack use; the number of paying partners; the number of times vaginal, oral, or anal sex was had with a paying partner; and sexual risks, such as trading sex for drugs, were reported over time. Significant ($p<0.05$) increases in male condom use with sex partners were observed, as well as decreases in casual partners' refusal of condoms. Findings suggest that combined components of our culturally appropriate, gender-tailored intervention may be most effective at enhancing preventive behavior among similar populations.

In 2004, Drs. DiClemente and Wingood, published the results of a randomized, two-arm, single blind, controlled trial of sexually experienced African American females ($N=522$), 14–18 years of age, conducted at a family medicine clinic (DiClemente et al., 2004). Participants in this study completed a self-administered survey, a personal interview, demonstrated condom application skills, and provided vaginal swab specimens for STD testing at baseline and at 6- and 12-months post-intervention. The intervention emphasized ethnic and gender pride, HIV prevention knowledge, communication and condom use skills, refusal and avoidance skills, and the benefits of healthy relationships. Using population-averaged generalized estimating equations (GEE) analyses for the entire 12-month follow-up period, adolescents in the intervention, in contrast to the comparison group, were nearly twice as likely to report using condoms consistently in the 30 days preceding assessments (OR=1.97; 95% CI=1.25, 3.10; $p=0.004$) and were more than twice as likely to report using condoms consistently in the 6 months preceding assessments (OR=2.28; 95% CI=1.50, 3.47; $p=0.0001$). Adolescents in the HIV intervention also had a lower incidence of laboratory-confirmed chlamydia infections (OR=0.17; 95% CI=0.03,

0.93; $p=0.04$) and trichomonas infections (OR$=0.19$; 95% CI$=0.03$, 1.16; $p=0.07$), though this latter finding did not achieve statistical significance. Adolescents in the HIV intervention were also more likely to use a condom at last sexual intercourse, less likely to have new sex partners, had a higher frequency of applying condoms to sex partners, had better condom application skills, had a higher proportion of condom-protected sex acts, and had fewer unprotected vaginal sex acts. Adolescents in the HIV intervention also had higher scores on measures of psychosocial mediators of HIV-preventive behaviors. This is one of the first HIV prevention trials to report a reduction in high-risk sexual behaviors and incident Chlamydia among African-American adolescent females.

In 2004, Dr. Wechsberg and colleagues published the results of a randomized, three-arm trial for out-of-drug treatment African-American women who used crack ($N=620$) and women were assessed at 3- and 6-months follow-up (Wechsberg, Lam, Zule, & Bobashev, 2004). Participants were randomized to one of three arms, a woman-focused HIV intervention for crack abusers, a revised National Institute on Drug Abuse standard intervention, and a control group. The woman-focused intervention addressed drug dependence as a form of "bondage" and was designed to facilitate greater independence and increase personal power and control over behavior choices as well as life circumstances. The intervention contained psycho-educational information and skills training on reducing HIV risk and drug use, presented within the context of African American women's lives in the inner city, where pervasive poverty and violence limit women's options and increase the likelihood of poor (i.e., high-risk) behavior choices. All three groups reported significant reductions in the proportion of women having any unprotected sex in the past 30 days between baseline and 3- and 6-month follow-up. Although the woman-focused group demonstrated greater reductions in unprotected sex than the standard-R and control groups at 3 months, these results were not statistically significant at the 0.05 level. However, at 6 months this trend was statistically significant relative to controls, with fewer woman-focused group participants reporting any unprotected sex in the past 30 days (odds ratio [OR]$=0.62$, $p=0.03$). All study conditions demonstrated significant reductions in the proportion of women reporting trading sex for money or drugs in the past 30 days between baseline and 3- and 6-month follow-up. Both intervention groups showed significant reductions in the percentage of women who traded sex compared with control subjects, with the standard-R group (OR$=0.48$, $p=0.007$) having slightly stronger effects than the woman-focused group (OR$=0.58$, $p=0.046$) at 3-month follow-up. At 6 months, these trends in reduction continued, although they were not statistically significant. At 3 months, the odds of being homeless were the lowest in the woman-focused group (OR$=0.35$, $p=0.0002$). In multiple logistic regression analysis controlling for full-time employment at baseline, the odds of being employed full time at 3 months were significantly higher in the woman-focused group relative to both controls (OR$=2.53$; $p=0.0027$) and the standard-R group (OR$=2.02$, $p=0.0175$). The study concluded that a woman-focused intervention can successfully reduce risk and facilitate employment and housing and may effectively reduce the frequency of unprotected sex in the longer term.

In 2004, Dr. Wingood and DiClemente published a randomized controlled trial of 366 women living with HIV in Alabama and Georgia (ref. 72, AJPH). The intervention emphasized gender pride, maintaining current and identifying new network members, HIV transmission knowledge, communication and condom use skills, and healthy relationships. Over the 12-month follow-up, women in the *WiLLOW* intervention, relative to the comparison, reported fewer episodes of unprotected vaginal intercourse (1.8 vs. 2.5; $p=0.022$), were less likely to report never using condoms (OR$=0.27$; $p=0.008$), had a lower incidence of bacterial infections (chlamydia and gonorrhea) (OR$=0.19$; $p=0.006$), reported higher HIV knowledge and condom use self-efficacy, and more network members, fewer beliefs that condoms interfere with sex, fewer partner-related barriers to condom use, demonstrated greater skill in using condoms. This is the first trial to demonstrate reductions in risky sexual behavior and incident bacterial STDs and enhance HIV-preventive psychosocial and structural factors among women living with HIV.

Disseminating HIV Prevention Interventions for African-American Women

While the design, implementation and evaluation of HIV prevention interventions for African-American women is important, perhaps even more critical is the dissemination of these studies. Through the Diffusion of Evidence-Based Intervention (DEBI) program, nationally, more than 650 agencies have received training in SiSTA (Prather, 2005), an evidence-based HIV prevention program for African-American women (DiClemente & Wingood, 1995). Agencies seeking certification in implementing SiSTA can send two staff members to participate in a week long training. The 1 week SiSTA training program is known as the SiSTA Institute. Trainees in the SiSTA Institute are provided training on the theoretical frameworks, core elements, intervention activities and evaluation methods that comprise SiSTA. Trainees graduating from the SiSTA Institute are certified to implement this intervention. A technical assistance program has been created to provide additional training and address questions and concerns that may arise during the implementation of SiSTA in the trainees' local communities. Individuals, who have been certified to implement SiSTA through the SiSTA Institute, are eligible to receive a 1-week training and certification to implement a newly published evidence-based HIV prevention program for African-American female adolescents, known as SiHLE (DiClemente et al., 2004) and an evidence-based HIV intervention for women living with HIV, known as WiLLOW (Wingood et al., 2004). All three programs, SiSTA, SiHLE and WiLLOW target African-American females, are designed to reduce HIV sexual risk behaviors and share similar theoretical, core and methodological elements. Given their similarities, these programs are being promoted as a suite of HIV interventions for African-American women.

In an effort to accommodate and expand the intervention suite to new and emerging subpopulations of African-American women, the designers of the suite (Drs. Gina Wingood and Ralph DiClemente) have tailored and are evaluating the efficacy of several of the interventions within this suite for use with other subgroups of African-American women (i.e., female adolescents attending STD clinics, and young adult women receiving care at health maintenance organizations). Moreover, in an attempt to reach women across the African Diaspora the original researchers are currently adapting and evaluating the efficacy of interventions within the suite for use with women in sub-Saharan Africa and the Caribbean. In an era when fiscal and human resources are severely constrained by competing public health priorities, it would be cost- and time-prohibitive for many public and private sector agencies to develop and evaluate a new program for each subgroup for which they desire to administer an HIV prevention program. Perhaps, promoting clusters of technological innovations, such as an HIV intervention suite, may serve to facilitate adoption and diffusion of evidence-based HIV prevention programs.

Future Directions

While notable research, programs and services designed to reduce HIV risk among African-American women have been developed, public health researchers have to expand their agenda. Among the new and emerging issues there is a need to:

1. Explore effective ways to design and implement social structural interventions to reduce African-American women's risk of HIV.
2. Explore how female controlled methods, such as microbicides, can be used as HIV risk reduction agents.
3. Explore how effective primary and secondary HIV prevention interventions for women can be more widely disseminated to African-American women at greatest risk.
4. Explore ways to design cost-effective HIV prevention interventions for African-American women that can reduce risky sexual practices as well as, biological outcomes, such as sexually transmitted infections.

Creating a new and expanded agenda to reduce and even halt the feminization of the HIV epidemic needs to be a public health priority. However, prior to creating a new agenda first requires an assessment of the lessons learned from our current prevention efforts conducted among women. Several meta-analyses and reviews of HIV prevention programs conducted among women research have demonstrated that HIV prevention programs with African-American women are effective. However, without a new vision and forward foresight the HIV epidemic will continue its devastating toll on the health of African-American women nationally.

References

Adimora, A. A., & Schoenbach, V. J. (2002). Contextual factors and the black-white disparity in heterosexual HIV transmission. *Epidemiology, 13*, 707–712.
Anderson, J. E., Brackbill, R., & Mosher, W. D. (1996). Condom use for disease prevention among unmarried U.S. women. *Family Planning Perspectives, 28*, 25–28.

Anderson, R. N., & Smith, B. L. (2005). Deaths: Leading causes for 2002. *National Vital Statistics Reports, 53*(17), 1–8.

Catania, J. A., Coates, T. J., Kegeles, S., Fullilove, M. T., Peterson, J., Marin, B., et al. (1992). Condom use in multi-ethnic neighborhoods of San Francisco: The population-based AMEN (AIDS in multi-ethnic neighborhoods) study. *American Journal of Public Health, 82*, 284–287.

Centers for Disease Control & Prevention. (2005a). Trends in HIV/AIDS diagnoses–33 states, 2001–2004. *Morbidity and Mortality Weekly Report, 54*, 1149–1153.

Centers for Disease Control & Prevention. (2005b). *HIV/AIDS surveillance report, 2004* (Vol. 16, pp. 1–46). Atlanta, GA: US Department of Health & Human Services.

Connell, R. W. (1987). *Gender and power*. Stanford, CA: Stanford University Press.

Diaz, T., Chu, S. Y., Buehler, J. W., Boyd, D., Checko, P. J., Conti, L., et al. (1994). Socioeconomic differences among people with AIDS: Results from a multistate surveillance project. *American Journal of Preventive Medicine, 10*, 217–222.

DiClemente, R. J., & Wingood, G. M. (1995). A randomized controlled social skills trial: An HIV sexual risk-reduction intervention among young adult African-American women. *Journal of the American Medical Association, 274*, 1271–1276.

DiClemente, R. J., Wingood, G. M., Harrington, K. F., Lang, D. L., Davies, S. L., Hook, E. W., III, et al. (2004). Efficacy of an HIV prevention intervention for African American adolescent girls: A randomized controlled trial. *Journal of the American Medical Association, 292*, 171–179.

Edlin, B. R., Erwin, K. L., Faruque, S., McCoy, C. B., Word, C., Serrano, Y., et al. (1994). Intersecting epidemics: Crack cocaine use and HIV infection among inner city young adults. Multicenter Crack Cocaine and HIV Infection Study Team. *New England Journal of Medicine, 24*, 1422–1427.

Ehrhardt, A. A., Exner, T. M., Hoffman, S., Silberman, I., Leu, C.-S., Miller, S., et al. (2002). A gender-specific HIV/STD risk reduction intervention for women in a health care setting: Short- and long-term results of a randomized clinical trial. *AIDS Care, 14*, 147–161.

Fullilove, R., Fullilove, M., Bowser, B., & Goss, S. (1990). Risk of sexually transmitted disease among black adolescent crack users in Oakland and San Francisco, Calif. *Journal of the American Medical Association, 263*, 851–855.

Ghani, A. C., Swinton, J., & Garnett, G. P. (1997). The role of sexual partnership networks in the epidemiology of gonorrhea. *Sexually Transmitted Diseases, 24*, 45–56.

Gorbach, P. M., Stoner, B. P., Aral, S. O., Whittington, W. L., & Holmes, K. K. (2002). "It takes a village": Understanding concurrent sexual partnerships in Seattle, Washington. *Sexually Transmitted Diseases, 29*, 453–462.

Graves, K. L., & Hines, A. M. (1997). Ethnic differences in the association between alcohol and risky sexual behavior with a new partner: An event-based analysis. *AIDS Education and Prevention, 9*, 219–237.

Jemmott, J. B., Jemmott, L. S., Spears, H., Hewitt, N., & Cruz-Collins, M. (1992). Self-efficacy, hedonistic expectanices, and condom-use intentions among inner-city black adolescent women: A social cognitive approach to AIDS risk behavior. *Journal of Adolescent Health, 13*, 512–519.

Koumans, E. H., Farley, T. A., Gibson, J. J., Langley, C., Ross, M. W., McFarlane, M., et al. (2001). Characteristics of persons with syphilis in areas of persisting syphilis in the United States: Sustained transmission associated with concurrent partnerships. *Sexually Transmitted Diseases, 28*(9), 497–503.

Laumann, E. O., Gagnon, J. H., Michael, R. T., & Michaels, S. (1994). *The social organization of sexuality*. Chicago, IL: The University of Chicago Press.

Miller, K., Clark, L., & Moore, J. S. (1997). Heterosexual risk for HIV among female adolescents: Sexual initiation with older male partners. *Family Planning Perspectives, 29*, 212–214.

Montgomery, J. P., Mokotoff, E. D., Gentry, A. C., & Blair, J. M. (2003). The extent of bisexual behaviour in HIV-infected men and implications for transmission to their female partners. *AIDS Care, 15*, 829–837.

Morris, M., & Kretzschmar, M. (1997). Concurrent partnerships and the spread of HIV. *AIDS, 11*, 641–648.

Nyamathi, A., Bennett, C., Leake, B., Lewis, C., & Flaskerud, J. (1993). AIDS-related knowledge, perceptions, and behaviors among impoverished minority women. *American Journal of Public Health, 83*, 65–71.

Peterson, J. L., Grinstead, O. A., Golden, E., Catania, J. A., Kegeles, S., & Coates, T. J. (1992). Correlates of HIV risk behaviors in black and white San Francisco heterosexuals: The population-based AIDS in multiethnic neighborhoods (AMEN) study. *Ethnicity & Disease, 2*(4), 361–370.

Potterat, J. J., Zimmerman-Rogers, H., Muth, S. Q., Rothenberg, R. B., Green, D. L., Taylor, J. E., et al. (1999). Chlamydia transmission: Concurrency, reproduction number, and the epidemic trajectory. *American Journal of Epidemiology, 150*(12), 1331–1339.

Prather, C. (2005). Personal communications regarding progress of CDC disseminating SiSTA.

Stephenson, J. (2000). Rural HIV/AIDS in the United States: Studies suggest presence, no rampant spread. *JAMA, 284*(2), 167–168.

Sterk, C. (1999). *Fast lives: Women who use crack cocaine.* Philadelphia, PA: Temple University Press.

Sterk, C. E. (2000). *Tricking and tripping: Prostitution in the era of AIDS.* Putnam Valley, NY: Social Change Press.

Sterk, C. E., Theall, K. P., & Elifson, K. W. (2003). Effectiveness of a risk reduction intervention among African American women who use crack cocaine. *AIDS Education and Prevention, 15,* 15–32.

U.S. Bureau of the Census. (1998). *Current population survey. Marital status and living arrangements: March 1998 [update] (P20-514).* Washington, DC: U.S. Bureau of the Census.

U.S. Census Bureau. (2003). *Poverty: 1999. Census 2000 Brief* (Issued May 2003).

Valleroy, L. A., MacKellar, D. A., Karon, J. M., Janssen, R. S., & Hayman, C. R. (1998). HIV infection in disadvantaged out-of-school youth: Prevalence for U.S. Job Corps entrants, 1990 through 1996. *Journal of Acquired Immune Deficiency Syndromes and Human Retrovirology, 19,* 67–73.

Wechsberg, W. M., Lam, W. K., Zule, W. A., & Bobashev, G. (2004). Efficacy of a woman-focused intervention to reduce HIV risk and increase self-sufficiency among African American crack abusers. *American Journal of Public Health, 94,* 1165–1173.

Wingood, G. M., & DiClemente, R. J. (1997). The effects of an abusive primary partner on the condom use and sexual negotiation practices of African-American women. *American Journal of Public Health, 87*(6), 1016–1018.

Wingood, G. M., & DiClemente, R. J. (1998a). Relationship characteristics associated with non-condom use among young adult African-American women. *American Journal of Community Psychology, 26,* 29–53.

Wingood, G. M., & DiClemente, R. J. (1998b). The influence of psychosocial factors, alcohol, drug use on African-American women's high-risk sexual behavior. *American Journal of Preventive Medicine, 15*(1), 54–59.

Wingood, G. M., & DiClemente, R. J. (1998c). Partner influences and gender-related factors associated with noncondom use among young adult African-American women. *American Journal of Community Psychology, 26*(1), 29–51.

Wingood, G. M., & DiClemente, R. J. (2001). Application of the theory of gender and power to examine HIV-related exposures, risk factors, and effective interventions for women. *Health Education & Behavior, 27*(5), 539–565.

Wingood, G. M., DiClemente, R. J., McCree, D. H., Harrington, K., & Davies, S. (2001). Dating violence and African-American adolescent females' sexual health. *Pediatrics, 107*(5), E72.

Wingood, G. M., DiClemente, R. J., Mikhail, I., Lang, D., McCree, D. H., Davies, S. L., et al. (2004). A randomized controlled trial to reduce HIV transmission risk behaviors and STDs among women living with HIV: The WiLLOW Program. *Journal of Acquired Immune Deficiency Syndromes, 37,* S58–S67.

Wyatt, G. E. (1992). The sociocultural context of African American and White American women's rape. *Journal of Social Issue, 48,* 77–91.

Chapter 12
Formulating the Stress and Severity Model of Minority Social Stress for Black Men Who Have Sex with Men

Kenneth Terrill Jones, Leo Wilton, Gregorio Millett, and Wayne D. Johnson

Introduction

Despite drastic declines in HIV in the United States (US) (Holtgrave, Hall, Rhodes, & Wolitski, 2008), communities of color and men who have sex with men (MSM) are still disproportionately infected. Nationally, MSM comprise 48% of people living with HIV (CDC, 2008a). For MSM of all age groups, 35% of new infections were in black MSM (CDC, 2008b). Epidemiological studies of MSM demonstrate that rates of HIV infection have been greater for black MSM as compared with other racial or ethnic groups of MSM (Harawa et al., 2004; Lemp et al., 1994; Mansergh et al., 2002; CDC, 2001). In fact, between 2001 and 2004, black MSM were the only subgroup of blacks for whom new HIV diagnoses actually increased rather than decreased (CDC, 2005a). HIV seroprevalence rates of black MSM in the US have been shown analogous to those in some resource-limited countries (CDC, 2002; CDC, 2005b).

HIV seroprevalence rates of younger black MSM may be even more pronounced. Nearly half of new infections in MSM ages 13–29 were in blacks (CDC, 2008b). A recent study of people in five US cities found that black MSM had the highest HIV prevalence (46%) of all MSM and that two-thirds of black MSM were unaware of their HIV infection (CDC, 2005b). A retrospective study conducted from January 2001 to May 2003 in North Carolina found that 88% (49/56) of new HIV cases in men aged 18–30 were in black men, a majority of whom reported same-sex sexual behavior (CDC, 2004). HIV behavioral studies have demonstrated that unprotected anal intercourse (UAI) has been a primary risk factor or acquiring and transmitting HIV between MSM (Vittinghoff et al., 1999). Two studies (Guenther-Grey et al., 2005; Valleroy et al., 2000) reported rates of UAI between 26 and 55%. A more recent study found that rates of UAI among black MSM were 34 and 47% for

K.T. Jones (✉)

Division of HIV/AIDS Prevention, Centers for Disease Control and Prevention, 1600 Clifton Road NE, MS E-37, Atlanta, GA 30333, USA

e-mail: KJones4@cdc.gov

D.H. McCree et al. (eds.), *African Americans and HIV/AIDS*,
DOI 10.1007/978-0-387-78321-5_12, © Springer Science+Business Media, LLC 2010

casual and for main male partners, respectively. By comparison, white MSM had rates of 39 and 64% for casual and main male partners, respectively (CDC, 2006).

The Paradox of Behavioral Risk Correlates

Black MSM report higher rates of HIV disease progression (Hall, Byers, Ling, & Espinoza, 2007) and AIDS mortality (Blair, Fleming, & Karon, 2002) among MSM in the US than the rates reported by MSM of other racial or ethnic backgrounds. However, commonly understood risk factors for HIV infection do not fully explain the disparate rates of the disease burden of black MSM. A recent review (Millett, Peterson, Wolitski, & Stall, 2006) found empirical support for potential explanations for increased HIV seroprevalence rates in black MSM compared with their white counterparts. These include (1) high rates of sexually transmitted infections (STIs) that facilitate acquisition and transmission of HIV (CDC, 2001); (2) less frequent HIV testing (CDC, 2002); and (3) higher rates of unrecognized HIV (Millett, Peterson, et al.).

Few studies have examined correlates of HIV infection or HIV risk of black MSM. A recent literature review reported that only 14 correlates were tested in multiple studies of black MSM (Millett, Flores, Peterson, & Bakeman, 2007). Of these, only four showed similar relationships across studies in their comparison of black MSM: first, those with a history of gonorrhea were more likely to be HIV-positive; second, those with low incomes engaged in more risky sexual behaviors; third, those who disclosed their MSM behavior were more likely to have been tested for HIV; and fourth, those who reported high psychological distress were more likely to engage in risky sexual behavior. Black MSM engages in fewer risk behaviors than do MSM of other races and ethnicities despite black MSM's having high rates of HIV infection (Millett, Flores, et al.).

The Effects of Psychological Distress and Social Stress

The contribution of psychological distress to black MSM's HIV sexual risk behavior has not been as adequately studied as it has been for other populations of MSM (Peterson & Jones, 2009; Wilton, 2009). In a study of 912 Latino gay men, Diaz, Ayala, and Bein (2004) found that those who experienced multiple forms of discrimination, including racism, homophobia, and poverty, were more likely to engage in risky sexual situations, which provided the context for HIV sexual risk behavior. These factors also were predictors of greater psychological distress in Latino gay men. The dearth of such research among black MSM has led investigators to advocate for studies that explore both interpersonal and societal determinants of the HIV risk of black MSM (Mays, Cochran, & Zamudio, 2004; Wilson, Cook, McGlaskey, Rowe, & Dennis, 2009). In a qualitative study, Woodyard,

Peterson, and Stokes (2000) found that young black MSM churchgoers experienced psychological distress because of homophobic messages they heard at church. Distress also was associated with "secret" same-sex activity, which in another study (Stokes and Peterson, 1998) was associated with internalized homophobia. Internalized homophobia has been associated with limited participation in HIV-prevention activities (Huebner, Davis, Nemeroff, & Aiken, 2002). Further, Jones et al., (2008a) found that young black MSM who had a family member disapprove of their same-sex activities were more likely to have been recently incarcerated, which was associated with recent risky sex. The same study found that black MSM who reported experiencing racial discrimination also reported favorable condom use peer norms, which were associated with decreased unprotected sex. Favorable condom peer norms were a predictor of protected anal sex among black MSM in another study (Hart & Peterson, 2004).

Formulating a Culturally Congruent Model for HIV Prevention

Negative associations of discrimination on physical and mental health have been well documented (Clark 2001; Clark, Moore, & Adams, 1998; Jones, Harrell, Morris-Prather, Thomas, & Omowale, 1996; Sellers, Caldwell, Schmeelk-Cone, Zimmerman, 2003; Sellers & Shelton, 2003; Sellers, Bonham, Neighbors, & Arnell, 2009; Williams, Neighbors, & Jackson, 2003; Williams, Yu, Jackson, & Anderson, 1997). However, Jackson et al. (1996) found that perceived racism may motivate some blacks to be protective of their own health when they believe that whites may hinder their chances for achievement. Racial socialization (Hughes et al., 2006) is offered as one culturally congruent strategy to explain this finding. Racial socialization is an umbrella term that refers to strategies used by parents to prepare their children to deal with racial discrimination and harassment. Racial socialization can be characterized by five strategies:

1. Cultural socialization – racial/ethnic history and customs, cultural traditions are promoted
2. Preparation for bias – individuals are taught to recognize and cope with racism and inequality
3. Promotion of distrust – distrust of people from other races, especially whites, is promoted
4. Egalitarianism – individual characteristics according to the principle of universal equality, regardless of race, is endorsed
5. Silence about race – the discussion of race is avoided, as such, individuals are not taught about differences or similarities between or among races

This process has been studied mainly in relation to messages transmitted from parents or caregivers to children (Hughes, 2003; Hughes et al., 2006) and has rarely been explored in relation to HIV risk in the peer-reviewed literature. However, Jones et al., (2008a) have argued that racial socialization might explain the reduced

HIV risk behaviors of some black MSM who reported perceived racial discrimination. Therefore, culturally congruent models that explore the impact of unique stressors based on black MSM's race and sexual behaviors deserve attention in prevention efforts.

Studies demonstrate that those who are racially socialized report better health and academic outcomes (Fischer & Shaw, 1999; Hughes et al., 2006). Resiliency has been shown among black children (Hughes and Johnson, 2001; Stevenson, Cameron, Herrero-Taylon, & Davis, 2002). Youth who were taught about race in an earlier study reported higher grades (Bowman & Howard, 1985). Data from a national longitudinal study of African American adolescents found increased academic motivation among those who anticipated future discrimination (Eccles, Wong, & Peck, 2006). Two studies found a reduction in prejudice when racial categories were highlighted (Richeson & Nussbaum, 2004; Wolsko, Park, Judd, & Winterbrink, 2000). Providing additional support to the importance of recognizing racial differences, LaVeist, Sellers, and Neighbors (2001) found that attributing negative life-events to external factors, such as societal racism, rather than to individual characteristics, was protective of black's health. Similarly, self-attribution of social discrimination was associated with increase HIV risk behaviors in a sample of Asian and Pacific Islander gay men (Wilson & Yoshikawa, 2004). This attribution technique has been explored decades earlier by Rotter (1966) in his locus of control theory.

The importance of transmitting messages, values, and symbolic rituals to children has also been examined in the literature (Bowman & Howard, 1985; Knight, Bernal, Cota, Garza, & Ocampo, 1993; Knight, Cota, & Bernal, 1993; Phinney & Chavira, 1995; Phinney & Rotheram, 1987; Sanders-Thompson, 1994; Thornton, Chatters, Taylor, & Allen, 1990). According to Omi and Winant (1996), cultural socialization is one of the ways in which race is formed in the US and it can facilitate collective identity (Ogbu, 2004). Collective identity refers to one's sense of belonging to a particular group or class. The importance of racial-ethnic group identification has been documented in the literature (Eccles et al., 2006; Sellers, Smith, Shelton, Rowley, & Chavous, 1998; Yip, Gee, & Takeuchi, 2008). Yip et al. (2008) report in the first national representative study of Asian Americans that identification with one's ethnic group was a protective factor of psychological distress. A similar finding was reported among African American adolescents and school achievement (Eccles et al.).

Unfortunately, unintended consequences may be encountered later in life as a result of specific strategies that black MSM experience as children. These consequences are discussed elsewhere in the manuscript. We first present a model in an attempt to explain how racial socialization and other culturally appropriate strategies might reduce the HIV risk of black MSM. Additionally, we propose "sexual socialization" along the lines of the just-described components of "racial socialization." In so doing, we hope to devise another strategy that may mitigate such risk. Sexual socialization has been defined as those strategies that are used to prepare lesbians, gay men, and bisexuals to deal with discrimination and harassment associated with being a sexual minority. Unfortunately, sexual socialization, especially parent-to-child socialization, may be unlikely to take place in today's society, given stigma, homophobia, and systematic discrimination against lesbian, gay, bisexual, and transgender populations in the US. We should note that these ideas are not entirely new but the present conceptualization specifically for black MSM may be. For example, Meyer (2003) offers a stress model for lesbian, gay, and bisexual men and women.

The Stress and Severity Model of Minority Social Stress

Similar to the Glanz and Schwartz (2008) (also see Lazarus and Folkman, 1984) Transactional Model of Stress and Coping, Fig. 12.1 depicts a model to help the reader understand the effects of social stress on the lives of black MSM and on their level of HIV risk. Figure 12.1 also depicts how different coping strategies, including racial and sexual socialization, might lessen HIV risk. This model has been termed the *Stress and Severity Model of Minority Social Stress (SMS)*. While many stressors affect the lives of black MSM, the application of the SMS currently focuses only on stress stemming from being a racial and sexual minority; however, the model can be applied to other social stressors that black MSM experience.

According to the SMS, black MSM experience social stressors that are harmful to their physical, emotional, and sexual health. Upon experiencing these stressors, black MSM will evaluate the significance of the stressors in their lives (*perceived severity*). The likelihood that maladaptive behaviors will take place will increase if black MSM who are under such stress perceive that they will pay a high social cost for their sexual practices. For example, if parental rejection is perceived to be significant in black MSM's lives then stress is elevated. In previous research, family rejection has been associated with feelings of loneliness, depression, anger, anxiety, and other adverse health outcomes in populations of gay men (Greene, 1994; Kreiss & Patterson, 1997; Loiacano, 1993; Mays & Cochran, 2001; Meyer, 2003; So, 2003). Zamboni and Crawford (2007) found that elevated levels of sexual problems were significantly associated with reduced levels of social support for African

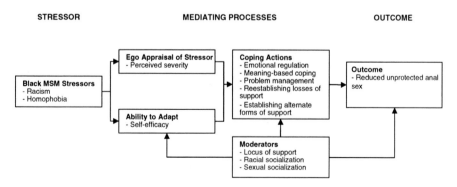

Fig. 12.1 Stress and severity model of minority social stress

American MSM. Therefore, family and community rejection may cause black MSM to feel unprotected and vulnerable when faced with a loss of expected assurance, support, and protection.

According to the SMS, and consistent with other ecological and theoretical approaches, severity of stress is differentially experienced, given the proximity and availability of perceived and actual sources of support and given the level of stress to the individual from these sources of support (referred to as *locus of support* in the SMS, see Fig. 12.2; also see Lazarus & Folkman, 1984 and Meyer, 2003 for additional discussions of the distal-proximal distinction). The larger black community is an important source of support for many black MSM (Kraft, Beeker, Stokes, & Peterson 2000; Mays, Chatters, Cochran, & Mackness, 1998). Most black gay men and lesbians live in black communities rather than in urban gay communities unlike their white counterparts (Dang & Frazer 2004). Black gay men and lesbians tend to have mostly black friends (Mays, Nardi, Cochran, & Taylor, 2000) and view their racial identity (rather than being gay or lesbian) as their primary identity (Battle, Cohen, Warren, Fergerson, & Audam, 2002; Greene, 1994). Mays et al., (1998) has also highlighted the importance of African American families as important social networks. Therefore, in some contexts, homophobia in the black community may be regarded differently from oppression experienced in the larger society or in the general "gay community," thus differentially affecting the perceived severity of the stressor in black MSM's lives. The same is true for experiences associated with racism. For example, individuals in racially homogeneous communities may not exhibit maladaptive behaviors when they perceive racism in those communities by non-black individuals. Further, one often unanswered question that can be addressed by this model is whether racism experienced in the broader gay community has differing effects on black MSM's risk-taking from the homophobia experienced in the broader black community. For example, Raymond and McFarland (2009) found in a recent study that black MSM in San Francisco were significantly more likely to engage in assortative sexual pairing than would be expected by chance. MSM from other racial groups viewed blacks

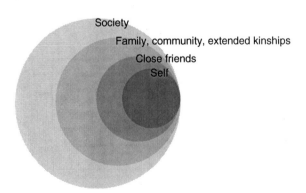

Fig. 12.2 Locus of support for Black MSM

as least desirable sexually or even as friends. Blacks were also viewed as least welcomed to MSM venues in these communities.

Whether conscious or unconscious, black MSM will appraise the severity of the stressor to themselves or their interests (ego appraisal) and make an additional appraisal of their ability to cope with the stressor. This appraisal may include a general evaluation of their *ability to adapt* or to choose the more healthful and potentially life-saving option. According to the model, rejection and not having the skills, or possessing decreased self-efficacy, can lead to negative health outcomes for black MSM. Therefore, it is vital to increase black MSM's self-efficacy. One particular quote from a black MSM in a contextually unrelated study nonetheless illuminates this point about risky sex and rejection. He states:

> Well, you know how some people, when they get depressed, eat food or go to sleep or do whatever? Well, I have sex. When things don't go well, the first thing I want to do is have sex. So I don't know if that makes me an addict, but [laughs], you know, it's something that I use as a crutch, you know. I mean it's just—and I think it has to do with—in the industry that I'm in there's a lot of rejection, you know... And, going and having anonymous sex with someone, it's like, you know, acceptance, you know (Vicioso, Parsons, Nanin, Purcell, & Woods, 2005, p. 16).

The task of helping black MSM realize that they can control their sexual practices by choosing more healthful responses to stress is only one component of reducing these men's HIV risk. It is important to prepare them through culturally appropriate skills-building activities to improve their self-efficacy, or agency, for making more healthful sexual and risk-reduction decisions. For example, one general goal of an HIV intervention might be to help diminish an HIV-negative black MSM's belief that he is predestined to become HIV-positive. However, these efforts are futile if the individual does not feel that he has the agency, or lacks self-efficacy, to practice more healthful behaviors that will keep him or his sex partners to remain HIV-negative especially given societal messages arguably reinforcing his inferiority.

There are several *coping efforts* that black MSM may use when faced with these stressors. One action is to give different meanings to the stressor. This *meaning-based* technique may be used to dispel negative emotions about the stressor and the reason it is occurring. These beliefs may be rooted in religious or spiritual contexts. For example, black MSM may view the stressor as a "test" to strengthen their character. Using this strategy, black MSM who experience homophobia in their family may exhibit persistent determination to be successful in order to disprove negative views that others may have about him. Also, common among many marginalized groups, including women, is the notion of having to be twice *as good* in order to warrant the same treatment accorded to non-marginalized people. In such situations, additional meaning may be given for the disparate behavior. This resiliency has been reported as one reason for the longevity and success of blacks (Bright, Duefield, & Caldwell, 1998; LaVeist et al., 2001).

Black MSM may take actions to personally modify the situation or the root cause of the stress (*problem management*). This could include individual approaches such as confronting or avoiding the stressor. It also may include collective activism to combat the stressor, similar to the activism used during the Civil Rights Movement and to strategies employed by AIDS Coalition to Unleash Power (ACT UP) in the 1980s and 1990s. Black MSM might engage in strategies to change they way they and others consider or actualize the situation. These strategies may include the invocation of social and behavioral scripts in order to regulate affect (*emotional regulation*). This could include constant monitoring and regulation of personal feelings of anger, of facial expressions, and of other biological markers. It should be noted that this constant self-monitoring of affect also may contribute to stress in black MSM. Emotional regulation also may involve talking to a close friend or other sources of support in order to process the stressful event.

Despite homophobia in some black communities, and homophobia and racism in some white communities against these men, black MSM may continue, or at least try, to maintain their roles in these communities and to reconnect to those causing the perceived stress. *Re-establishment* is defined as a coping technique that black MSM invoke so as to allow themselves to maintain or re-establish connections to those sources of stress in order to receive a portion of the desired support. Disruption of black MSM's roles and of their refuge in these communities is a source of psychological distress and of social stress and will likely increase their risk for unhealthful behaviors (Bowleg, Craig, & Burkholder, 2004). One black MSM described this loss of support thus: "Being in the black community, the only thing you got is each other. And [if you are gay], you really don't have them, so you don't have nothing" (Kraft et al., 2000, p. 433).

The act of re-*establishment* is important in the lives of black MSM. However, *establishing* alternative sources of support, when re-establishment is not a viable option, also is as important for black MSM. Examples may include attendance at gay-affirming churches or membership in the House Ballroom community popular among black and Latino gay men and women (Arnold & Bailey, 2009). The House Ballroom community consists of recreated family structures led by a "mother" or "father." These individuals provide leadership and mentorship typical of that given by a parent or caregiver. Members of these communities tend to engage in fashion and dance competitions referred to as balls (Marks et al., 2008). Unfortunately, high rates of HIV have been reported in the House Ballroom community (Murrill et al., 2005), suggesting that recreating social support alone may be necessary but not sufficient for HIV prevention.

Finally, racial and sexual socialization strategies moderate the relationship between social stressors and black MSM HIV risk. Certain strategies unfortunately may have unintended consequences for black MSM and may require certain revision in order to be effective in reducing HIV among black MSM and other multiply stigmatized individuals. For example, Preparing youth to recognize discrimination may lead them to anticipate discrimination in their daily lives. High levels of depressive symptoms and low self-esteem were reported in one study (Rumbaut, 1994). Biafora, Warheit, Zimmerman, & Gil (1993) earlier reported that racial mistrust was predictive of maladaptive behaviors in a sample of black children. Racial mistrust has also been examined in relation to black's utilization of mental heath services. In a systematic review, Whaley (2001) found that mistrust explained black's underutilization of mental health services. Promoting distrust of whites may also fuel conspiracy beliefs about HIV. While these beliefs are reasonable given historic unethical medical practices against blacks (Washington, 2006), conspiracy beliefs have nonetheless been associated with inconsistent condom use among black men generally (Bogart and Thorburn, 2005; Klonoff and Landrine, 1999) and black MSM specifically (Hutchinson et al., 2007).

Research has shown that not talking about race and egalitarian approaches do not always relieve experiences of discrimination or prejudice (Park & Judd, 2005). Bowman and Howard (1985) earlier reported that silence about race was associated with lower grades. For black MSM, silence about race may leave black MSM ill prepared to even understand the potential risk of HIV from partner selection choices. Selecting sexual partners from high prevalence populations, including black MSM, increases the probability of HIV transmission or acquisition especially when risky sexy occurs (Peterson & Jones, 2009; Raymond & McFarland, 2009). Silence about race and egalitarian stances, very similar to color-blind racism (Bonilla-Silva, 2006), may be associated with barriers to governmental interventions meant to reduce racial inequalities.

Black cultural transmission may be a source of psychological distress for black MSM. Constantine-Simms (2001) examines notions that equate homosexuality as an imposition of white cultural values on black men and women. In these instances, the exclusion of contributions from lesbian, gay, bisexual, and transgender men and women to black culture and society can be expected. Excluding these contributions may lead black MSM to question their larger role in the black community, decrease identification with the black community, may lead to inaccurate assessments about black MSM's capabilities, and may result in a lack of positive LGBT role models. The lack of such role models has been associated with increased HIV risk behaviors among Latino MSM (Diaz & Ayala, 2001).

Future Directions

There is a critical need to provide effective and culturally appropriate interventions that prevent HIV transmission and progression to AIDS for black MSM (Wilton, 2009). Only three HIV prevention interventions developed for, and tested solely among, black MSM have been published in the peer-reviewed literature (Jones et al., 2008b; Peterson et al., 1996, Wilton et al., 2009).

Peterson and colleagues (1996) conducted the first evaluation. Participants were randomized to one of three conditions: (1) three weekly 3 h sessions on AIDS risk education, cognitive behavioral self-management training, assertion training, and attempts to develop self-identity and social support; (2) a single 3 h session of the same content; or (3) a wait-list control condition. At 12- and 18-month follow-ups, those assigned to the three-session condition, reported less unprotected sex than those assigned to the single session. Unfortunately, neither of the groups differed significantly from the control condition. However, lessons learned and strategies from this study have been used as the basis for developing behavior interventions for black MSM (see Jones et al., 2008b and Wilton et al., 2009).

Many Men, Many Voices (3MV) is an innovative, group-level, integrated HIV/STI prevention intervention for black MSM who self-identify as HIV-negative or status unknown. The primary objectives of the 3MV intervention are as follows: (1) to prevent HIV /STI transmission through an increase in the practice of safer sexual behaviors and a decrease in unprotected anal and vaginal intercourse; (2) to increase their seeking health care (e.g., testing for HIV and for other STIs and obtaining the results); (3) to encourage mutually monogamous relationships with an uninfected partner; and (4) to promote key behavior-influencing factors that include HIV/STI knowledge, perception of HIV/STI risk, identity and self-value, self-efficacy skills, and behavioral intentions for safer sexual behaviors.

In a recent randomized controlled trial (Wilton et al., 2009), men in the intervention group, as compared with the comparison group, significantly reduced unprotected anal intercourse (UAI) with their casual male sex partners and they reduced the number of male sex partners. Men in the intervention group also were tested for HIV more often than those in the comparison group. Furthermore, a trend toward significance was established for consistent condom use during receptive anal intercourse with casual male sex partners.

In 2004, CDC funded the North Carolina Department of Health to adapt Kelly et al. (1991) community-level intervention, Popular Opinion Leader, in three North Carolina cities (Jones et al., 2008b). The adapted intervention included discussions about racism, homophobia, bisexuality, employment, poverty, and religion. Through culturally relevant role-play exercises, opinion leaders learn how to address these social factors if encountered as an obstacle to their peer's safer-sex practices.

Serial cross-sectional community surveys were conducted in the same night-clubs where opinion leaders were recruited, first at baseline (before any interven-tion activity) and then repeated at 4, 8, and 12 months. At baseline, 32.4% of black MSM reported unprotected receptive anal intercourse (URAI) in the 2 months prior; 29.3% reported unprotected insertive anal intercourse (UIAI); and 42.1% reported any UAI ($n=284$). After implementing the intervention over the course of 1 year, URAI decreased by 44.1% from baseline measures, 35.2% for UIAI, and 31.8% for any UAI. Overall, these findings provide evidence that adapting interven-tions already proven effective for other groups of MSM also may be an effective strategy in reducing black MSM's HIV risk.

Within the context of HIV prevention research, a considerable amount of schol-arly work still needs to be conducted, and appropriate strategies developed and implemented for black MSM (Peterson & Jones, 2009). Based on the SMS and available interventions with demonstrated and suggestive efficacy for this popula-tion, there are several implications of this model that can serve as the basis for further adaptations and the creation of additional interventions.

First, the SMS can inform how social stress is perceived and managed by black MSM. This understanding will assist interventionists in developing additional appropriate stress coping strategies. Using this model, interventionists will be prepared to assist black MSM in understanding the possible courses of actions available to them, based on the perceived stressor and with an emphasis on more healthful courses of action. As suggested by Durantini, Albarracin, Mitchell, Earl, & Gillette, (2006), black MSM serving as interventionists may be more effective at delivering these types of interventions and at leading evaluation efforts.

Interventionists using this model also can assist black MSM in improving their self-efficacy. This may involve providing culturally appropriate skills for black MSM to improve their ability to make more healthful sexual and risk-reduction decisions in relation to social stress. It also may involve strategies to provide different meaning to discrimination and to re-establish support. One option is the location, or creation, of alternative forms of healthy support where supportive behaviors and norms are reinforced. Finally, interventionists using this model should be prepared to help black MSM seek to ameliorate stressors including racism, homophobia, poverty, and incarceration. While the latter is an ambitious goal, it is nonetheless important from a social justice perspective that is inherent throughout the conceptualizations of the SMS.

Ultimately, interventions that strengthen black MSM's individual support systems and the acceptance of same-sex behaviors within familial and communal support networks should be explored because they may prove to be effective strategies for reducing the men's HIV risk (Bowleg et al., 2004; Jones et al., 2008a; Mays et al., 1998; Mays et al., 2004). The value of social support has been demonstrated in the scientific literature generally (House, 1981; Langford, Bowsher, Maloney, & Lillis, 1997; McColl, Lei, & Skinner, 1995), specifically in those parts of the literature that focus on people living with HIV (Kadushin, 1999; Reeves, 2001; Renwick, Halpen, Rudman & Friedland, 1999). The SMS can serve as an impetus for the development of future interventions for black MSM and for the potential to optimize different strategies in response to different social stressors (Cutrona and Russell, 1990).

Conclusion

Discrimination and various forms of social stress have negative consequences on the lives of black MSM. This discrimination can limit access to health care and increase exposure to poverty and incarceration. Theoretical models are needed to offer an explanation of black MSM's interactions with these forms of social stress and with unprotected anal sex. The SMS is offered as one such theoretical model to explain this behavior and how it can contribute to our understanding of disparate rates of individual HIV risk of black MSM. The SMS can serve as a theoretical framework that will inform the development of interventions for black MSM.

Acknowledgements The findings and conclusions in this manuscript are those of the authors and do not necessarily represent the views of the Centers for Disease Control and Prevention. The authors sincerely thank Drs. Pilgrim Spikes and Leigh Willis and Mr. Kevin T. Jones for their support and critical review of this manuscript.

References

Arnold, E. A., & Bailey, M. M. (2009). Constructing home and family: How the Ballroom Community supports African American GLBTQ youth in the face of HIV/AIDS. *Journal of Gay and Lesbian Social Services, 21*, 171–188.

Battle, J., Cohen, C. J., Warren, D., Fergerson, G., & Audam, S. (2002). *Say it loud, I'm Black and I'm Proud: Black Pride Survey 2000*. Washington, DC: Policy Institute of the National Gay and Lesbian Task Force.

Biafora, F. A., Warheit, G. J., Zimmerman, R. S., & Gil, A. G. (1993). Racial mistrust and deviant behaviors among ethnically diverse Black adolescent boys. *Journal of Applied Social Psychology, 23*, 891–910.

Blair, J. M., Fleming, P. L., & Karon, J. M. (2002). Trends in AIDS incidence and survival among racial/ethnic minority men who have sex with men, United States, 1990–1999. *Journal of Acquired Immune Deficiency Syndrome, 31*, 339–347.

Bogart, L. M., & Thorburn, S. (2005). HIV/AIDS conspiracy beliefs a barrier to HIV prevention among African Americans? *Journal of Acquired Immune Deficiency Syndrome, 38*, 213–218.

Bonilla-Silva, E. (2006). *Racism without racists: Color-blind racism and the persistence of racial inequality in the United States*. Lanham, Maryland: Rowman and Littlefield.

Bowleg, L., Craig, M. L., & Burkholder, G. (2004). Rising and Surviving: A conceptual model of acting coping among black lesbians. *Cultural Diversity & Ethnic Minority Psychology, 3*, 229–240.

Bowman, P. J., & Howard, C. (1985). Race related socialization, motivation, and academic achievement: A study of Black youths in three-generation families. *Journal of the American Academy of Child Psychiatry, 24*, 134–141.

Bright, C. M., Duefield, C. A., & Caldwell, C. (1998). Perceived barriers and biases in medical education experience by gender and race. *Journal of the National Medical Association, 90*, 681–688.

CDC. (2001). HIV incidence among young men who have sex with men – seven U.S. cities, 1994–2000. *MMWR Morbidity & Mortality Weekly Report, 50*, 440–444.

CDC. (2002). Unrecognized HIV Infection, risk behaviors, and perceptions of risk among young black men who have sex with men – six U.S. cities, 1994–1998. *MMWR Morbidity & Mortality Weekly Report, 51*, 733–736.

CDC. (2004). HIV transmission among black college student and non-student men who have sex with men – North Carolina, 2003. *MMWR Morbidity & Mortality Weekly Report, 53*, 731–734.

CDC. (2005a). Trends in HIV/AIDS diagnoses – 33 states, 2001–2004. *MMWR Morbidity & Mortality Weekly Report, 54*, 1149–1153.

CDC. (2005b). HIV prevalence, unrecognized infection, and HIV testing among men who have sex with men – five U.S. cities, June 2004–April 2005. *MMWR Morbidity & Mortality Weekly Report, 54*, 597–601.

CDC. (2006). Human immunodeficiency virus (HIV) risk, prevention, and testing behaviors – United States, national HIV behavioral surveillance system: Men who have sex with men, November 2003–April 2005. *MMWR Morbidity & Mortality Weekly Report, 55*, 1–20.

CDC. (2008a). HIV prevalence estimates – United States, 2006. *MMWR Morbidity & Mortality Weekly Report, 57*, 1073–1076.

CDC. (2008b). Subpopulation estimates from the HIV incidence surveillance system – United States, 2006. *MMWR Morbidity & Mortality Weekly Report, 57*, 985–989.

Clark, V. R. (2001). The perilous effects of racism on blacks. *Ethnicity & Disease, 11*, 769–772.

Clark, V. R., Moore, C. L., & Adams, J. H. (1998). Cholesterol concentrations and cardiovascular reactivity to stress in African-American college volunteers. *Journal of Behavior & Medicine, 21*, 505–515.

Constantine-Simms, D. (2001). (Ed). *The Greatest Taboo: Homosexuality in Black Communities*. New York: Alyson Books.

Cutrona, C. E., & Russell, D. (1990). Type of social support and specific stress: Toward a theory of optimal matching. In I. G. Sarason, B. R. Sarason, & G. R. Pierce (Eds.), *Social support: An interactional view* (pp. 319–366). New York: Wiley.

Dang, A., & Frazer, S. (2004). *Black same-sex households in the United States: A report from the 2000 Census*. New York: National Gay and Lesbian Task Force Policy Institute & the National Black Justice Coalition.

Diaz, R. M., & Ayala, G. (2001). *Social discrimination and health: The case of Latino gay men*. New York: The Policy Institute of the National Gay and Lesbian Task Force.

Diaz, R. M., Ayala, G., & Bein, E. (2004). Sexual risk as an outcome of social oppression: Data from a probability sample of Latino gay men in three U.S. cities. *Cultural Diversity & Ethnic Minority Psychology, 10,* 255–267.

Durantini, M. R., Albarracin, D., Mitchell, A. L., Earl, N. A., & Gillette, J. C. (2006). Conceptualizing the influence of social agents of behavior change: A meta-analysis of the effectiveness of HIV-prevention interventionists for different groups. *Psychological Bulletin, 132,* 212–248.

Eccles, J. S., Wong, C. A., & Peck, S. (2006). Ethnicity as a context for the development of African-American adolescents. *Journal of School Psychology, 44,* 407–426.

Fischer, A. R., & Shaw, C. M. (1999). African Americans' mental health and perceptions of racist discrimination: The moderating effects of racial socialization experiences and self-esteem. *Journal of Counseling Psychology, 62,* 243–251.

Glanz, K., & Schwartz, M. D. (2008). Stress, coping, and health behavior. In K. Glanz, B. K. Rimer, & K. Viswanath (Eds.), *Health behavior and health education: Theory, research, and practice* (4th ed., pp. 211–236). San Francisco, CA: Jossey-Bass.

Greene, B. (1994). Ethnic-minority lesbians and gay men: Mental health and treatment issues. *Journal of Consulting and Clinical Psychology, 62,* 243–251.

Guenther-Grey, C. A., Varnell, S., Weiser, J. I., Mathy, R. M., O'Donnell, L. O., Stueve, A., et al. (2005). Trends in sexual risk-taking among urban young men who have sex with men, 1999–2002. *Journal of the National Medical Association, 97,* 38–43.

Hall, I., Byers, R. H., Ling, Q., & Espinoza, L. (2007). Racial/ethnic and age disparities in HIV prevalence and disease progression among men who have sex with men in the United States. *American Journal of Public Health, 97,* 1060–1066.

Harawa, N. T., Greenland, S., Bingham, T. A., Johnson, D. F., Cochran, S. D., Cunningham, W. E., et al. (2004). Associations of race/ethnicity with HIV prevalence and HIV-related behaviors among young men who have sex with men in 7 urban centers in the United States. *Journal of Acquired Immune Deficiency Syndrome, 35,* 526–536.

Hart, T., Peterson, J. L., & Community Intervention Trial for Youth (CITY) Study Team. (2004). Predictors of risky sexual behavior among young African-American men who have sex with men. *American Journal of Public Health, 94,* 1122–1123.

Holtgrave, D. R., Hall, H. I., Rhodes, P. H., & Wolitski, R. J. (2008). Updated annual HIV transmission rates in the United States, 1997–2006. *Journal of Acquired Immune Deficiency Syndromes, 50*(2), 236–238.

House, J. S. (1981). *Work stress and social support.* Reading, MA: Addison-Wesley.

Huebner, D. M., Davis, M. C., Nemeroff, C. J., & Aiken, L. S. (2002). The impact of internalized homophobia on HIV prevention interventions. *American Journal of Community Psychology, 30,* 327–348.

Hughes, D. (2003). Correlates of African American and Latino parents' messages to children about ethnicity and race: A comparative study of racial socialization. *American Journal of Community Psychology, 31,* 15–33.

Hughes, D., & Johnson, D. (2001). Correlates in children's experiences of parents' racial socialization behaviors. *Journal of Marriage and Family, 63,* 981–995.

Hughes, D., Rodriguez, J., Smith, E. P., Johnson, D. J., Stevenson, H. C., & Spicer, P. (2006). Parents' ethnic-racial socialization practices: A review of research and directions for future study. *Developmental Psychology, 42,* 747–770.

Hutchinson, A. B., Begley, E. B., Sullivan, P., Clark, H. A., Boyett, B. C., & Kellerman, S. C. (2007). Conspiracy beliefs and trust in information about HIV/AIDS among minority men who have sex with men, [Letter]. *Journal of Acquired Immune Deficiency Syndrome, 45,* 603–605.

Jackson, J. S., Brown, T. N., Williams, D. R., Torres, M., Sellers, S. L., & Brown, K. (1996). Racism and the physical and mental health status of African Americans: A thirteen-year national panel study. *Ethnicity and Disease, 6,* 132–147.

Jones, K. T., Gray, P., Whiteside, Y. O., Wang, T., Bost, D., Dunbar, E., et al. (2008). Evaluation of an HIV prevention intervention adapted for black men who have sex with men. *American Journal of Public Health, 98,* 1043–1050.

Jones, D. R., Harrell, J. P., Morris-Prather, C. E., Thomas, J., & Omowale, N. (1996). Affective and physiological responses to racism: The roles of Afrocentrism and mode of presentation. *Ethnicity & Disease, 6*, 109–122.

Jones, K. T., Johnson, W. D., Wheeler, D. P., Gray, P., Foust, E., & Gaiter, J. (2008). Nonsupportive peer norms and incarceration as HIV risk correlates for young black men who have sex with men. *AIDS & Behavior, 12*, 41–50.

Kadushin, G. (1999). Barriers to social support and support received from their families of origin among gay men with HIV/AIDS. *Health and Social Work, 24*, 198–209.

Kelly, J. A., St Lawrence, J. S., Diaz, Y. E., Stevenson, L. Y., Hauth, A. C., Brasfield, T. L., et al. (1991). HIV risk behavior reduction following intervention with key opinion leaders of a population: An experimental analysis. *American Journal of Public Health, 81*, 168–171.

Klonoff, E. A., & Landrine, H. (1999). Do blacks believe that HIV/AIDS is a government conspiracy against them? *Preventive Medicine, 28*, 451–457.

Knight, G. P., Bernal, M. E., Cota, M. K., Garza, C. A., & Ocampo, K. A. (1993). Family socialization and Mexican American identity and behavior. In G. P. Knight & M. E. Bernal (Eds.), *Ethnic identity*. Albany, NY: State University of New York Press.

Knight, G. P., Cota, M. K., & Bernal, M. E. (1993). The socialization of cooperative, competitive, and individualistic preferences among Mexican American children: The mediating role of ethnic identity. *Hispanic Journal of Behavioral Sciences, 15*, 291–309.

Kraft, J. M., Beeker, C., Stokes, J., & Peterson, J. L. (2000). Finding the "community" in community-level HIV/AIDS interventions: Formative research with young African-American men who have sex with men. *Health Education & Behavior, 27*, 430–441.

Kreiss, J. L., & Patterson, D. L. (1997). Psychosocial issues in primary care of lesbian, gay, bisexual, and transgender youth. *Journal of Pediatric Health Care, 11*, 266–274.

Langford, C. P. H., Bowsher, J., Maloney, J. P., & Lillis, P. P. (1997). Social support: A conceptual analysis. *Journal of Advanced Nursing, 25*, 95–100.

LaVeist, T. A., Sellers, R., & Neighbors, H. W. (2001). Perceived racism and self and system blame attribution: Consequences for longevity. *Ethnicity & Disease, 11*, 711–721.

Lazarus, R. S., & Folkman, S. (1984). *Stress, appraisal, and coping*. New York: Springer.

Lemp, G. F., Hirozawa, A. M., Givertz, D., Nieri, G. N., Anderson, L., Lindegren, M. L., et al. (1994). Seroprevalence of HIV and risk behaviors among young homosexual and bisexual men: The San Francisco/Berkeley Young Men's Survey. *Journal of the American Medical Association, 272*, 449–454.

Loiacano, D. K. (1993). Gay identity among black Americans: Racism, homophobia, and the need for validation. In L. D. Garnets & D. C. Kimmel (Eds.), *Psychological perspectives on lesbian and gay male experiences* (pp. 364–375). New York: Columbia University Press.

Mansergh, G., Marks, G., Colfax, G. N., Guzman, R., Rader, M., & Buchbinder, S. (2002). "Barebacking" in a diverse sample of men who have sex with men. *AIDS, 14*, 653–659.

Marks, S. M., Murrill, C., Sanchez, T., Liu, K., Finlayson, T., & Guilin, V. (2008). Self-reported tuberculosis disease and tuberculin skin testing in the New York City House Ballroom community. *American Journal of Public Health, 98*, 1–6.

Mays, V. M., Chatters, L. M., Cochran, S. D., & Mackness, J. (1998). African-American families in diversity: Gay men and lesbians as participants in family networks. *Journal of Comparative Family Studies, 29*, 73–87.

Mays, V. M., & Cochran, S. D. (2001). Mental health correlates of perceived discrimination among lesbian, gay, and bisexual adults in the United States. *American Journal of Public Health, 91*, 1869–1876.

Mays, V. M., Cochran, S. D., & Zamudio, A. (2004). HIV prevention research: are we meeting the needs of African-American men who have sex with men? *Journal of Black Psychology, 30*, 78–105.

Mays, V. M., Nardi, P. M., Cochran, S. D., & Taylor, R. J. (2000). *The importance of friendship networks in HIV prevention among African-American gay men*. Paper presented at the Thirteenth International Conference on AIDS, Durban, South Africa.

McColl, M. A., Lei, H., & Skinner, H. (1995). Structural relationship between social support and coping. *Social Science and Medicine, 41*, 395–407.

Meyer, I. H. (2003). Prejudice, social stress, and mental health in lesbian, gay, and bisexual populations: Conceptual issues and research evidence. *Psychological Bulletin, 129*, 674–697.

Millett, G. A., Flores, S. A., Peterson, J. L., & Bakeman, R. (2007). Explaining disparities in HIV infection among black and white men who have sex with men: A meta-analysis of HIV risk behaviors. *AIDS, 1*, 2083–2091.

Millett, G. A., Peterson, J. L., Wolitski, R. J., & Stall, R. (2006). Greater risk for HIV infection of black men who have sex with men: A critical literature review. *American Journal of Public Health, 96*, 1007–1019.

Murrill, C., Guilin, V., Dean, L., Liu-K., Junquera, Y., Asencio, R., et al. (2005, September). *HIV prevalence and risk behaviors among persons active in the New York City house ball community*. Paper presented at the National HIV Prevention Conference, Atlanta, GA.

Ogbu, J. U. (2004). Collective identity and the burden of "acting white" in black history, community, and education. *The Urban Review, 36*, 1–35.

Omi, M., & Winant, H. (1996). *Racial formation in the United States: From the 1960s to the 1990s*. New York: Routledge.

Park, B., & Judd, C. M. (2005). Rethinking the link between categorization and prejudice within the social cognition perspective. *Personality and Social Psychological Review, 9*, 108–130.

Peterson, J. L., Coates, T. J., Catania, J. A., Hauck, W. W., Acree, M., & Daigle, D. (1996). Evaluation of an HIV risk reduction intervention among African American homosexual and bisexual men. *AIDS, 10*, 319–325.

Peterson, J. L., & Jones, K. T. (2009). HIV prevention for Black men who have sex with men in the United States. *American Journal of Public Health, 99*, 1–5.

Phinney, J. S., & Chavira, V. (1995). Parental ethnic socialization and adolescent coping with problems related to ethnicity. *Journal of Research on Adolescent, 5*, 31–53.

Phinney, J. S., & Rotheram, M. J. (1987). *Children's ethnic socialization*. New York: Lawrence Erlbaum.

Raymond, H. F., & McFarland, W. (2009). Racial mixing and HIV risk among men who have sex with men. *AIDS and Behavior, 13*, 630–637.

Reeves, P. M. (2001). How individuals coping with HIV/AIDS use the Internet. *Health Education Research, 16*, 709–719.

Renwick, R., Halpen, T., Rudman, D., & Friedland, J. (1999). Description and validation of a measure of received support specific to HIV. *Psychological Reports, 84*, 663–673.

Richeson, J. A., & Nussbaum, R. J. (2004). The impact of multiculturalism versus color-blindness on racial bias. *Journal of Experimental Social Psychology, 40*, 417–423.

Rotter, J. B. (1966). Generalized expectancies for internal versus external control of reinforcement. Psychological Monographs, 80. (Whole No. 609).

Rumbaut, R. G. (1994). The crucible within: Ethnic identity, self-esteem, and segmented assimilation among children of immigrants. *International Migration Review, 28*, 748–794.

Sanders-Thompson, V. L. (1994). Socialization to race and its relationship to racial identification among African Americans. *Journal of Black Psychology, 20*, 175–188.

Sellers, S. L., Bonham, V., Neighbors, H. W., & Arnell, J. W. (2009). Effects of racial discrimination and health behaviors on mental and physical health of middle-class African American men. *American Journal of Public Health, 36*, 31–44.

Sellers, R. M., Caldwell, C. H., Schmeelk-Cone, K. H., & Zimmerman, M. A. (2003). Racial identity, racial discrimination, perceived stress, and psychological distress among African American young adults. *Journal of Health and Social Behavior, 43*, 302–317.

Sellers, R. M., & Shelton, J. N. (2003). The role of racial identity in perceived racial discrimination. *Journal of Personality and Social Psychology, 84*, 1079–1092.

Sellers, R. M., Smith, M. A., Shelton, J. N., Rowley, S. A. J., & Chavous, T. M. (1998). Multidimensional model of racial identity: A reconceptualization of African American racial identity. *Personality and Social Psychology Review, 2*, 18–39.

So, D. W. (2003). Psychosocial HIV/AIDS prevention for high-risk African-American men: Guiding principles for clinical psychologist. *Clinical Psychology: Science and Practice, 10*, 468–480.

Stevenson, H. C., Cameron, R., Herrero-Taylon, T., & Davis, G. Y. (2002). Development of the teenage experience of racial socialization scale: Correlates of race-related socialization frequency from the perspective of black youth. *Journal of Black Psychology, 28*, 84–106.

Stokes, J. P., & Peterson, J. L. (1998). Homophobia, self-esteem, and risk for HIV among African-American men who have sex with men. *AIDS Education and Prevention, 10*, 278–292.

Thornton, M. C., Chatters, L. M., Taylor, R. J., & Allen, W. R. (1990). Sociodemographic and environmental correlates of racial socialization by Black parents. *Child Development, 61*, 401–409.

Valleroy, L. A., MacKellar, D. A., Karon, J. M., Rosen, D. H., McFarland, W., Shehan, D. A., et al. (2000). HIV prevalence and associated risks in young men who have sex with men. *Journal of the American Medical Association, 284*, 198–204.

Vicioso, K. J., Parsons, J. T., Nanin, J. E., Purcell, D. W., & Woods, W. E. (2005). Experiencing release: Sex environments and escapism for HIV-positive men who have sex with men. *Journal of Sex Research, 42*, 13–19.

Vittinghoff, E., Douglas, J., Judson, F., McKirnan, D., MacQuee, K., Buchbinder, S. P. (1999). Per-contact risk of human immunodeficiency virus transmission between male sexual partners. *American Journal of Epidemiology, 150*, 306–311.

Washington, H. A. (2006). *Medical apartheid: The dark history of medical experimentation on Black Americans from colonial times to the present*. New York: Harlem Moon.

Whaley, A. L. (2001). Cultural mistrust and mental health services for African Americans: a review and meta-analysis. *Counseling Psychology, 29*, 513–531.

Williams, D. R., Neighbors, H. W., & Jackson, J. S. (2003). Racial/ethnic discrimination and health: Findings from community studies. *American Journal of Public Health, 93*, 200–208.

Williams, D. R., Yu, Y., Jackson, J. S., & Anderson, N. B. (1997). Racial differences in physical and mental health. *Journal of Health Psychology, 2*, 335–351.

Wilson, P. A., Cook, S., McGaskey, J., Rowe, N., & Dennis, N. (2009). Situational predictors of sexual risk episodes among men with HIV who have sex with men. *Sexually Transmitted Infections, 84*, 506–508.

Wilson, P. A., & Yoshikawa, H. (2004). Experiences of and responses to social discrimination among Asian and Pacific Islander gay men: Their relationship to HIV risk. *AIDS Education and Prevention, 16*, 68–83.

Wilton, L. (2009). Men who have sex with men of color in the age of AIDS: The sociocultural contexts of stigma, marginalization, and structural inequalities. In V. Stone, B. Ojikutu, K. Rawlings, & K. Smith (Eds.), *HIV/AIDS in communities of color*. New York: Springer.

Wilton, L., Herbst, J. H., Coury-Doniger, P., Painter, T. M., English, G., Alvarez, M. E., et al. (2009). Efficacy of an HIV/STI prevention intervention for black men who have sex with men: Findings from the Many Men, Many Voices (3MV) project. *AIDS & Behavior, 13*(3), 532–544.

Wolsko, C., Park, B., Judd, C. M., & Winterbrink, B. (2000). Framing interethnic ideology: Effects of multicultural and color-blind perspectives on judgments of groups and individuals. *Journal of Personality and Social Psychology, 78*, 635–654.

Woodyard, J. L., Peterson, J. L., & Stokes, J. P. (2000). 'Let us go into the house of the Lord': Participation in African-American churches among young African-American men who have sex with men. *Journal of Pastoral Care, 54*, 451–460.

Yip, T., Gilbert, G. C., & Takeuchi, D. T. (2008). Racial discrimination and psychological distress: The impact of ethnic identity and age among immigrant and United States-born Asian adults. *Development Psychology, 44*, 787–800.

Zamboni, B. D., & Crawford, I. (2007). Minority stress and sexual problems among African-American gay and bisexual men. *Archives of Sexual Behavior, 36*, 569–578.

Chapter 13
HIV Prevention Interventions for African American Injection Drug Users

David W. Purcell, Yuko Mizuno, and Cynthia M. Lyles

Background

Injection drug use has been a major risk factor for transmission of HIV in the United States since the beginning of the HIV epidemic (Des Jarlais & Semaan, 2008) and is a major risk factor for African Americans. While the proportion of injection drug users (IDUs) among HIV-positive persons has decreased over time, the Centers for Disease Control and Prevention (CDC) reported that, at the end of 2007, IDUs accounted for 23% of existing AIDS cases in the United States (30% if men who have sex with men (MSM) and inject drugs are included) (CDC, 2009). By gender, 35% of overall AIDS cases among women and 20% among men are attributed to drug injection (29% among men if MSM/IDUs are included) (CDC, 2009). African Americans are disproportionately affected by HIV and AIDS – in 2006 African American accounted for approximately 12% of the population and 46% of the persons estimated to be living with HIV (CDC, 2008). When looking at the percent of reported AIDS cases attributed to injection drug use within race and gender, it is much higher among African American men (29%) than among white, non Hispanics men (9%) while the percent of AIDS cases attributed to IDUs is similarly high for African American women (33%) and white women (40%) and also is similar among MSM/IDUs for African American men (8%) and white men (9%) (CDC, 2009). For both African American men and women, IDU is the second leading transmission risk category (CDC, 2009).

Many studies describe IDUs and non-IDU substance users as socio-economically marginalized and often struggling with a variety of complex challenges including mental health problems, substance abuse, incarceration, discrimination, marginal housing, poverty, and family conflict (Mizuno et al., 2006). With such a background,

D.W. Purcell (✉)
Division of HIV/AIDS Prevention, Centers for Disease Control,
1600 Clifton Road MS E-37, Atlanta, GA 30333, USA
e-mail: dpurcell@cdc.gov

D.H. McCree et al. (eds.), *African Americans and HIV/AIDS*,
DOI 10.1007/978-0-387-78321-5_13,

HIV can easily become a competing life priority that is given limited attention or importance (Mizuno, Purcell, Borkowski, Knight & the SUDIS Team, 2003). Similarly, due to historical and on-going stigmatization and marginalization and other structural and social determinants of health, African Americans IDUs are more likely to struggle with elevated rates of infectious diseases as well as other complex psychosocial challenges than other racial and ethnic groups (Blankenship, Smoyer, Bray, & Mattocks, 2005; Estrada, 2005; Hogben & Leichliter, 2008; Mays, Chochran, & Barnes, 2007). In addition to their contextual vulnerability to poor health outcomes in general, IDUs are vulnerable to HIV infection from injection-related risk (e.g., sharing of needles or other injection equipment) and sex-related risk behaviors (e.g., unprotected sex, trading sex for money or drugs, having a large number of sexual partners). HIV-positive IDUs also may struggle with accessing HIV-related health care and adhering to HIV medications (Purcell et al., 2004).

Intravenous injection is an efficient source for viral transmission which contributed to rapid spread of HIV among IDUs in the United States early in the epidemic. But also contributing were factors that made it hard for IDUs to protect themselves (e.g., lack of information about HIV and AIDS, restricted access to sterile needles and paraphernalia), and factors that increased the likelihood of HIV transmission (e.g., rapid exchange of injection partner in some situations such as "shooting galleries," and high infectiousness among newly infected persons) (Des Jarlais & Semaan, 2008). Because IDUs were one of the earliest groups identified as affected by the HIV/AIDS epidemic, community-based organizations and research-ers began developing interventions for IDUs early in the epidemic. Research shows that effective prevention of HIV among IDUs can both prevent epidemics and con-tain existing epidemics (Des Jarlais & Semaan).

Before discussing the interventions designed to reduce HIV risk among IDUs, and particularly African American IDUs, there is an important emerging historical trend that is important to note. It appears that African Americans are increasingly turning away from injection as a route of administration for heroin, the primary injection drug used by African Americans (Broz & Ouellet, 2008). Evidence from multiple studies and datasets indicate a very large decline in young African American heroin injectors entering drug treatment and enrolling in research studies, even in cities with large African American populations. For example, in cohorts born before 1955, African Americans had a higher lifetime probability of drug injection than whites, but the reverse is true for later born cohorts (Armstrong, 2007). Recent evi-dence shows a slower, later, and smaller transition from snorting to injecting heroin among African Americans compared to whites (Broz & Ouellet). Potential explana-tions include avoidance of heroin injection due to the severe impact of HIV in the African American community, changes in social conditions and identity that may impact choices about drug use, and increases in drug quality leading to movement away from injection. While reduced injection among African Americans is good news for injection risk, African American IDUs are still at increased sexual and injection risk because of higher background prevalence of HIV infection in their community, and interventions are needed for this vulnerable population.

Interventions to Prevent HIV Among IDUs

In this chapter, we briefly describe the response to the HIV epidemic among IDUs, and the various broad types of interventions that have been developed to try to decrease HIV, as well as other blood-born infections among this heavily affected population. Then we focus on evidence-based behavioral interventions designed to reduce sexual or drug injection risk among IDUs, and particularly individual-, group-, and community-level interventions designed for African American IDUs. We also will discuss interventions for IDUs and non-injection substance users that might be adapted for African American IDUs. Finally we will indicate next directions for HIV prevention interventions for African American IDUs.

Responses to the HIV Epidemic Among IDUs

Due to very high rates of prevalent and incident HIV infection among IDUs, particularly in New York City, a variety of projects and programs were developed and tested to respond to the public health challenges. Education, community outreach, drug treatment, and risk reduction programs were among the earliest efforts. One of the first large-scale behavioral intervention studies was the National AIDS Demonstration Research (NADR) project funded by the National Institute on Drug Abuse (NIDA) designed to reach and intervene with IDUs and their partners (Weissman & Brown, 1995). Reviews have found a variety of interventions to be effective in reducing sexual risk including community outreach to IDUs, individual and group interventions, and drug treatment programs (Copenhaver, Johnson, Lee, Harman, Carey, & the SHARP Research Team, 2006; Des Jarlais & Semaan, 2005, 2008; Farrell, Gowing, Marsden, Ling, & Ali, 2005; Metzger, Navaline, & Woody, 1998; Needle et al., 2005). As with other populations, HIV counseling and testing also is effective in reducing the risk behaviors of IDUs found to be HIV-positive (but generally not those found to be HIV-negative) (Weinhardt, Carey, Johnson, & Bickham, 1999). In general, interventions with IDUs have been more successful at reducing injection risk than sexual risk (Kotranski et al., 1998; McMahon, Malow, Jennings, & Gomez, 2001; Prendergast, Urada, & Podus, 2001; Semaan et al., 2002). This is important because more recent studies have shown that unprotected sexual behavior is a strong independent predictor of HIV seroconversion among IDUs (Kral et al., 2001; Strathdee & Sherman, 2003).

In the late 1980s and throughout the 1990s, public health officials, community members, and researchers also examined structural interventions. For example, syringe exchange programs (SEPs) were developed to decrease barriers for IDUs to access sterile syringes by allowing the exchange of used needles for free, new sterile syringes to reduce the transmission of bloodborne infections (CDC, 2007; Des Jarlais & Friedman, 1996). As of late 2007, 185 SEPs were part of the North American Syringe Exchange network and were operating in 36 states, the District of Columbia, and Puerto Rico (CDC, 2007). SEPs often offer other services such as HIV testing and access to other HIV risk reduction interventions and drug treatment resources. Although the research designs have not always been optimal, the weight of the evidence on SEPs indicates that they reduce injection risk behaviors and incident infections while not leading to increased drug use (Gibson, Flynn, & Perales, 2001; Huo & Ouellet, 2007; Ksobiech, 2003). Communities also sought easier access to sterile syringes through changing laws to decriminalize selling of syringes by pharmacists and possession and disposal by IDUs (Jones & Coffin, 2002). There is evidence of reduced syringe sharing in those locales undertaking some or all of these policy or legal changes (Rich, Hogan, Wolf, DeLong, Zaller, Mehrotra, & Reinert, 2007).

Given the broad range of possible interventions for IDUs, a multi-level approach is often suggested. Research suggests that HIV prevalence is related to the amount and breadth of services provided to IDUs (Watters, Bluthenthal, & Kral, 1995). In this study, wide variance in HIV prevalence rates between IDUs in different areas within a large metropolitan area were not explained by individual-level variables but instead by structural and systems variables such as low resources and the lack of IDU-targeted programs and services (Watters et al., 1995). In fact, a comprehensive package of interventions for IDUs has been recommended by the Joint United Nations Programme on HIV/AIDS (UNAIDS), the United Nations Office on Drug Policy (UNODP), and the World Health Organization (WHO) (Donoghoe, Verster, Pervilhac, & Williams, 2008). The comprehensive package recommended for consideration in countries around the world includes the following: SEPs, opioid substitution therapy (methadone maintenance treatment programs), voluntary HIV counseling and testing, anti-retroviral treatment, prevention and treatment of sexually transmitted infections, condom programs for IDUs and their partners, education and communication for IDUs and their partners, hepatitis diagnosis, treatment (Hepatitis A, B, and C), and vaccination (Hepatitis A and B), and tuberculosis prevention, diagnosis, and treatment (Donoghoe et al., 2008). The focus for the rest of this review will be on one part of such a comprehensive package – namely behavioral interventions for IDUs designed to reduce injection or sexual risk. In a given community, the success of these interventions may partly depend on the other contextual and resource-related issues that have been discussed.

Reviews of HIV Prevention Behavioral Interventions for IDUs

Copenhaver et al. (2006) examined 37 randomized controlled trials evaluating 49 independent HIV risk reduction interventions targeting IDUs (51% of overall study participants were African American). Through meta-analyses, the authors concluded that the interventions facilitated condom use, promoted entry into drug treatment, and helped to reduce injection and non-injection drug use and sex trading. Stratified analyses showed that behavioral interventions were more successful at reducing injection risk when participants were non-white, when the content focused equivalently on drug-related and sex-related risks, and when the content included interpersonal skills training specific for safer needle use. For sexual risk, condom use outcomes improved when two intervention facilitators were used instead of one. These analyses also showed that reductions in injection risk did not tend to decay over time while sexual risk outcomes did decay. This latter finding suggested the need for booster sessions for sexual risk after an intervention ends (Copenhaver et al.) and indicates the challenge facing interventionists in trying to make lasting changes to sexual risk after a relatively brief behavioral intervention.

In a meta-analysis of interventions to reduce sexual risk among IDUs, Semaan et al. (2002) examined the effectiveness of 33 US-based HIV intervention studies identified as of June 1998 (58% of the studies included 66% or more minority participants). The overall meta-analysis showed that IDUs in the intervention groups were more likely to reduce sexual risk behaviors than those in the comparison groups. However, when the results were stratified, three studies in which the comparison groups received no intervention had a significantly stronger effect compared to the 30 studies in which the comparison condition received some HIV prevention intervention. Studies in which both the experimental and the comparison groups received an HIV-related intervention had a small but statistically non-significant average effect size. Semaan et al. interpreted these results to show that providing some intervention is better than providing nothing for IDUs, although these results also could be due to socially desirable responding. A recent intervention study for HIV-positive IDUs found similar results. In a randomized controlled trial that included 66% African Americans, participants in both the 10-session intervention condition and the 8-session video discussion comparison group reported similar decreases in sexual and injection risk behaviors (Purcell et al., 2007).

In sum, meta-analyses of HIV prevention interventions suggest that interventions can reduce the injection and sexual risk behaviors of IDUs, however, the effect size for sexual risk is modest (Semaan et al., 2002) and the effects tends to decay over time more quickly for sexual risk compared to injection risk (Copenhaver et al., 2006).

Evidence-Based Interventions Relevant for African American IDUs

While meta-analyses indicate a modest effect of behavioral interventions on injection and sexual risk (Copenhaver et al., 2006; Semaan et al., 2002), these papers also provide evidence that a small number of interventions individually have significant effects on the outcomes of interest. For example, graphs show that only 4 of the 33 effect sizes calculated by Semaan et al. for reductions in unsafe sexual behaviors were significant. Similarly, Copenhaver et al. showed that only 4 of 30 effect sizes for injection risk and 6 of 15 effects sizes for condom use were significant. When moving from research to practice, it is important to identify strong interventions for IDUs so that they can be packaged and disseminated to health departments and community based organizations (Lyles, Crepaz, Herbst, & Kay for the HIV/AIDS Prevention Research Synthesis Team, 2006).

CDC's Division of HIV/AIDS Prevention has developed a research-to-practice model to identify, package, and disseminate evidence-based HIV risk reduction interventions for all groups, including African American IDUs. First, evidence-based interventions (EBIs) are identified by the Prevention Research Synthesis (PRS) project through systematic efficacy reviews of the intervention literature and applying standards related to study design, study implementation, statistical analyses, and strength of findings (CDC, 2010a; Lyles et al., 2006). By mid-2009, CDC had identified 63 EBIs and 58 focus on individuals or small groups. After identification by PRS, intervention developers have the opportunity to apply for funding to package their intervention into user friendly materials through the Replicating Effective Programs (REP) project (Eke et al., 2006). Finally, CDC provides training and technical assistance through its Diffusion of Effective Behavioral Interventions (DEBI) program for a number of HIV prevention interventions that are implemented by health departments and community-based organizations (AED, 2009; Collins et al., 2006).

To date, CDC has identified 12 evidence-based behavioral interventions for IDUs that have been shown to reduce either injection or sexual risk or reduce STDs – one community-level intervention and the rest individual or small-group interventions (CDC, 2010a). Some group-level interventions included only IDUs and some included a combination of IDUs and non-IDUs. Similarly, many interventions focus on IDUs without regard to race, leading to most studies including a racially mixed sample. We first focus on interventions that include a majority IDUs and a majority African Americans. Then we discuss other interventions that are relevant to African American IDUs and might be adapted if existing interventions do not meet local needs.

Female and Culturally Specific Negotiation Intervention

This intervention was tested with HIV-negative, heterosexual, African American women who were either crack cocaine smokers or active IDUs (Sterk, Theall, Elifson, & Kidder 2003). The goal of the intervention, which was developed after extensive formative work with the target population, was to reduce sexual and injection risk through four individual sessions focusing on the social context of the women's daily lives. Sessions included exploring gender dynamics, the meaning of behaviors and social interactions, gender-specific norms and values, and power and control. The intervention sessions also emphasized the extent of the local HIV epidemic, sex and drug-related risk behaviors, HIV risk reduction strategies, correct condom use, safer injection, communication and assertiveness skills, and the importance of race and gender on HIV risk and protective behaviors.

This negotiation intervention was tested against a standard intervention and against a motivation intervention that did not include skills building for negotiation. Results at the 6-month follow-up showed that the negotiation intervention group reported significantly greater reductions in the proportion of women who had a paying sex partner ($p < 0.05$), the proportion of women who traded sex for money or drugs ($p < 0.01$), and the mean number of injections ($p < 0.05$) than women who received the standard intervention. The women in the negotiation intervention also reported significantly greater reductions in frequency of alcohol use during sex ($p < 0.001$) than women receiving the motivation intervention at 6 months. Unfortunately, frequency of use of male condoms did not differ between groups, again indicating the challenge of changing sexual risk behavior among IDUs. This outcome may have been a particular challenge in this study because women usually do not control application of the male condom.

This intervention is a good choice for agencies that work with African American female IDUs or crack users and who have the staffing that would allow for four individual sessions per clients. Part of the success of the intervention may be due to the formative research as well at the theoretical basis (social cognitive theory, theory of reasoned action, theory of planned behavior, transtheoretical model of change, and theory of gender and power). The authors also report that a key component of this intervention is the focus on the social context of the women's lives, which allowed for the intervention to be sensitive to each woman's needs (Sterk et al., 2003). A CDC-supported package is not available for this intervention but materials may be requested from the primary author, Dr. Claire Sterk.

Self-Help in Eliminating Life-Threatening Diseases

The second evidence-based intervention most relevant to African American IDUs is the SHIELD intervention which was tested in Baltimore with IDUs who were primarily African American (94%) and male (61%) (Latkin, Sherman, & Knowlton, 2003). This intervention, based on social identity theory and peer outreach, consisted of ten small-group interactive sessions that relied on peer networks to reduce drug and sex risk behaviors. The intervention included training and skills building sessions that involved goal setting, role plays, demonstrations, and group discussions. In the groups, participants were asked to make a public commitment to increase their health behaviors and to promote HIV prevention among their networks and community contacts. In addition, one session occurred in the community and provided a "street outreach" practice session. Overall, the sessions instructed on techniques for personal risk reduction including injection drug and sexual risk, the development of correct condom use and safer sex negotiation skills, and the avoidance of risky situations.

Positive results were found for the SHIELD intervention for both drug and sex risks. At the 6-months follow-up, IDUs receiving the SHIELD intervention reported significantly greater reductions in needle sharing ($p < 0.05$) and IDU frequency ($p < 0.05$) and were more likely to stop injecting drugs ($p < 0.05$) than participants in the control group. Among sexually active IDUs, those receiving the SHIELD intervention reported significantly greater increases in condom use with casual sex partners ($p < 0.05$), but no differences with main partners, than those in the control group. Latkin et al. (2003) noted that outreach to peers is a prosocial role that fits with the historical experiences and communal values of African Americans.

Developing such a role for African American IDUs in an HIV prevention intervention may be meaningful as well because of its association with religious outreach and with the advocacy for drug abstinence that is characteristic of 12-step drug treatment programs. Finally, peer outreach may be especially effective for African American inner-city IDUs because it provides one of few available prosocial roles and is culturally familiar. SHIELD recently completed the REP process, and a package will be available for dissemination through DEBI in late 2009 (Academy for Educational Development, 2009).

Other interventions, such as the Intervention for Seropositive Injectors: Research and Evaluation (INSPIRE) study, used the same notion of promoting a prosocial, peer mentoring role in a group setting, in this case with disenfranchised HIV-positive IDUs (66% African American) (Purcell et al., 2004). While those in the 10-session intervention group reported decreased sexual and injection risk over time, so did participants in the 8-session control group (Purcell et al., 2007). One finding coming from qualitative interviews of participants who attended at least four sessions of the intervention or the comparison group was that HIV-positive IDUs in both conditions felt very positively about their time spent with other people like them. The findings from this study are also consistent with conclusions from a meta-analysis described above – that IDUs may benefit from any active intervention (Semaan et al., 2002). While this reduction of reported risk behaviors in both conditions could be due to the effect of participating in multiple assessments, or due to socially desirable responding, this finding also would support the explanation that general attention and support can benefit marginalized populations such as African American IDS across various domains.

Peers Reaching Out and Modeling Intervention Strategies (Community PROMISE)

Community PROMISE is a community-level intervention (CLI) that included a majority African Americans (54%) and a majority who reported lifetime IDU (53%), but it was designed to apply to a broad range of community members who were underserved and at risk for HIV infection including IDUs and their female sex partners, sex workers, non-gay-identified MSM, high-risk youth, and residents of areas with high rates of sexually transmitted diseases (The CDC AIDS Community Demonstration Projects Research Group, 1999). In CLIs, the goal is to change community norms among a substantial portion of the target population so that behavior change can be observed among the population. By their very nature, these interventions target a broad physical community, and thus do not target African Americans except to the extent the population of the intervention community is made up of African Americans. Community Promise begins with the development of role model stories based on the real experiences of members of the target population who have made positive HIV/STD behavior change. Peer advocates from the target populations then are recruited and trained to distribute the role model stories and prevention materials (condoms and bleach kits) within their social networks. The role model stories, using true-to-life information, show fictional community members in different stages of change from the Transtheoretical model (Prochaska, DiClemente, & Norcross, 1992). The intervention was conducted in ten communities and each community had a comparison community that did not receive the intervention. Using an assessment of stage-of-change scores for the community-level assessment, they found greater movement toward consistent condom use with main ($p<0.05$) and non-main partners ($p<0.05$), as well as increased condom carrying ($p<0.0001$), in intervention than in comparison communities (The CDC AIDS Community Demonstration Projects Research Group, 1999). At the individual level, participants recently exposed to the intervention were more likely to carry condoms and to have higher stage-of-change scores for condom and bleach use. This intervention has some similarity to SHIELD (Latkin et al., 2003) in its use of peers to disseminate important public health information to close peers and community members. In this case, using a large number and type of community volunteers to deliver the intervention led to a high level of community exposure and made it possible to reach many more persons than could have been reached by paid staff. In addition, these volunteers reached community members who might not have participated if they had to travel to an organization to attend a prevention program. Furthermore, the presence of these volunteers served as an ongoing reminder of the risk reduction messages disseminated by the project and provided ongoing reinforcement of behavior change efforts (The CDC AIDS Community Demonstration Projects Research Group). This intervention has been packaged into a community-friendly format, and trainings can be provided through various CDC-supported mechanisms (Academy for Educational Development, 2009)

Other Evidence-Based Interventions Relevant for African American IDUs

There are some group and individual interventions that were tested on substance users in general that either excluded IDUs or include both IDU and non-IDUs. These are relevant for potential adaptation for IDUs, particularly those interventions that were successful at reducing sexual risk among substance users. Similarly, there are some interventions tested among IDUs other than African Americans that could potentially be adapted for African American IDUs. Adaptation is generally best suited for situations when an EBI does not exist for a particular target population or if the existing EBIs are not relevant for some contextual reasons. One relevant adaptation model has been described by McKelroy et al. (2006). Generally, adaptation of an EBI requires fidelity to the defined core elements of an intervention while key characteristics can be changed to meet population needs (Academy for Educational Development, 2009; CDC, 2010b).

The Women's Co-Op intervention is an evidence-based intervention (CDC, 2010a) that was developed for and tested with crack-abusing African American women (Wechsberg, Lam, Zule, & Bobashev, 2004). This woman-focused intervention is grounded in women's empowerment theory and consists of two individual sessions focusing on a personal HIV risk assessment and skills building around HIV protective behaviors and then two small group sessions to help women further develop these skills with the support of peers. Wechsberg et al. (2004) argue interventions targeting African American women need to address power differentials in society and partner influences in relationships that may affect a woman's sexual behavior and negotiation practices. This intervention is unique in its attention to the potential role that women's economic empowerment (e.g., employment) may play in reducing their sexual risk behavior (Stratford, Mizuno, Williams, Courtenay-Quirk, & O'Leary, 2008) Although the mechanism through which economic empowerment is associated with sexual risk reduction was not clearly delineated in the study, the study lends credence to an approach that moves beyond standard skill-building interventions based in social cognitive theories. This intervention is not yet packaged but information is available from the original researcher.

Modelo de Intervention Psicomedia (MIP) is an evidence-based intervention that targeted Hispanic IDUs who were not currently in drug treatment and could be adapted for African American IDUs. MIP is an intensive intervention including standard HIV counseling and testing, six weekly one-on-one counseling sessions by a registered nurse, and ongoing case management. The counseling sessions use motivational interviewing strategies to engage and motivate clients for behavior change. The sessions focus on developing a work plan and goal setting to facilitate behavior change, encouraging the client to enter drug treatment, discussing relapse prevention strategies, including how to refuse needle sharing, providing skills building activities for safer sex negotiation and correct condom use, and improving self-efficacy around reducing injection behaviors. The case manager helps the client get through the intervention, provides access to drug treatment, health care services, and other legal or social welfare services as needed. When compared to the comparison group, this intervention found significant decline in participants continuing injection drug use and in reporting needle sharing at a 3.5 months follow-up after the intervention. The MIP intervention was packaged by the CDC's DEBI project (Academy for Educational Development, 2009).

Four other evidence-based interventions for substance users also have relevance for IDUs. The Intensive AIDS Education Intervention was tested with predominantly African American (66%) incarcerated drug using youth (Magura, Kang, & Shapiro, 1994). The intervention consisted of four small-group sessions that focused on health issues relevant to male adolescent drug users, with emphasis on HIV/AIDS. Intervention topics included HIV/AIDS knowledge, drug abuse, sexual behavior, ways to reduce AIDS risk, and how to seek health and social services and drug abuse treatment in the community. The discussions were facilitated using techniques drawn from Problem-Solving Therapy. Information about this intervention is available from its developer (See CDC, 2010a) and adaptation for IDUs should be feasible using general adaptation guidelines (McKelroy et al., 2006).

Safety Counts is an EBI that has been packaged by CDC's DEBI program. The intervention was designed for crack and injection drug users (injectors, crack smokers, and smoking injectors) that included nearly a majority of African Americans (47%) (Hershberger, Wood, & Fisher, 2003). This theory-based cognitive-behavioral intervention consisted of two group sessions, one individual counseling session, at least two social events focused on HIV risk reduction, and at least two field-based follow-up outreach contacts in addition to the two-session standard counseling and testing intervention developed by the National Institute on Drug Abuse (NIDA). Research evaluating the Safety Counts intervention concluded that the intervention had limited advantage over the NIDA standard intervention as participants in both conditions significantly reduced their HIV risk behaviors. One of the few significant effects of the Safety Count intervention was found on the percentage who had injected within the last 30 days. Although Safety Counts participants who were injectors used their own injection equipments more frequently, the sample of injectors consisted of relatively fewer African Americans (14%). The limited intervention effects suggest that Safety Counts did not reduce most risk behaviors more than the NIDA standard intervention did. Hershberger et al. (2003) speculate that the NIDA intervention might have already been strong, and they note that the study findings are consistent with conclusion of meta-analysis by Semaan et al. (2002) that interventions effects are more likely to be significant when a comparison group receives no intervention.

DUIT is an intervention that has recently been identified as EBI although the RCT that tested this intervention included a minority African Americans (8%) (Garfein et al., 2007). The intervention was designed for young (age 15–30 years old) IDUs who were seronegative for HIV and Hepatitis C. This six-session, small group intervention was based on social learning theory and the information, motivation, and behavioral skills models and taught young IDUs how to educate peers about HIV and HCV risk reduction. The intervention had a significant effect on overall injection risk (a 29% greater reduction among intervention participants compared to the control participants at 6 months post intervention). Like INSPIRE, however, participants reported declines in sexual risk behaviors in both study arms. As mentioned earlier, the RCT did not include a sufficient number of African Americans to fully assess the efficacy of this intervention for young African American IDUs, partly due to the decreased number of young African American IDUs (Broz & Ouellet, 2008). However, the use of a peer mentoring approach may be relevant for this population to reduce injection risk (Latkin et al., 2003).

STRIVE is another intervention developed by the investigators of DUIT. It targets HIV-negative IDUs who are seropositive for Hepatitis C [HCV] (Latka et al., 2008). This intervention has also been identified as an EBI, however, only a minority of participants in the research were African Americans (7%). The format of STRIVE is similar to that of DUIT; it is a six-session, small group intervention that taught participants to educate peers about safer injection practices to reduce transmission of HCV. The intervention also included sessions aimed to help participants manage their HCV health care. The intervention had a significant effect on overall injection risk and also sharing of drug preparation equipment and might be considered for adaptation if relevant (CDC, 2010a; McKelroy et al., 2006).

Other Interventions to Consider for IDUs

Holistic Health Recovery Program (HHRP+) is an intervention that was tested in a small study and has been packaged by the CDC's DEBI program, although it did not meet CDC criteria to be an EBI because of its small sample size (CDC, 2010a).

The intervention was designed for HIV-positive IDUs entering methadone maintenance treatment (MMT) and included nearly a majority African Americans (49%) (Margolin, Avants, Warburton, Hawkins, & Shi, 2003). Participants were assigned to either a control group (daily methadone + weekly individualized substance abuse counseling and case management + a six-session HIV risk reduction intervention) or the HIV Harm Reduction Program (HHRP+) (which added twice weekly manual-guided group therapy to the control group activities). The content of the HHRP + was comprehensive and addressed the medical, emotional, and spiritual needs of HIV-positive persons. The intervention activities were specifically designed to take into account potential problems that HIV-positive IDUs might have with memory, self-regulation, and foresight and planning, which are required to enact risk reduction. Because these capacities might be impaired in HIV-positive IDUs because of chronic drug use or HIV disease, the intervention used cognitive remediation strategies to facilitate learning and retention of theoretically important elements of the intervention. Participants in the HHRP + intervention were significantly less likely to have engaged in either unprotected sex or needle sharing during the post-treatment follow-up than participants in the comparison condition. HHRP + participants also reported a significantly greater decrease in illicit opiate use, greater reduction in addiction severity, and better adherence to HIV medications (Margolin et al., 2003). HHRP + may be relevant for HIV-positive African American IDUs who are entering MMT.

Conclusions

Although fewer young African Americans appear to be injecting heroin and the proportion of injection drug users (IDUs) among HIV-positive persons has decreased over time, IDU is still the second leading transmission risk category among African Americans (CDC, 2009), and sexual transmission appears to be an increasing factor for infection. But for IDUs in general, and for African American IDUs, an examination of existing EBIs indicates that challenges remain in reducing the sexual risk behaviors among IDUs in a meaningful and long-lasting manner. Clearly, finding effective ways to reduce sexual risk behaviors must continue to be the focus of intervention developers who are targeting IDUs. Evidence suggests that individual, group, and community interventions that have a peer support element have been effective in changing the risk behaviors of African American IDUs. Thus, this appears to be an important component for future interventions to consider. Another important issue to address is the myriad of psychosocial issues that IDUs struggle with that can make HIV prevention a lower priority. Addressing structural issues of housing, mental health, addiction, parenting concerns (including regaining custody), incarceration, and poverty may be necessary to support behavioral interventions for African American IDUs (Kotranski et al., 1998; Mizuno et al., 2003).

In addition to existing EBIs for African American IDUs, there are IDU interventions that could be successfully adapted if caution is taken regarding intervention selection. But adaptation should not be undertaken lightly – it is not necessarily easy and the science of adaptation is still in its infancy. In thinking about how to adapt an EBI that was not developed for African Americans or tested with majority African Americans, the issue of whether and how to add cultural specificity is likely to arise. This issue may be particularly important when a given EBI does not address African American cultural elements because a recent meta-analysis found that cultural specificity is associated with intervention efficacy for African American women (Crepaz et al., 2009). The good news is that we do have existing EBIs for African American IDUs, and these interventions along with carefully tailored adaptation should be provided to the community while the search for stronger and more durable interventions continues.

References

Academy for Educational Development. (2009). DEBI – Diffusion of Effective behavioral interventions website. Accessed March 16, 2009 from http://www.effectiveinterventions.org.

Armstrong, G. L. (2007). Injection drug users in the United States, 1979–2002: An aging population. *Archives of Internal Medicine, 167*, 166–173.

Blankenship, K. M., Smoyer, A. B., Bray, S. J., & Mattocks, K. (2005). Black-White disparities in HIV/AIDS: The role of drug policy and the corrections system. *Journal of Health Care for Poor and Underserved, 16*(4 Suppl B), 140–156.

Broz, D., & Ouellet, L. J. (2008). Racial and ethnic changes in heroin injection in the United States: Implications for the HIV/AIDS epidemic. *Drug and Alcohol Dependence, 94*, 221–233.

Centers for Disease Control and Prevention. (2007). Syringe exchange programs – United States, 2005. *MMWR. Morbidity and Mortality Weekly Report, 56*, 1164–1167.

Centers for Disease Control and Prevention. (2008). HIV prevalence estimates – United States, 2006. *MMWR. Morbidity and Mortality Weekly Report, 57*, 1073–1076.

Centers for Disease Control and Prevention. (2009). *HIV/AIDS Surveillance Report, 2007* (Vol. 19). Atlanta, GA: US Department of Health and Human Services, Centers for Disease Control and Prevention.

Centers for Disease Control and Prevention. (2010a). *Compendium of evidence-based HIV prevention interventions*. Atlanta, GA: Centers for Disease Control and Prevention. (July 19, 2010). http://www.cdc.gov/hiv/topics/research/prs/evidence-based-interventions.htm.

Centers for Disease Control and Prevention. (2010b). *Provisional procedural guidance for community based organizations*. Atlanta, GA: Centers for Disease Control and Prevention. (July 10, 2010). http://www.cdc.gov/hiv/topics/prev_prog/AHP/resources/guidelines/pro_guidance.htm.

Collins, C., Harshbarger, C., Sawyer, R., & Hamdallah, M. (2006). The diffusion of effective behavioral interventions project: Development, implementation, and lessons learned. *AIDS Education and Prevention, 18*(Suppl A), 5–20.

Copenhaver, M. M., Johnson, B. T., Lee, I.-C., Harman, J. J., Carey, M. P., & SHARP Research Team. (2006). Behavioral HIV risk reduction among people who inject drugs: Meta-analytic evidence of efficacy. *Journal of Substance Abuse Treatment, 31*, 163–171.

Crepaz, N., Marshall, K. J., Aupont, L. W., Jacobs, E. D., Mizuno, Y., Kay, L. S., et al. (2009). The efficacy of HIV/STI behavioral interventions for African-American females in the United States: A meta-analysis. *American Journal of Public Health, 99*, 1–10.

Des Jarlais, D. C., & Friedman, S. R. (1996). HIV epidemiology and interventions among injection drug users. *International Journal of STDs and AIDS, 7*(Suppl 2), 57–61.

Des Jarlais, D. C., & Semaan, S. (2005). Interventions to reduce the sexual risk behaviour of injection drug users. *International Journal of Drug Policy, 16S*, S58–S66.

Des Jarlais, D. C., & Semaan, S. (2008). HIV prevention for injection drug users: The first 25 years and counting. *Psychosomatic Medicine, 70*, 606–611.

Donoghoe, M. C., Verster, A., Pervilhac, C., & Williams P. (2008). Setting targets for universal access to HIV prevention, treatment and care for injecting drug users (IDUs): Towards consensus and improved guidance. *International Journal of Drug Policy, 19*(Suppl 1) 1, S5–S14.

Eke, A. N., Neumann, M. S., Wilkes, A. L., & Jones, P. L. (2006). Preparing effective behavioral interventions to be used by prevention providers: The role of researchers during HIV prevention research trials. *AIDS Education and Prevention, 18*(Suppl A), 44–58.

Estrada, A. L. (2005). Health disparities among African-American and Hispanic drug injectors – HIV, AIDS, hepatitis B virus and hepatitis C virus: a review. *AIDS, 19*(Suppl 3), S47–S52.

Farrell, M., Gowing, L., Marsden, J., Ling, W., & Ali, R. (2005). Effectiveness of drug dependence treatment in HIV prevention. *International Journal of Drug Policy, 16*, 67–75.

Garfein, R. S., Golub, E. T., Greenberg, A. E., Hagan, H., Hanson, D. L., Hudson, S. M., Kapadia, F., Latka, M. H., Ouellet, L. J., Purcell, D. W., Strathdee, S. A., Thiede, H., for the DUIT Study Team. (2007). A peer-education intervention to reduce injection risk behaviors for HIV and hepatitis C virus infection in young injection drug users. *AIDS, 21*, 1923–1932.

Gibson, D. R., Flynn, N. R., & Perales, D. (2001). Effectiveness of syringe exchange programs in reducing HIV risk behavior and HIV seroconversion among injecting drug users. *AIDS, 15*, 1329–1341.

Hershberger, S. L., Wood, M. M., & Fisher, D. G. (2003). A cognitive-behavioral intervention to reduce HIV risk behaviors in crack and injection drug users. *AIDS and Behavior, 7*, 229–243.

Hogben, M., & Leichliter, J. S. (2008). Social determinants and sexually transmitted disparities. *Sexually Transmitted Diseases, 35*, S13–S18.

Huo, D., & Ouellet, L. J. (2007). Needle exchange and injection-related risk behaviors in Chicago: A longitudinal study. *Journal of Acquired Immune Deficiency Syndromes, 45*, 108–114.

Jones, T. S., & Coffin, P. O. (2002). Preventing blood-borne infections through pharmacy syringe sales and safe community syringe disposal. *Journal of the American Pharmaceutical Association, 42*(Suppl 2), S6–S9.

Kotranski, L., Semaan, S., Collier, K., Lauby, J., Halbert, J., & Feighan, K. (1998). Effectiveness of an HIV risk reduction counseling intervention for out-of-treatment drug users. *AIDS Education and Prevention, 10*, 19–33.

Kral, A. H., Bluthenthal, R. N., Lorvick, J., Gee, L., Bacchetti, P., & Edlin, B. R. (2001). Sexual transmission of HIV-1 among injection drug users in San Francisco, USA: Risk-factor analysis. *Lancet, 357*, 1397–1401.

Ksobiech, K. (2003). A meta-analysis of needle sharing, lending, and borrowing behaviors of needle exchange program attenders. *AIDS Education and Prevention, 15*, 257–268.

Latka, M. H., Hagan, H., Kapadia, F., Golub, E. T., Bonner, S., Campbell, J. V., Coady, M., Garfein, R. S., Pu, M., Thomas, D. L., Thiel, T. K., & Strathdee, S. A. (2008). A randomized intervention trial to reduce the lending of used injection equipment among injection drug users infected with hepatitis C. *American Journal of Public Health, 98*, 853–861.

Latkin, C. A., Sherman, S., & Knowlton, A. (2003). HIV prevention among drug users: Outcome of a network-oriented peer outreach intervention. *Health Psychology, 22*, 332–339.

Lyles, C. M., Crepaz, N., Herbst, J. H., Kay, L. S., & HIV/AIDS Prevention Research Synthesis Team. (2006). Evidence-based HIV behavioral prevention from the perspective of CDC's HIV/AIDS Prevention Research Synthesis Team. *AIDS Education and Prevention, 18*(Suppl A), 21–31.

Magura, S., Kang, S. Y., & Shapiro, J. L. (1994). Outcomes of intensive AIDS education for male adolescent drug users in jail. *Journal of Adolescent Health, 15*, 457–463.

Margolin, A., Avants, S. K., Warburton, L. A., Hawkins, K. A., & Shi, J. (2003). A randomized clinical trial of a manual-guided risk reduction intervention for HIV-positive injection drug users. *Health Psychology, 22*, 223–228.

Mays, V. M., Cochran, S. D., & Barnes, N. W. (2007). Race, race-based discrimination, and health outcomes among African Americans. *Annual Review of Psychology, 58*, 201–225.

McKleroy, V. S., Galbraith, J. S., Cummings, B., Jones, P., Harshbarger, C., Collins, C., Gelaude, D., Carey, J. W., & the ADAPT Team. Adapting evidence-based behavioral interventions for new settings and target populations. *AIDS Education and Prevention, 18*(Suppl A), 59–73.

McMahon, R. C., Malow, R. M., Jennings, T. E., & Gomez, C. J. (2001). Effects of a cognitive-behavioral HIV prevention intervention among HIV negative male substance abusers in VA residential treatment. *AIDS Education and Prevention, 13*, 91–107.

Metzger, D., Navaline, H., & Woody, G. (1998). Drug abuse treatment as AIDS prevention. *Public Health Reports, 113*(Suppl 1), 97–106.

Mizuno, Y., Purcell, D., Borkowski, T. M., Knight, K., & SUDIS Team. (2003). The life priorities of HIV-seropositive injection drug users: Findings from a community-based sample. *AIDS and Behavior, 7*, 395–403.

Mizuno, Y., Wilkinson, J. D., Santibanez, S., Dawson Rose, C., Knowlton, A., Handley, K., et al. (2006). Correlates of health care utilization among HIV-seropositive injection drug users. *AIDS Care, 18*, 417–425.

Needle, R. H., Burrows, D., Friedman, S. R., Dorabjee, J., Touze, G., Badrieva, L., et al. (2005). Effectiveness of community-based outreach in preventing HIV/AIDS among injection drug users. *International Journal of Drug Policy, 16S*, S45–S57.

Prendergast, M. L., Urada, D., & Podus, D. J. (2001). Meta-analysis of HIV risk-reduction interventions within drug abuse treatment programs. *Journal of Consulting and Clinical Psychology, 69*, 389–405.

Prochaska, J. O., DiClemente, C. C., & Norcross, J. C. (1992). In search of how people change. *American Psychologist, 47*, 1101–1113.

Purcell, D. W., Latka, M. H., Metsch, L. R., Latkin, C. A., Gomez, C. A., Mizuno, Y., et al. (2007). Results from a randomized controlled trial of a peer-mentoring intervention to reduce HIV transmission and increase access to care and adherence to HIV medications among HIV-seropositive injection drug users. *Journal of Acquired Immune Deficiency Syndromes, 46*(Suppl 2), S35–S47.

Purcell, D. W., Metsch, L., Latka, M., Santibanez, S., Eldred, L., Gomez, C. A., et al. (2004). Behavioral prevention trial with HIV-seropositive injection drug users: Rationale and methods of the INSPIRE Study. *Journal of Acquired Immune Deficiency Syndromes, 37*(Suppl 2), S110–S118.

Rich, J. D., Hogan, J. W., Wolf, F., DeLong, A., Zaller, N. D., Mehrotra, M., & Reinhert, S. (2007). Lower syringe sharing and re-use after syringe legalization in Rhode Island. *Drug and Alcohol Dependence, 89*, 292–297.

Semaan, S., Des Jarlais, D. C., Sogolow, E., Johnson, W. D., Hedges, L. V., Ramirez, G., et al. (2002). A meta-analysis of the effect of HIV prevention interventions on the sex behaviors of drug users in the United States. *Journal of Acquired Immune Deficiency Syndromes, 30*, S73–S93.

Sterk, C. E., Theall, K. P., Elifson, K. W., & Kidder, D. (2003). HIV risk reduction among African American women who inject drugs: A randomized controlled trial. *AIDS and Behavior, 7*, 73–86.

Stratford, D., Mizuno, Y., Williams, K., Courtenay-Quirk, C., & O'Leary, A. (2008). Addressing poverty as a risk for disease: Recommendations from the CDC's consultation on microenterprise as HIV prevention. *Public Health Reports, 123*, 9–20.

Strathdee, S. A., & Sherman, S. G. (2003). The role of sexual transmission of HIV infection among injection and non-injection drug users. *Journal of Urban Health, 2003*(80), 7–14.

The CDC AIDS Community Demonstration Projects Research Group. (1999). Community-level HIV intervention in 5 cities: Final outcome data from the CDC AIDS community demonstration projects. *American Journal of Public Health, 89*, 336–345.

Watters, J. K., Bluthenthal, R. N., & Kral, A. H. (1995). HIV seroprevalence in injection drug users. *Journal of the American Medical Association, 273*, 1178.

Wechsberg, W. M., Lam, W. K., Zule, W. A., & Bobashev, G. (2004). Efficacy of a woman focused intervention to reduce HIV risk and increase self-sufficiency among African American crack abusers. *American Journal of Public Health, 94*, 1165–1173.

Weinhardt, L., Carey, M., Johnson, B., & Bickham, N. (1999). Effects of HIV counseling and testing on sexual risk behavior: A meta-analytic review of published research, 1985–1997. *American Journal of Public Health, 89*, 1397–1404.

Weissman, G., & Brown, V. (1995). Drug using women and HIV risk reduction and prevention issues. In A. O'Leary & L. S. Jemmott (Eds.), *Women at risk: Issues in the primary prevention of AIDS* (pp. 175–193). New York: Plenum.

Chapter 14
Structural Interventions with an Emphasis on Poverty and Racism

Renata Arrington Sanders and Jonathan M. Ellen

HIV/AIDS continues to disproportionately affect African Americans. While African Americans represent 13% of the U.S. population, they account for nearly 50% of new HIV/AIDS infections (Centers for Disease Control and Prevention (CDC), 2008; McKinnon, 2003). Disproportionate rates are seen most among African American men who have sex with men (MSM) and women. Many African Americans at risk for acquiring HIV or other STIs disproportionately live in poverty and are plagued by communities with high rates of homelessness, unemployment, incarceration and substance abuse/dependence (Adimora & Schoenbach, 2005). How such factors increase the probability of exposure is very complex.

Epidemiologic risk associated with HIV results from the probability that an individual is exposed to the virus and the efficiency of transmission once exposed. Factors associated with increased probability of exposure may result from individual, population and structural level determinants. Structural factors that affect an individual's HIV risk may include physical, social, cultural, political, community and economic forces that may impede or facilitate ones likelihood to avoid HIV infection.

In this chapter, we focus on the structural factors or determinants that may facilitate transmission of HIV and present structural interventions that either historically have been associated with reducing HIV transmission or might impact the HIV epidemic.

Definition of Structural Factors

What defines structural factors? Structural factors have been broadly defined as features of the environment outside an individual's control that may serve as a barrier to, or facilitator of, an individual's ability to prevent acquisition of HIV

R.A. Sanders (✉)
Division of General Pediatrics & Adolescent Medicine,
Johns Hopkins School of Medicine, 200 North Wolfe Street, Baltimore, MD 21287, USA
e-mail: rarring3@jhmi.edu

D.H. McCree et al. (eds.), *African Americans and HIV/AIDS*,
DOI 10.1007/978-0-387-78321-5_14, © Springer Science+Business Media, LLC 2010

(Gupta, Parkhurst, Ogden, Aggleton, & Mahal, 2008; Sumartojo, Doll, Holtgrave, Gayle, & Merson, 2000). These factors are "built" into an individual's surroundings, creating the structure for which people operate. Imbedded in the complex system of structure, policies, practices and norms, are tangible features of the environment that make excellent targets for change. These include the availability of resources, physical structures in the environment, organizational structures and laws and policies. These structural features mediate the impact of large social forces associated with HIV such as poverty, gender inequality, racism, mobility and stigma by affecting the distribution of STIs, behavior, networks and risk of exposure to infection.

Structural Factors and HIV

Poverty

It is estimated that approximately one-quarter (24.3%) of all African-Americans in 2006, live in poverty (US Census Bureau, 2003). Poverty, socioeconomic factors and income are important co-factors in HIV and STI transmission (Sumartojo, 2000). Residential instability, which can result from poverty, was identified as a key contributor to rising HIV rates in African Americans (Nicholas et al., 2005). Recent research by Krieger, Chen, Waterman, Rehkopf, and Subramanian (2005) found that 50% of the cases of STIs and HIV would not have occurred if the population poverty rates had equaled those of the persons residing in the least impoverished census tracks. Additionally, recent work has demonstrated that social capital, poverty and income inequality influence sexual risk and protective behaviors, prevalence of STIs and AIDS case rates (Cohen et al., 2000; Crosby, Holtgrave, DiClemente, Wingwood, & Gayle, 2003). One theory is that social environmental factors, such as housing quality, abandoned cars, graffiti, trash and public school deterioration may reflect deteriorating communities and foster sexual risk behavior that would not be as common in intact communities (Cohen et al. 2000).

Poverty also contributes to the high rates of HIV in certain populations by creating low sex ratios and destabilizing long term relationships in black communities. High rates of morbidity, mortality, unemployment and incarceration rates among young black adults can create a low ratio of men to women that supports partner concurrency (sexual relationships that overlap in time) and rapid spread of infection in a community (Adimora & Schoenbach, 2002). Multiple concurrent sexual relationships have been shown to contribute to the spread of STIs (Koumans et al., 2001; Potterat et al., 1999) and found to be a risk factor for heterosexual HIV transmission among African Americans who were otherwise low risk (Adimora et al., 2006).

High incarceration rates among African American males contribute to a system of poverty in the black community. In 2007, black persons were almost three times more likely than Hispanics and five times more likely than whites to be in jail (815 per 100,000 U.S. residents for non-Hispanic Blacks versus, 170 for non-Hispanic whites and 276 for Hispanics) (U.S. Department of Justice, Office of Justice Programs, Bureau of Justice Statistics, 2009). Incarceration results in high unemployment rates in poor minority communities which may predispose individuals to pursue alternative employment prospects that are illegal and socially disruptive (Adimora, & Schoenbach, 2005). By directly disrupting partner relationships and contributing to the low male to female sexual ratio, incarceration may have indirect effects on social (and sexual) networks by predisposing the partner left behind to concurrent relationships (Gorbach, Ryan, Saphonn, & Detels, 2002) and the incarcerated partner to a group of individuals where the prevalence of HIV infection, high risk behavior and STIs are high (Heimberger et al., 1993; Hellard & Aitken, 2004; Khan et al., 2008; Wolfe et al., 2001). Furthermore, as a result of racism and segregation, socioeconomic status, poverty, and geography often parallel racial disparities in health (Baicker, Chandra, & Skinner, 2005).

Racial Disparities

Despite advancements made with the civil rights movement and diversity initiatives, racial gaps exist in educational institutions, many occupations, health care services, income, housing and government services. In fact, for many African Americans, racism and discrimination predict access to political power, neighborhoods, and most life resources. One example of this is residential segregation. Residential segregation persists in many urban areas. It results from individual actions but also by a long-standing historical mechanism of discrimination in mortgage rates and by realtors (Massey & Denton, 1993). Neighborhood segregation by socioeconomic group concentrates poverty and its social influence. This predisposes individuals to the deleterious effects of social and economic isolation, such as violence, poverty, drugs and high teenage pregnancy rates which increases the risk of socioeconomic failure of the segregated group (Massey & Denton, 1993). And because, people choose partners from the neighborhoods they live, and residence determines the school district one attends, residence can strongly contribute to the social (and sexual) networks in individuals (Zenilman, Ellish, Fresia, & Glass, 1999).

Differential access to high quality care contributes to co-morbidities associated with many chronic illnesses. Racial disparities contribute to unequal distribution of care among African Americans when compared to Whites. African Americans are more uninsured than whites and as a group and encounter greater barriers to obtaining health insurance, and access to care even when insured (Doty & Holmgren, 2006). Krieger (2005) describes five pathways that discrimination can harm health – economic and social deprivation, residential segregation, targeted marketing of legal and illegal psychoactive substances and inadequate health care. Delay in care for STIs and HIV can lead to higher rates of transmission, potentially poorer immune restoration (Kaufmann et al., 2000) and can inhibit linking HIV infected persons to care. Limited accessibility, acceptability and poor quality of care may serve as important social determinants in who is able to receive early STI-related care. As Baicker et al. (2005) and colleagues demonstrated because geographic disparities result in African Americans being concentrated in areas or seeking care in regions in which health-care quality is low for all patients, insuring equal access to care on the local level without implementing national policies designed to improve quality of care to all patients, will not reduce such disparities.

Structural Interventions in Practice

Structural interventions are approaches that target the physical, environmental, sociocultural, economic, political and organizational factors that affect individual risk and vulnerability to HIV. Effective policy interventions include reducing perinatal HIV transmission by providing HIV medications to HIV positive pregnant mothers (Mofenson & Centers for Disease Control and Prevention, U.S. Public Health Service Task Force, 2002), screening the blood supply for HIV (Dodd, 2004) and needle and syringe exchange programs. Needle/syringe exchange and methadone programs are interventions that have worked because of policy shifts away from prohibition to harm minimization (Des Jarlais, 2000; Drucker, Lurie, Wodak, & Alcabes, 1998). Successful national or country level policies that promote HIV prevention have been the ABC (abstinence, be faithful, condom) policy in Uganda; (Parkhurst, 2001; Stoneburner & Low-Beer, 2004; Watson, 1988) and Australia's success of managing epidemics of HIV among men who have sex with men and injection drug users by collective involvement of affected communities, supportive policy and research (Bernard, Kippax, & Baxter, 2008; Kippax & Race, 2003).

Two commonly referenced structural approaches that target the cultural, political and organizational factors that help to reduce the risk and vulnerability of sex workers are the condom use policies implemented in Thailand and the Dominican Republic. In each approach both brothel or bar managers and police had a key role in promoting condom use (Gupta et al., 2008; Kerrigan et al., 2006). Other programs have worked at the community level. The Sonagachi project in Calcutta, India worked at the community level to mobilize sex workers to design and implement activities and enable participants to make their own decisions, including those that protected them from HIV infection (Basu et al., 2004; Cohen 2004; Jana, Basu, Rotheram-Borus, & Newman, 2004). An effective environmental level intervention in bathhouses has been to have condoms, lubricant, HIV testing and screening on site at gay bathhouses (Woods, 2003).

Some interventions have attempted to target the issues of poverty and racism. In Table 12.1, we present interventions implemented that impact features of poverty and racism and articles that suggest areas that can be targeted in the United States.

Table 14.1 Structural Interventions that impact poverty and racism

Structural intervention	Reference
Housing	
RCT designed to evaluate the effects of providing rental housing assistance to homeless and unstably housed PLWHA	Kidder, Wolitski, and Royal et al. (2007)
Reductions in rates of sex and drug risk behaviors among homeless or unstably housed PLWHA whose housing status improved compared to those whose housing did not change	Aidala, Cross, Stall, Harre, and Sumartojo (2005)
Housing is a cost-saving strategy whereby HIV transmissions can be averted	Holtgrave et al. (2007)
Neighborhood revitalization as a structural intervention to target drug injection behavior and high risk sexual partners	Latkin, Williams, Wang, and Curry (2005) Latkin, Curry, Hua, and Davey (2007)
Economic Independence	
Micro-credit loan programs for poor women	Schuler and Hashemi (1994), Pronyk et al. (2008), Ashburn, Kerrigan, and Sweat et al. (2008)
Pilot among drug using and sex trading women in Baltimore, Maryland, pre/post test design taught HIV prevention and risk reduction combined with making, marketing and selling of jewelry in six two-hour sessions	Sherman, German, Cheng, Marks, and Bailey-Kloche (2006)
AIDS prevention and care for STIs at work sites for migrant laborers and mentoring programs at migrant work sites to facilitate social integration of new arrivals	Sweat and Denison (1995)
Access	
Co-located substance use treatment and HIV prevention and primary care services, New York State, 1990–2002: a model for effective service delivery to a high-risk population	Rothman et al. (2007)
Hired community members who worked with the AIDS Office of the California Department of Health and Human Services to link HIV positive persons of color to IDUs to needed services for HIV care and treatment	Molitor et al. (2005)
Improved access to care for HIV and AIDS in a statewide Medicaid managed care system	Bailey, Van Brunt, Raffanti, Long, and Jenkins (2003)
Modeled Expansion of the Medicaid eligibility would increase access to antiretroviral therapy and have substantial health benefits at affordable costs	Kahn, Haile, Kates, and Chang (2001)

(continued)

Table 14.1 (continued)

Structural intervention	Reference
Free access to condoms	Cohen (1999)
	Harvey (1994)
Program improved access to preventive services (i.e., HIV testing) for adolescents	Klein et al. (2003)
Improved access to clean needles and needle exchange sites; Increasing safe syringe collection sites	Neaigus et al. (2008), Groseclose et al. (1995) Klein et al. (2008)
Interventions to prevent HIV-related stigma and discrimination: findings and recommendations for public health practice	Klein, Karachner, and O'Connell (2002)

Criminal Justice & Policy Changes

Interagency collaboration to provide a continuum of care for New York State prison inmates (including HIV education/VCT, outreach to inmates, peer training, condom distribution for family visits, HIV primary care, referrals, support groups for HIV positive inmates and case management for HIV infected inmates upon release)	Klein, O'Connell, Devore, Wright, and Birkhead et al. (2002)
Condom availability to inmates in Washington, D.C. prisons	May and Williams (2002)
Therapeutic community programs in the context of imprisonment	Martin, Butzin, and Inciardi (1995)
Screening and treatment of women in jails for chlamydial and gonococcal infection	Mertz et al. (2002)
Health Link intervention assisted drug-using incarcerated women to reintegrate into their communities, decrease STIs and avoid re-arrest	Richie, Freudenberg, and Page (2001)
Massachusetts' policy initiatives to facilitate the integration of HIV and AIDS services with alcoholism and drug abuse treatment and prevention programs	McCarty, LaPrade, and Botticelli (1996)
Nevada law required condom use in legal brothels	Albert et al. (1998)
Name-based reporting improved testing rates in six states	Nakashima et al. (1998)
Partner contact and tracing	Rutherford et al. (1991)
Anonymous testing improved testing in 25 Oregon counties	Fehrs et al. (1988)

Proposed Structural Interventions

In order to change the structural factors that impact risk of HIV and other STIs, a multifaceted approach must occur that will affect national and local policies to improve access to housing, microenterprise, HIV prevention strategies and to health care services for African Americans. Structural programs that improve access to housing have demonstrated that access to housing helps to avert HIV transmission, promotes medication adherence and health outcomes among persons living with

HIV and AIDS (PLWHA) (Wolitski, Kidder, & Fenton, 2007). Work done by Aidala et al. (2005) demonstrated that stable housing has been associated with reduced rates of sex and drug risk behaviors among homeless or unstably housed PLWHA whose housing status improved compared to those whose housing did not change. Other work has demonstrated that stable housing is associated with better health as indicated by CD4 counts and viral load (Kidder, Wolitski, Campsmith, & Nakamura, 2007; Knowlton et al., 2006). Stable housing also has the potential to be cost-effective and cost-saving in the long run (Holtgrave et al., 2007). The National Minority AIDS Council recommended in the 2006 Fullilove Report that the nation as a whole "support the strengthening of stable black communities by addressing the need for more affordable housing." (Fullilove & National Minority AIDS Council, 2006) Programs that focus on improving housing resources for marginalized communities have high retention rates and create sustainable community-level change. (Dasinger & Speiglman, 2007; Kidder et al. 2007).

Microenterprise, another intervention that has been used effectively to target individual risk and vulnerability to HIV, provides financial and social welfare support to at-risk or vulnerable populations. As a result, individuals are more likely to choose positive alternatives to high risk behaviors. In Baltimore, a pilot study for women who used drugs and traded sex for drugs, combined HIV prevention and risk reduction with making, marketing and selling jewelry (Sherman et al., 2006). In follow up, after six 2-hour sessions, women reported fewer sex trade partners; receiving less drugs or money for sex; less daily drug use; and less daily crack use and money spent on drugs. The study demonstrated the efficacy of economic empowerment and HIV prevention programs in lowering risk for acquisition of HIV. Economic empowerment can be expanded by using programs like the Job Corps to create job training programs and jobs for commercial sex workers, adolescents, and former and active drug users. In addition to developing trades and skills in individuals, programs could provide integrative services that include drug treatment, HIV prevention, and General Educational Development (or GED) services. Alternatively, Job Corps programs could be introduced as part of drug treatment, incarceration, dropout or rehabilitation programs.

Expansion of condoms and HIV testing programs in hard to reach vulnerable communities is also needed. Low cost or free access to condoms has been shown to increase utilization of condoms (Cohen, 1999). Venue-based HIV testing is an effective strategy that reaches undiagnosed HIV positive men who have sex with men and high-risk heterosexuals (CDC, 2005; Towe et al. 2010). Condoms and HIV testing need to be accessible in settings such as bars, bathhouses, restaurants and hotels, where sexual contact between strangers is likely to occur. HIV prevention programs that help private enterprises, such as hotels, beauty/barbershops and bathhouses provide low-cost HIV testing and condoms to clients is needed.

There are data that show comprehensive sex and HIV education programs can be effective in delaying or decreasing high risk sexual behaviors and increasing condom or contraceptive use (Kirby 1999; Kirby, Laris, & Rolleri, 2007). Age-appropriate comprehensive sexuality education and condom availability needs to be expanded in state and local school districts. Currently, 35 states and the District of Columbia require the provision of STI/HIV education, but many states place requirements on how abstinence and contraception are treated (Guttmacher

Institute, 2009). For example, 26 states require that abstinence be stressed when taught as part of STD/HIV education, while 11 require that it be covered. Seventeen states require that STI/HIV programs cover contraception but no state requires that it be stressed. Most curricula are heavily weighted toward stressing abstinence; in contrast, while many states allow or require that contraception be covered, none require that it be stressed. Additionally, parental consent requirements or "opt-out" clauses, which allow parents to remove students from instruction, further affect whether students receive adequate instruction on sex or STI/HIV prevention. Federal funding to expand sexual education programs in the school and to evaluate the success of comprehensive sex and HIV education programs are needed. Programs in African American communities will need to be within a cultural and religious context. Collaboration with foundations and private organizations, such as the Kaiser Family Foundation, SIECUS (Sexuality Information and Education Council of the U.S.), and the Guttmacher Institute, is needed to develop, research and promote sexuality and HIV/STD education in the schools.

Condom distribution and STI testing programs should also be expanded. Low cost or free access to condoms has been shown to increase utilization of condoms (Cohen, 1999) Condoms should be accessible in settings such as bars, bathhouses, restaurants and hotels, where sexual contact between strangers is likely to occur. Condom distribution programs should partner with private enterprises, such as hotel and bathhouse owners to purchase condoms at low costs directly from the manufacturer and actively distribute them to clients, where condoms are provided as part of check-in to hotels or visible in bars.

HIV prevention and education programs, including expansion of condom distribution and universal screening for STIs, including HIV, in jails and drug treatment programs is necessary to change the epidemic in African American communities. The period of incarceration and subsequent parole provides a unique opportunity to implement HIV prevention and risk reduction programs in prisons and link newly released inmates to community services and assist in the process of community reintegration. Braithwaite and Arriola (2003), in their review of city and state projects funded by the Centers for Disease Control and Prevention (CDC) and Health Resources and Services Administration (HRSA) Corrections Demonstration Project to provide HIV prevention programs in correctional settings, recommend the following risk reduction policy initiatives: adoption of mandatory HIV testing, reinforcement of continuity of care for HIV-infected inmates returning to the community, and improvement of access to incarcerated populations for community-based organizations and AIDS Services Organizations (ASOs) for delivery of HIV prevention and education programs. The correctional system creates an environment for high rates of concurrency in the African-American community by removing a high percentage of African-American men, but such programs that collaborate with CBOs to reintegrate inmates into the community after release and promote health in jails and prisons can have a positive effect on health in urban African American populations where many individuals live.

Although state-level laws on STD screening, name-based reporting of STDs/ HIV, and partner notification have been used to target prevention and treatment of HIV and STDs, laws can sometimes act as pathways for social determinants that impact HIV risk. Drucker et al., (1998) suggests that drug use control policies act as a barrier to medical and social services which can foster behavior such as sharing equipment and commercial sex work, both of which increase transmission of HIV. Additionally, drug control laws that result in longer sentences and higher rates of incarceration for minorities can theoretically translate into increased HIV risk in prison by creating a system whereby simultaneous inadequate drug treatment and disrupted social and sexual networks results in high risk behavior. A review of needle exchange programs have found evidence of efficacy without associated adverse events (Huo & Outellet, 2007, 2009; Huo, Bailey, Hershow, & Ouellet, 1998; Vlahov & Junge, 1998). Efforts are needed to educate law enforcement, policy makers and legislators of the benefit of destigmitizing drug users. For example, the presence of clean needles should not indicate possession of drugs or result in police harassment or jail time. Drug control laws that encourage alternatives to incarceration for non-violent drug users will help to destigmatize drug users and will impact the racially disparate rates of minority arrests and incarcerations.

Laws can also serve to weaken the social capital and cohesion of communities by limiting access to housing (mandatory residency requirements), federal student loans (ineligible if convicted of drug offense), and voting rights in certain states (Cason et al., 2002). Additional programs are needed that provide drug treatment, housing and job placement in order to decrease risk of transmission of HIV by addressing the primary condition and also improving the social capital of families and communities.

HIV disproportionately affects African American adolescents. School-based HIV education and testing is one reasonable strategy to promote HIV prevention in this group. There are data that show comprehensive sex and HIV education programs can be effective in delaying or decreasing high-risk sexual behaviors and increasing condom or contraceptive use. (Kirby 1999; Kirby et al., 2007) Age-appropriate comprehensive sexuality education and condom availability needs to be expanded in state and local school districts. Currently, 35 states and the District of Columbia require the provision of STI/HIV education, but many states place requirements on how abstinence and contraception are treated. (Guttmacher Institute, 2009) For example, 26 states require that abstinence be stressed when taught as part of STD/HIV education, while 11 require that it be covered. Seventeen states require that STI/HIV programs cover contraception but no state requires that it be stressed. Most curricula are heavily weighted toward stressing abstinence; in contrast, while many states allow or require that contraception be covered, none require that it be stressed. Additionally, parental consent requirements or "opt-out" clauses, which allow parents to remove students from instruction, further affect whether students receive adequate instruction on sex or STI/HIV prevention. Federal funding to expand sexual education programs in the school and to evaluate the success of comprehensive sex and HIV education programs are needed.

Programs in African American communities will need to be within a culturally and developmentally appropriate media in order to be effective. Collaboration with foundations and private organizations, such as the Kaiser Family Foundation, SIECUS (Sexuality Information and Education Council of the U.S.), and the Guttmacher Institute, is needed to develop, research and promote sexuality and HIV/STD education in the schools.

Sexually active African American adolescents have low rates of HIV testing despite being disproportionately affected by the disease. (Swenson et al. 2009) HIV testing still occurs primarily as part of risk-based STI and pregnancy-related screening, thus limiting the cases of HIV detected in health-care settings (Arrington-Sanders, Ellen, Trent 2008; Arrington-Sanders, Ellen 2009; Swenson et al. 2009). Moreover, Swenson (2009) demonstrated that African American adolescents in high-risk urban communities continue to report low rates of HIV testing. This finding suggests that HIV testing needs to reach non-care seeking adolescents tested in venues where HIV rates are high. (Barnes et al. 2010) Structural interventions that increase the availability of free or low-cost HIV testing in settings that are youth-friendly and convenient, such as school-based health centers and malls, may help to reduce barriers to testing and improve testing rates in sexually active minority adolescents.

On the national level, differential access to high-quality health care must be eliminated. Baicker et al., (2005) demonstrated that African American and white patients are treated differently within provider groups and health systems and that African Americans tend to live in areas with low health care quality. When timeliness of diagnosis and treatment are important in limiting the spread and transmission of infectious diseases, improving access is crucial to eliminating disparities of care that contribute to HIV. In order to simultaneously assure equal access to and high-quality of care, programs that expand health insurance and create clinical benchmarks that insure high-quality care will need to be created. One way to eliminate disparities is for funding agencies such as the CDC and National Institutes of Health (NIH) to collaborate with African American community coalitions, churches, historically black colleges and universities to build culturally sensitive, community focused research and programs that mobilize African American communities. Another structural change is to promote prevention research and the development of African American researchers and community based organizations to expand culturally relevant research that develops such programs. These programs or interventions should target social networks, individuals, couples and families while addressing the socio-cultural and economic concerns most relevant to African Americans such as limited health care access, social/economic isolation and partner availability (Aral, Adimora, & Fenton, 2008). Research is also needed that understands and describes African-American sexuality which develops mostly during adolescence. Currently, paradigms to explain adolescent African American sexuality use a pathology-based paradigm that can promote stigma as it relates to the acceptance of sexual diversity within African American communities and can limit HIV prevention efforts (Giordano, Manning, & Longmore, 2005; McLoyd & Steinberg, 1998). Programming will need to work to promote anti-discrimination by partnering with gay-straight alliances, hiring sexual minority, and funding programs/research that focuses on reducing stigma of sexual minorities.

Additional efforts need to expand name-based reporting, universal testing, highly active antiretroviral therapy (HAART), and promote the use of evidence-based medicine in underserved neighborhoods. Resources need to be distributed to communities that have the greatest need. One approach is to improve collaboration across federal agencies in order to build a consensus and develop a plan around the social determinants of the HIV epidemic in African Americans. Aral et al. (2008) provides one example of how the public-health system could strengthen collaboration with the Departments of Justice and Education. In this example, by strengthening such collaboration and coordination, the public health system works with the Department of Justice to reduce the adverse health effects of incarceration and works with the Department of Education to increase high school graduation rates among African Americans.

Closing Paragraph

The sustained racial/ethnic and socioeconomic disparities in STIs including HIV point to the profound effect of racism and poverty on shaping risk for STIs. While racism and poverty need to be addressed within society, we have proposed that it may be more expeditious to focus on structural features of the environment that affect risk and mediate the impact of racism and poverty. Many of structural features of the environment originate and are maintained by policies, programs and practice patterns that at times are obvious and at times hidden. Fortunately, the growing emphasis on "upstream" causes of STIs including HIV has shed new light on important structures and efforts to address them. The intent of this review was to describe structural interventions designed to decrease STIs and review their effectiveness. In summary, the body of science focused on structural intervention is not extensive but, nonetheless suggest that there is reason to be optimistic that a structural approach to STI/HIV prevention will reduce incidence and prevalence of STIs including HIV.

References

Adimora, A. A., & Schoenbach, V. J. (2002). Contextual factors and the black-white disparity in heterosexual HIV transmission. *Epidemiology, 13*, 707–712.

Adimora, A. A., & Schoenbach, V. J. (2005). Social context, sexual networks, and racial disparities in rates of sexually transmitted infections. *The Journal of Infectious Diseases, 191*, S115–S122.

Adimora, A. A., Schoenbach, V. J., Martinson, F. E., Coyne-Beasley, T., Doherty, I., et al. (2006). Heterosexually transmitted HIV infection among African Americans in North Carolina. *Journal of Acquired Immune Deficiency Syndromes, 41*, 616–623.

Aidala, A., Cross, J. E., Stall, R., Harre, D., & Sumartojo, E. (2005). Housing status and HIV risk behaviors: Implications for prevention and policy. *AIDS and Behavior, 9*, 251–265.

Albert, A. E., Warner, D. L., & Hatcher, R. A. (1998). Facilitating condom use with clients during commercial sex in Nevada's legal brothels. *American Journal of Public Health, 88*, 643–646.

Aral, S. O., Adimora, A., & Fenton, K. (2008). Understanding and responding to disparities in HIV and other sexually transmitted infections in African Americans. *Lancet, 372*, 337–340.

Arrington-Sanders, R., Ellen, J., Trent, M. (2008). HIV testing in adolescents and young adults receiving STI testing in an urban primary care setting. *Sex Transm Dis, 35*, 686–688.

Arrington-Sanders, R., Ellen, J. (2009). Prevalence of self-reported human immunodeficiency virus testing among a population-based sample of urban African-American adolescents. *J Adolesc Health, 43*, 306–308.

Ashburn, K., Kerrigan, D., & Sweat, M. (2008). Micro-credit, women's groups, control of own money: HIV-related negotiation among partnered Dominican women. *AIDS and Behavior, 12*, 396–403.

Baicker, K., Chandra, A., & Skinner, J. S. (2005). Geographic variation in health care and the problem of measuring racial disparities. *Perspectives in Biology and Medicine, 48*, S42–S53.

Bailey, J. E., Van Brunt, D. L., Raffanti, S. P., Long, W. J., & Jenkins, P. H. (2003). Improvements in access to care for HIV and AIDS in a statewide Medicaid managed care system. *The American Journal of Managed Care, 9*, 595–602.

Barnes, W., D'Angelo, L., Yamazaki, M., Belzer, M., Schroeder, S., et al. (2010). Identification of HIV-infected 12- to 24-year-old men and women in 15 US cities through venue-based testing. *Arch Pediatr Adolesc Med, 164*, 273–276.

Basu, I., Jana, S., Rotheram-Borus, M. J., Swendeman, D., Lee, S. J., et al. (2004). HIV prevention among sex workers in India. *Journal of Acquired Immune Deficiency Syndromes, 36*, 845–852.

Bernard, D., Kippax, S., & Baxter, D. (2008). Effective partnership and adequate investment underpin a successful response: Key factors in dealing with HIV increases. *Sexual Health, 5*, 193–201.

Braithwaite, R. L., & Arriola, K. R. (2003). Male prisoners and HIV prevention: A call for action ignored. *American Journal of Public Health, 93*, 759–763.

Cason, C., Orrock, N., Schmitt, K., Tesoriero, J., Lazzarini, Z., & Sumartojo, E. (2002). The impact of laws on HIV and STD prevention. *The Journal of Law, Medicine & Ethics, 30*, 139–145.

Centers for Disease Control and Prevention. (2005). HIV prevalence, unrecognized infection and HIV testing among men who have sex with men–five US cities, June 2004-April 2005. *MMWR Morb Mortal Wkly Rep, 54*, 597–601.

Centers for Disease Control and Prevention. (2008). HIV prevalence estimates – United States, 2006. *Morbidity and Mortality Weekly Report, 57*, 1073–1076.

Cohen, D. (1999). Cost as a barrier to condom use: The evidence for condom subsidies in the United States. *American Journal of Public Health, 89*, 567–568.

Cohen, J. (2004). HIV/AIDS in India. Sonagachi sex workers stymie HIV. *Science, 304*, 560.

Cohen, D., Spear, S., Scibner, R., Kissinger, P., Mason, K., & Wildgen, J. (2000). "Broken windows" and the risk of gonorrhea. *American Journal of Public Health, 90*, 230–236.

Crosby, R. A., Holtgrave, D. R., DiClemente, R. J., Wingwood, G. M., & Gayle, J. A. (2003). Social capital as a predictor of adolescents' sexual risk behavior: A state-level exploratory study. *AIDS and Behavior, 7*, 245–252.

Dasinger, L. K., & Speiglman, R. (2007). Homelessness prevention: The effect of a shallow rent subsidy program on housing outcomes among people with HIV or AIDS. *AIDS and Behavior, 11*, 128–139.

Des Jarlais, D. C. (2000). Structural interventions to reduce HIV transmission among injection drug users. *AIDS, 14*, 46.

Dodd, R. Y. (2004). Current safety of the blood supply in the United States. *International Journal of Hematology, 80*, 301–305.

Doty, M. M., & Holmgren, A. L. (2006). Health care disconnect: Gaps in coverage and care for minority adults. Findings from the commonwealth fund biennial health insurance survey (2005). *Issue Brief – Commonwealth Fund, 21*, 1–12.

Drucker, E., Lurie, P., Wodak, A., & Alcabes, P. (1998). Measuring harm reduction: The effects of needle and syringe exchange programs and methadone maintenance on the ecology of HIV. *AIDS, 12*, S217–S230.

Fehrs, L. J., Fleming, D., Foster, L. R., McAlister, R. O., Fox, V., et al. (1988). Trial of anonymous versus confidential human immunodeficiency virus testing. *Lancet, 8607*, 379–382.

Fehrs, L. J., Foster, L. R., Fox, V., et al. (1988). Trial of anonymous versus confidential human immunodeficiency virus testing. *Lancet, 332*, 379–382.

Fullilove, R.E., & National Minority AIDS Council. (2006). *African Americans, health disparities and HIV/AIDS: Recommendations for confronting the epidemic in Black America: 2006 Fullilove report.* Retrieved April 27, 2009 from http://www.nmac.org/index/cms-filesystem action?file=grpp/african%20americans,%20health%20disparities%20and%20hiv/aids.pdf

Giordano, P. C., Manning, W. D., & Longmore, M. A. (2005). The romantic relationships of African-American and white adolescents. *The Sociological Quarterly, 46*, 545–568.

Gorbach, P. M., Ryan, C., Saphonn, V., & Detels, R. (2002). The impact of social, economic and political forces on emerging HIV epidemics. *AIDS, 16*, 35–43.

Groseclose, S. L., Weinstein, B., Jones, S. T., Valleroy, L. A., Fehrs, L. J., & Kassler, W. J. (1995). Impact of increased legal access to needles and syringes on practices of injecting-drug users and police officers- Connecticut, 1992–1993. *Journal of Acquired Immune Deficiency Syndromes and Human Retrovirology, 10*, 82–89.

Gupta, G. R., Parkhurst, J. O., Ogden, J. A., Aggleton, P., & Mahal, A. (2008). Structural approaches to HIV prevention. *Lancet, 372*, 764–775.

Guttmacher Institute. *State policies in brief: Sex and STI/HIV education. Retrieved April 27, 2009 from* http://www.guttmacher.org/statecenter/spibs/spib_SE.pdf

Harvey, P. D. (1994). The impact of condom prices on sales in social marketing programs. *Studies in Family Planning, 25*, 52–58.

Heimberger, T. S., Chang, H. G., Birkhead, G. S., DiFerdinando, G. D., Greenberg, A. J., et al. (1993). High prevalence of syphilis detected through a jail screening program. A potential public health measure to address the syphilis epidemic. *Archives of Internal Medicine, 153*, 1799–1804.

Hellard, M. E., & Aitken, C. K. (2004). HIV in prison: What are the risks and what can be done? *Sexual Health, 1*, 107–113.

Holtgrave, D. R., Briddell, K., Little, E., Bendixen, A. V., Hooper, M., et al. (2007). Cost and threshold analysis of housing as an HIV prevention intervention. *AIDS and Behavior, 11*, S162–S166.

Huo, D., Bailey, S. L., Hershow, R. C., & Ouellet, L. (1998). Drug use and HIV risk practices of secondary and primary needle exchange users. *AIDS Education and Prevention, 17*, 170–184.

Huo, D., & Ouellet, L. J. (2007). Needle exchange and injection-related risk behaviors in Chicago: A longitudinal study. *Journal of Acquired Immune Deficiency Syndromes, 45*, 108–114.

Huo, D., & Ouellet, L. J. (2009). Needle exchange and sexual risk behaviors among a cohort of injection drug users in Chicago, Illinois. *Sexually Transmitted Diseases, 36*, 35–40.

Jana, S., Basu, I., Rotheram-Borus, M. J., & Newman, P. A. (2004). The Sonagachi project: A sustainable community intervention program. *AIDS Education and Prevention, 16*, 405–414.

Kahn, J. G., Haile, B., Kates, J., & Chang, S. (2001). Health and federal budgetary effects of increasing access to antiretroviral medications for HIV by expanding Medicaid. *American Journal of Public Health, 91*, 1464–1473.

Kaufmann, G. R., Zaunders, J. J., Cunningham, P., Kelleher, A. D., Grey, P., et al. (2000). Rapid restoration of CD4 T cell subsets in subjects receiving antiretroviral therapy during primary HIV-1 infection. *AIDS, 14*, 2643–2651.

Kerrigan, D., Moreno, L., Rosario, S., Gomez, B., Jerez, H., et al. (2006). Environmental-structural interventions to reduce HIV/STI risk among female sex workers in the Dominican Republic. *American Journal of Public Health, 96*, 120–125.

Khan, M. R., Miller, W. C., Shoenbach, V. J., Weir, S. S., Kaufman, J. S., et al. (2008). Timing and duration of incarceration and high-risk sexual partnerships among African Americans in North Carolina. *Annals of Epidemiology, 18*, 403–410.

Kidder, D. P., Wolitski, R. J., Campsmith, M. L., & Nakamura, G. V. (2007). Health status, health care use, medication use, and medication adherence among homeless and housed people living with HIV/AIDS. *American Journal of Public Health, 97*, 2238–2245.

Kidder, D. P., Wolitski, R. J., Royal, S., Aidala, A., Courtenay-Quirk, C., et al. (2007). Access to housing as a structural intervention for homeless and unstably housed people living with HIV: Rationale, methods, and implementation of the housing and health study. *AIDS and Behavior, 11*, 149–161.

Kippax, S., & Race, K. (2003). Sustaining safe practice: Twenty years on. *Social Science & Medicine, 57*, 1–12.

Kirby, D. (1999). Sexuality education: It can reduce unprotected intercourse. *SIECUS Report, 21*, 19–25.

Kirby, D. B., Laris, B. A., & Rolleri, L. A. (2007). Sex and HIV education programs: Their impact on sexual behaviors of young people throughout the world. *The Journal of Adolescent Health, 40*, 206–217.

Klein, S. J., Candelas, A. R., Cooper, J. G., Badillo, W. E., Tesoriero, J. M., et al. (2008). Increasing safe syringe collection sites in New York State. *Public Health Rep, 123*, 433–440.

Klein, S. J., Karachner, W. D., & O'Connell, D. A. (2002). Interventions to prevent HIV-related stigma and discrimination: Findings and recommendations for public health practice. *Journal of Public Health Management and Practice, 8*, 44–53.

Klein, S. J., O'Connell, D. A., Devore, B. S., Wright, L. N., & Birkhead, G. S. (2002). Building an HIV Continuum for inmates: New York State's criminal justice initiative. *AIDS Education and Prevention, 14*, 114–123.

Klein, J. D., Sesselberg, T. S., Gawronski, B., Handerwerker, L., Gestern, F., & Schetine, A. (2003). Improving adolescent preventive services through state, managed care, and community partnerships. *The Journal of Adolescent Health, 32*, 91–97.

Knowlton, A., Arnsten, J., Eldred, L., Wilkinson, J., Gourevitch, M., et al. (2006). Individual, interpersonal, and structural correlates of effective HAART use among urban active injection drug users. *Journal of Acquired Immune Deficiency Syndromes, 41*, 486–492.

Koumans, E. H., Farley, T. A., Gibson, J. J., Langley, C., Ross, M. W., et al. (2001). Characteristics of persons with syphilis in areas of persisting syphilis in the United States: Sustained transmission associated with concurrent partnerships. *Sexually Transmitted Diseases, 28*, 497–503.

Krieger, N., Chen, J. T., Waterman, P. D., Rehkopf, D. H., & Subramanian, S. V. (2005). Painting a truer picture of U.S. socioeconomic and Racial/Ethnic health inequalities: The public health disparities geocoding project. *American Journal of Public Health, 95*, 312–323.

Latkin, C. A., Curry, A. D., Hua, W., & Davey, M. A. (2007). Direct and indirect associations of neighborhood disorder with drug use and high-risk sexual partners. *American Journal of Preventive Medicine, 32*, S234–S241.

Latkin, C. A., Williams, C. T., Wang, J., & Curry, A. D. (2005). Neighborhood social disorder as a determinant of drug injection behaviors: A structural equation modeling approach. *Health Psychology, 24*, 96–100.

Martin, S. S., Butzin, C. A., & Inciardi, J. A. (1995). Assessment of a multistage therapeutic community for drug-involved offenders. *Journal of Psychoactive Drugs, 27*, 109–116.

Massey, D. S., & Denton, N. A. (1993). *American apartheid: Segregation and the making of the underclass.* Cambridge, MA: Harvard University Press.

May, J. P., & Williams, E. L. (2002). Acceptability of condom availability in a U.S. jail. *AIDS Education and Prevention, 14*, 85–91.

McCarty, D., LaPrade, J., & Botticelli, M. (1996). Substance abuse treatment and HIV services: Massachusetts' policies and programs. *Journal of Substance Abuse Treatment, 13*, 429–438.

McKinnon J. (2003). The black population in the United States: March 2002. In Washington: U.S. Census Bureau (Ed.) *Current Population Reports,* Series P20-541.

McLoyd, V. C., & Steinberg, L. (1998). *Studying minority adolescents: Conceptual, methodological, and theoretical issues.* Mahwah, NJ: Lawrence Erlbaum Associates.

Mertz, K. J., Schwebke, J. R., Gaydos, C. A., Beidinger, H. A., Tulloch, S. D., & Levine, W. C. (2002). Screening women in jails for chlamydial and gonoccocal infection using urine tests: Feasibility, acceptability, prevalence, and treatment rates. *Sexually Transmitted Diseases, 29*, 271–276.

Mofenson, L. M., & Centers for Disease Control and Prevention, U.S. Public Health Service Task Force. (2002). U.S. public health service task force recommendations for use of antiretroviral drugs in Pregnant HIV-1-infected women for maternal health and interventions to reduce Perinatal HIV-1 TRANSMISSION in the United States. *MMWR: Recommendations and Reports, 51*, 1–38.

Molitor, F., Kuenneth, C., Waltermeyer, J., Mendoza, M., Aguirre, A., et al. (2005). Linking HIV-infected persons of color and injection drug users to HIV medical and other services: The California bridge project. *AIDS Patient Care, 19*, 406–412.

Nakashima, A. K., Horsley, R., Frey, R. L., Sweeney, P. A., Weber, J. T., & Fleming, P. L. (1998). Effect of HIV reporting by name on use of HIV testing in publicly funded counseling and testing programs. *The Journal of the American Medical Association, 280*, 1421–1426.

Neaigus, A., Zhao, M., Gyarmathy, V. A., Cisek, L., Friedman, S. R., & Baxter, R. C. (2008). *Journal of Urban Health, 85*, 309–322.

Nicholas, S. W., Jean-Louis, B., Oritz, B., Northridge, M., Shoemaker, K., et al. (2005). Addressing the childhood asthma crisis in Harlem: The Harlem children's zone asthma initiative. *American Journal of Public Health, 95*, 245–249.

Parkhurst, J. O. (2001). The crisis of AIDS and the politics of response: The case of Uganda. *International Relations, 15*, 69–87.

Potterat, J. J., Zimmerman-Rogers, H., Muth, S. Q., Rothenberg, R. B., Green, D. L., et al. (1999). Chlamydia transmission: Concurrency, reproduction number, and the epidemic trajectory. *American Journal of Epidemiology, 150*, 1331–1339.

Pronyk, P. M., Kim, J. C., Abramsky, T., Phetla, G., Hargreaves, J. R., Morison, L. A., et al. (2008). A combined microfinance and training intervention can reduce HIV risk behaviour in young female participants. *AIDS, 22*, 1659–1665.

Richie, B. E., Freudenberg, N., & Page, J. (2001). Reintegrating women leaving jail into urban communities: A description of a model program. *Journal of Urban Health, 78*, 290–303.

Rothman, J., Rudnick, D., Slifer, M., Agins, B., Heiner, K., & Birkhead, G. (2007). Co-located substance use treatment and HIV prevention and primary care services, New York State, 1990–2002: A model for effective service delivery to a high-risk population. *Journal of Urban Health, 84*, 226–242.

Rutherford, G. W., Woo, J. M., Neal, D. P., Rauch, K. J., Geoghegan, C., McKinney, K. C., et al. (1991). Partner notification and the control of human immunodeficiency virus infection. Two years of experience in San Francisco. *Sexually Transmitted Diseases, 18*, 107–110.

Schuler, S. R., & Hashemi, S. M. (1994). Credit programs, women's empowerment, and contraceptive use in rural Bangladesh. *Studies in Family Planning, 25*, 65–76.

Sherman, S. G., German, D., Cheng, Y., Marks, M., & Bailey-Kloche, M. (2006). The evaluation of the JEWEL project: An innovative economic enhancement and HIV prevention intervention study targeting drug using women involved in prostitution. *AIDS Care, 18*, 1–11.

Stoneburner, R., & Low-Beer, D. (2004). Population-level HIV declines and behavioral risk avoidance in Uganda. *Science, 302*, 714–718.

Sumartojo, E. (2000). Structural and environmental factors in HIV prevention: Concepts, examples, and implications for research. *AIDS, 14*, S3–S10.

Sumartojo, E., Doll, L., Holtgrave, D., Gayle, H., & Merson, M. (2000). Enriching the mix: Incorporating structural factors in HIV prevention. *AIDS, 14*, S1–S2.

Sweat, M. D., & Denison, J. A. (1995). Reducing HIV incidence in developing countries with structural and environmental interventions. *AIDS, 9*, S251–S257.

Swenson, R. R., Rizzo, C. J., Brown, L. K., Payne, N., DiClemente, R. J., et al. (2009). Prevalence and correlates of HIV testing among sexually active African American adolescents in 4 US cities. *Sex Transm Dis, 36*, 584–591.

Towe, V. L., Sifakis, F., Gindi, R. M., Sherman, S. G., Flynn, C., et al. (2010) Prevalence of HIV Infection and Sexual Risk Behaviors Among Individuals Having Heterosexual Sex in Low Income Neighborhoods in Baltimore, MD: The BESURE Study. *JAIDS Journal of Acquired Immune Deficiency Syndromes, 53*, 522–528.

U.S. Department of Justice, Office of Justice Programs, Bureau of Justice Statistics. *Demographic trends in jail populations*. Retrieved April 27, 2009 from http://www.ojp.usdoj.gov/bjs/glance/tables/jailrairtab.htm

US Census Bureau. (2003). *Poverty: 1999. Census 2000 Brief.* Retrieved April 27, 2009 from http://www.census.gov/prod/2003pubs/c2kbr-19.pdf

Vlahov, D., & Junge, B. (1998). The role of needle exchange programs in HIV prevention. *Public Health Reports, 113*, S75–S80.

Watson, C. (1988). An open approach to AIDS. *Africe Report, 33*, 32–34.

Wolfe, M. I., Xu, F., Patel, P., O'Cain, M., Schillinger, J. A., et al. (2001). An outbreak of syphilis in Alabama prisons: Correctional health policy and communicable disease control. *American Journal of Public Health, 91*, 1220–1225.

Wolitski, R. J., Kidder, D. P., & Fenton, K. A. (2007). HIV, homelessness, and public health: Critical issues and a call for increased action. *AIDS and Behavior, 11*, S167–S171.

Woods, W. J. (2003). Public health policy and gay bathhouses. *Journal of Homosexuality, 44*, 1–21.

Zenilman, J. M., Ellish, N., Fresia, A., & Glass, G. (1999). The geography of sexual partnerships in Baltimore: Applications of core theory dynamics using a geographic information system. *Sexually Transmitted Diseases, 26*, 75–81.

Chapter 15
HIV Behavioral Interventions for Incarcerated Populations in the United States: A Critical Review*

David Wyatt Seal, Robin J. MacGowan, Gloria D. Eldridge, Mahnaz R. Charania, and Andrew D. Margolis

Background

Over 2.3 million adults were incarcerated in the United States (U.S.) at mid-year 2008, the majority of whom were male and a racial or ethnic minority (West & Sabol, 2009). African Americans and Latinos were more than six times and twice as likely, respectively, as whites to be incarcerated (West & Sabol). HIV prevalence and confirmed AIDS cases are higher among incarcerated populations than among the general U.S. population, with the highest rates observed among Latinos and African Americans and among women (Maruschak, 2008). Elevated rates of hepatitis and other STIs also have been documented among both adolescent (Kelly, Bair, Baillargeon, & Gerrman, 2000; Oh et al., 1998) and adult (Baillargeon, Black, Pulvino, & Dunn, 2000; Mertz et al., 2002) correctional populations.

Both adolescents and adults who are or have been incarcerated in the U.S. report frequent behaviors in the community that place them and their partners at considerable risk for HIV, hepatitis, and other STIs, including unprotected sex with multiple and high-risk sex partners, sex and substance use co-occurrence, and injection drug use with needle sharing. These risk behaviors have been documented both in the period immediately prior to incarceration (Hogben, St. Lawrence, & Eldridge, 2001; Margolis et al., 2006; Morris et al., 1995; Morris, Baker, Valentine, & Pennisi, 1998; Teplin, Mericle, McClelland, & Abram, 2003), and in the period immediately following release from a correctional facility (Belenko, Langley, Crimmins, & Chaple, 2004; Grinstead et al., 2005; MacGowan et al., 2003; Morrow et al., 2007).

---

*The findings and conclusions in this chapter are those of the authors and do not necessarily represent the views of the Centers for Disease Control and Prevention.

D.W. Seal (✉)
Center for AIDS Intervention Research, Medical College of Wisconsin,
2071 N. Summit Avenue, Milwaukee, WI USA
e-mail: dseal@mcw.edu

D.H. McCree et al. (eds.), *African Americans and HIV/AIDS*,
DOI 10.1007/978-0-387-78321-5_15,

271

Other studies have documented the occurrence of HIV risk behavior among adults during incarceration, including injection and other drug use (Clarke, Stein, Hanna, Sobota, & Rich, 2001; Seal et al., 2004, Seal et al., 2008) and coercive and non-coercive sexual behavior (Beck & Harrison, 2006; Moseley & Tewksbury, 2006; Seal et al., 2004, Seal et al., 2008; Struckman-Johnson & Struckman-Johnson, 2006). These studies also found that HIV prevention methods available in the community are rarely utilized in correctional settings. Further, infectious disease transmission within U.S. correctional facilities has been documented (e.g., CDC, 2001; Taussig et al., 2006; Wolfe et al., 2001).

Collectively, these data highlight an urgent need to develop effective and feasible risk reduction interventions specifically designed to meet the unique needs of incarcerated populations. Yet, few rigorously designed and evaluated intervention studies with correctional populations have appeared in the scientific literature. In this chapter, we critically review behavioral HIV risk reduction interventions and programs that have been published to date, summarize key findings, and offer programmatic and scientific recommendations.

Methods

The review was limited to indexed and non-indexed publications from 1983 through 2008 identified through the following databases: AIDSLine, CINAHL, Criminal Justice Abstracts, Medline (indexed and non-indexed), National Criminal Justice Resource Service, OVID (books and journals), and PsycInfo. Combinations of the following search terms were used: [HIV or AIDS] AND [prevention or intervention or program or adherence or testing] AND [corrections or correctional or jails or prison or detention or penal or penitentiary or incarcerated or prisoner or inmate or offender or detainee or probation or parole or juvenile or delinquency or delinquent]. Our review excluded published reports of preventive HIV counseling and testing, medical care or treatment services, which were beyond the scope of this chapter. We also excluded from our analyses studies which were conducted outside the U.S., although we draw upon these studies in our discussion. We located and summarized 48 articles describing 44 studies in the U.S. that were conducted with a correctional population.

Our review is organized around three primary subgroups: adolescents, adult drug users, and other adult populations (see Table 15.1 for complete summary). We further sorted the studies into intervention descriptions that reported (a) HIV risk reduction behavioral outcomes (n = 22), (b) non-behavioral outcomes only (such as increased knowledge, self-esteem, perceived self-efficacy) (n = 15), and (c) descriptive reports without an evaluation (n = 7). None reported biological outcomes. For brevity, we discuss primarily the articles that provided behavioral outcome data. Finally, we note that although this book is focused on prevention of AIDS among African Americans, none of the identified studies specifically targeted this population. Nonetheless, given the disproportionate rate of incarceration among African Americans in the U.S., a review of interventions with correctional populations is warranted.

Table 15.1 Summary of published HIV prevention interventions for people under correctional jurisdiction in the United States, 1983–2008

Study author and journal citation	Evaluation design	Sample description	Intervention description	Significant intervention effects (p≤0.05)
Adolescents (N=16)				
Behavioral (n=6)				
Gillmore et al. (1997). AIDS Education and Prevention, 9 (Suppl. A), 22–43	Design: Non-biased weekly block assignment Comparison: Test of 3 interventions Follow-up: Immediate post, 3- and 6-month postrelease Retention: Intervention completion (228/282 youth who completed baseline: 81%) FU among youth who completed intervention: 3m (161/228: 71%), 6m (174/228: 76%)	N: 228 Pop: Youth who completed intervention Site: Detention center Male: 54% African American: 52% (Study also included 168 youth recruited from public health STD clinics or other similar clinics)	Level: Individual or Group Duration: Group (8 h delivered in 1–4 sessions: four 2-h modules); Individual (<1 h) Content: All 3 interventions provided factual information and skills for communicating and negotiating condom use; varied in degree of instruction, modeling, role-play, and rehearsal (1) 1-page comic book with condom negotiation vignettes (2) 27-min videotape with peer actors couples negotiating condom use (3) Small group delivered by peer tutors with active role-play and rehearsal	• No significant behavioral outcomes reported • Increased comfort among group participants in talking with casual (3m) and steady (6m) partners

(continued)

Table 15.1 (continued)

Study author and journal citation	Evaluation design	Sample description	Intervention description	Significant intervention effects (p≤0.05)
Magura et al. (1994). *Journal of Adolescent Health, 15,* 457–463	*Design:* Non-biased weekly block assignment. *Comparison:* Wait-control youth released prior to intervention receipt. *Follow-up:* 5-month postrelease. *Retention:* (157/411 who completed baseline: 38%) (58/110 who received intervention: 53%) (Overall FU: 66%)	*N:* 157. *Pop:* First 99 wait-control and first 58 intervention youth who were released. *Site:* Detention center. *Male:* 100%. *African American:* 65%	*Level:* Group. *Duration:* Four 1-h sessions over 2 weeks. *Content:* Health education issues relevant to male drug users, with emphasis on HIV/AIDS (delivered by male counselor)	Intervention participants reported • Increased condom use frequency for vaginal, oral, and anal sex • Greater acceptability of condoms
Needels et al. (2005). *Journal of Urban Health: Bulletin of the New York Academy of Medicine, 82,* 420–433	*Design:* Random assignment based on who was willing to meet conditions of enhanced intervention. *Comparison:* Standard discharge planning services. *Follow-up:* 15-month postrelease. *Retention:* Adolescents (537/706: 76%) (Intervention: 60% had any postrelease contact, 42% retained at 6 months, 29% for full year)	*N:* 1,410. *Pop:* General (adult women=704; adolescent males=706). *Site:* Jail. *Adolescents:* *Male:* 100%. *African American:* NR	*Level:* Individual. *Duration:* Adolescents averaged 9.5 h of contact during 1-year postrelease period. *Content:* All participants received standard discharge planning (individual counseling+voluntary empowerment group meetings). Enhanced intervention also included community case management to help people successfully reintegrate and avoid problem behavior (in-jail services provided by jail caseworkers; community services provided by CBO case managers).	Adolescent males: • No significant behavioral outcomes. Adult women: See Adult Behavioral section below

Rosengard et al. (2008). *Journal of HIV/AIDS Prevention in Children and Youth*, 8, 45–64	*Design:* Random assignment *Comparison:* Test of two interventions *Follow-up:* 3-month postrelease *Retention:* Adolescents (114/117: 97%)	*N:* 117 *Pop:* Youth confined to the facility *Site:* Detention center *Male:* 90% *African American:* 34%	*Level:* Individual *Duration:* Both interventions were 2-sessions (length unspecified) – one session was post-baseline shortly after being admitted to the facility; the other session was a booster session conducted shortly prior to release *Content:* All participants received standard substance abuse treatment and other supplementary services offered to all residents in the facility. The Relaxation Training focused on progressive-muscle relaxation and visualizing a pleasant scene combined with generalized advice about abstinence from criminal, risky, and substance use activities. The Motivational Enhancement (ME) intervention centered on developing an individual plan to reduce substance use and associated risk behaviors (e.g., sexual activity, illegal behavior).	At 3-month post-release follow-up (97% retention), the strongest predictor of sexual risk was increased sexual risk prior to incarceration.Among participants who reported lower levels of depression at baseline, those in the ME condition, compared to those in the RT condition, reported: • Less condom non-use • Less condom non-use in conjunction with the use of marijuana

(continued)

Table 15.1 (continued)

Study author and journal citation	Evaluation design	Sample description	Intervention description	Significant intervention effects (p ≤ 0.05)
Slonim-Nevo and Auslander (1996). *Adolescence*, *31*, 409–421	*Design:* Random assignment *Comparison:* Discussion-only or wait-control group *Follow-up:* Immediate post and 9–12 month postrelease *Retention:* (Post-test: 268/358 of youth who completed pre-test: 75%) (9–12m FU: 218/268 who completed post-test: 81%)	*N:* 218 *Pop:* Youth affected by juvenile delinquency, child abuse or neglect, or mental health problems *Site:* Residential center *Male:* 56% *African American:* 46%	*Level:* Group *Duration:* Both groups consisted of nine 1.5–2 h sessions over 3 weeks *Content:* Intensive AIDS prevention program using interactive learning techniques; compared to attention-control discussion-only group focused on same topics and to a wait-control intervention (co-delivered by people who received at least 40 h of AIDS prevention training)	Compared to control, both group conditions showed • Increased AIDS knowledge and coping with AIDS-risk situations at immediate post-test (not sustained at 9–12 month FU) • No significant behavioral outcomes reported at either FU

St. Lawrence et al. (1999). *Journal of Sex Education and Therapy*, 24, 9–17	*Design:* Random assignment *Comparison:* Attention-control anger management intervention *Follow-up:* Immediate post and 6-month postrelease *Retention:* Intervention completion (361/430 youth who completed baseline: 84%) FU among youth who completed intervention: Post-test (349/361: 97%), 6m postrelease (312/361: 86%)	*N:* 361 *Pop:* Youth who completed intervention *Site:* State reformatory *Male:* 54% *African American:* 52%	*Level:* Group *Duration:* Six sessions over 3-week period lasting 1 h each *Content:* Informational and skills building HIV prevention curriculum, including peer modeling videos and dyadic role-play; comparison intervention was similarly structured, but focused on anger management skills (co-facilitated by trained male and trained female)	No significant between-group differences in behavioral outcomes reported at 6m FU: • Youth in both groups reported a lower number of sex partners and a lower frequency of oral sex acts and unprotected vaginal and anal sex acts • Youth in both groups reported fewer casual sex encounters, coercions into unwanted sexual activity, and occasions of exchanging drugs for sex • Youth in both groups reported decreased alcohol and marijuana use • Youth in both groups had showed less reliance on conflict in interpersonal interactions, fewer court appearances, and spent less days incarcerated • Youth in both groups increased their perceived risk for HIV/STI infection, with a larger increase in the HIV condition • Youth in HIV intervention had increased AIDS knowledge, more favorable attitudes toward condoms, enhanced self-efficacy for safer sex, and increased condom-use skills

(continued)

Table 15.1 (continued)

Study author and journal citation	Evaluation design	Sample description	Intervention description	Significant intervention effects (p ≤ 0.05)
Non-behavioral (n = 8)				
Clark et al. (2000). *Journal of Criminal Justice, 28*, 415–433	*Design:* 1-Group *Comparison:* NA *Follow-up:* Immediate post, 6-week postrelease (NR) *Retention:* (99/99: 100%)	*N:* 99 *Pop:* General *Site:* Detention Center *Male:* 65% *African American:* 65%	*Level:* Group *Duration:* 24 h over 4-day period *Content:* Curriculum designed to prevent HIV, STI, and pregnancy risk behavior (delivered by youth experts)	Immediate post-test: • Increased self-esteem • Increased efficacy for communication and listening skills • Increased HIV/AIDS-related knowledge • Increased perceived susceptibility to HIV/AIDS
Kelly et al. (2004). *Journal of Correctional Health Care, 11*, 45–58	*Design:* Non-biased block assignment by incarceration period *Comparison:* Attention-control delivery of same content delivered via video and lecture *Follow-up:* Immediate post *Retention:* (54/54: 100%)	*N:* 54 *Pop:* General *Site:* Detention Center *Male:* 0% *African American:* 15%	*Level:* Group *Duration:* 8 h over a weekend *Content:* Girls Talk-2 used social-cognitive theory to focus on precursors of behavior change, including self-efficacy, communication skills demonstration, positive condom attitudes, and knowledge of local resources (delivered by trained 18–22 year-old college students of similar ethnicity/race)	Intervention participants reported • Increased self-efficacy on a scale of HIV/STI risk knowledge, attitudes, and practices
Lanier and McCarthy (1989). *Criminal Justice and Behavior, 16*, 395–411	*Design:* Non-biased assignment by incarceration setting *Comparison:* No-intervention control *Follow-up:* Several weeks post-intervention *FU Response Rate:* (363/415 youth who completed intervention: 87%) (no pre-intervention baseline)	*N:* 363 *Pop:* Youth who completed FU survey *Site:* Delinquency center *Male:* NR *African American:* NR	*Level:* Group *Duration:* 2 sites – 1 h per day for 5 days; 1 site – 1 h per day for 3 days *Content:* State required AIDS education curriculum, including discussion and handouts about at-risk populations, transmission modes, medical terminology, and promotion of abstinence (facilitators not specified)	Intervention participants reported • Increased knowledge about AIDS • Increased perceived importance of the AIDS epidemic

Schlapman and Cass (2000). *Community Health Nursing*, 17, 151–158	*Design:* 1 Group *Comparison:* NA *Follow-up:* Immediate post *Retention:* (69/146: 47%)	*N:* 146 *Pop:* Youth who completed pre-test *Site:* Juvenile Center *Male:* 0% *African American:* NR	*Level:* Group *Duration:* 4 sessions were offered over a 7-month period on a rotating basis (session length not specified); 91 sessions in all were held *Content:* Interactive HIV education intervention aimed at reducing high-risk sexual behavior (delivered by a public health nurse)	Immediate post-test: • Increased percent of people answered 4 specific items correctly (out of 40) on an HIV/AIDS knowledge test
Shelton (2001). *Issues in Mental Health Nursing*, 22, 159–172	*Design:* 1 Group *Comparison:* NA *Follow-up:* Immediate post *Retention:* (36/36: 100%)	*N:* 36 *Pop:* General *Site:* 90-day community-based juvenile justice substance abuse treatment program *Male:* 100% *African American:* 100%	*Level:* Group *Duration:* 16 sessions provided weekly (session length not specified); post-intervention reinforcement provided in substance use treatment groups *Content:* Aimed at reducing drug use and high-risk sexual behavior; drew upon peer counseling and cross-cultural sensitivity training models (facilitators not specified)	Immediate post-test: • Increased knowledge about appropriate use of condoms, safer sex practices, and AIDS/HIV

(continued)

Table 15.1 (continued)

Study author and journal citation	Evaluation design	Sample description	Intervention description	Significant intervention effects ($p \leq 0.05$)
Ward and Waters (1999). *Journal of HIV/AIDS Prevention and Education for Adolescents and Children, 3,* 51–77	*Design:* 1 Group *Comparison:* NA *Follow-up:* Immediate post *Retention:* NR (Study also included youth recruited from a welfare program for teen mothers, county welfare offices, and county welfare hotels; total study sample size: 3,460)	*N:* 514 *Pop:* General *Site:* Detention Center *Male:* 96% *African American:* NR	*Level:* HIV prevention program within context of a Therapeutic Community *Duration:* 4 sessions over a 4-week period lasting 2 h each *Content:* HIV prevention program included modeling, media presentations, discussion group topics, and role-play to provide educational information, skills building, realization of substance use–HIV risk relationship, and development of realistic individual risk reduction plan (delivered by part-time peer educators and full-time health educators)	• No outcomes were reported separately for detention center participants; nor were between-site analyses conducted
Waters et al. (1996). *Crisis Intervention, 3,* 85–96	*Design:* 1 Group *Comparison:* NA *Follow-up:* Immediate post *Retention:* (189/556: 34%)	*N:* 556 *Pop:* Analyses limited to Black males who completed pre- and post-tests *Site:* Detention Center *Male:* 100% *African American:* 86%	*Level:* HIV prevention program within context of a Therapeutic Community *Duration:* 4 h per day for 5 days in a 1-week period; participants attend an advanced phase of the same duration at a later time *Content:* Prevention program designed to reduce HIV transmission risk, reduce drug abuse incidence, develop positive lifestyle alternatives to violence and crime (delivered by a male or female facilitator, 2 of whom were in recovery)	Immediate post-test: • Authors report some increases in HIV/AIDS knowledge and some decrease in perceived AIDS risk among program participants; however, statistical analyses not presented

Citation	Design	Sample	Intervention	Findings
Witte and Morrison (1995). *Journal of Applied Communication Research*, 23, 128–142	*Design:* Random assignment *Comparison:* High- versus low-threat HIV prevention message *Follow-up:* Immediate post *Retention:* (31/31: 100%)	*N:* 31 *Pop:* General *Site:* Detention Center *Male:* 65% *African American:* 52% (Study also included 92 high school teens)	*Level:* Group *Duration:* One 30-min session *Content:* Participants received a live, peer-facilitated health educator presentation with visual aids that was either high-threat or low-threat (delivered by trained peer educators)	• Low sensation seekers persuaded to adopt safer sex behaviors regardless of message threat; high sensation seekers unaffected by either message • Above finding did not interact with recruitment setting (detention center versus high school)
Descriptive (n = 2) Setzer et al. (1991). *Journal of Prison and Jail Health, 10,* 91–115	*Design:* NA *Comparison:* NA *Follow-up:* NA *Retention:* NA	*N:* NR *Pop:* General *Site:* Juvenile probation department *Male:* NR *African American:* NR	*Level:* Systemic Intervention *Duration:* NR *Content:* Describes a prevention model that integrates HIV risk assessment and reduction planning with provision of medical and substance use treatment services	• No formal evaluations reported
Zibalese-Crawford (1997). *Social Work in Health Care, 25,* 73–88	*Design:* NA *Comparison:* NA *Follow-up:* NA *Retention:* NA	*N:* NR *Pop:* General *Site:* Youth housed in alternative settings: both detention and non-detention facilities *Male:* NR *African American:* NR	*Level:* Group *Duration:* NR *Content:* Describes an empowerment-oriented approach to HIV/AIDS prevention	• No formal evaluations reported

(continued)

Table 15.1 (continued)

Study author and journal citation	Evaluation design	Sample description	Intervention description	Significant intervention effects (p ≤ 0.05)
Adult drug users (N = 7)				
Behavioral (n = 7)				
Baxter (1991). *Crime and Delinquency*, 37, 48–63	*Design*: Random assignment *Comparison*: No-intervention control *Follow-up*: 3-, 6-, 12-month post-intervention *Retention*: Can't calculate – baseline sample size not reported (3m FU: n=200; 6m FU: n=134; 12m FU: NR)	*N*: 134 at 6m FU *Pop*: People who injected drugs in the prior 6 months *Site*: Jail *Male*: 30% *African American*: 11%	*Level*: Group *Duration*: 8-h delivered in 5 modules over 2-week period *Content*: HIV/AIDS information, personal risk sensitization, promotion of sexual and needle risk reduction behavior (facilitator not specified)	3m FU (data not shown): • Author reported minimal changes in knowledge, attitudes, or behavior for either group 6m FU: • Education group had a higher risk behavior score for needle sharing Control group had a higher risk behavior score for number of IDU sexual partners
El-Bassel et al. (1995). *Social Work Research*, 19, 131–141	*Design*: Random assignment *Comparison*: AIDS information session *Follow-up*: 1-month postrelease *Retention*: Intervention completion (145/159 women who completed pre-test: 91%) FU among women who completed intervention: (101/145: 70%)	*N*: 145 *Pop*: Women who used cocaine, heroin, or crack 3+ times/week prior to arrest *Site*: Jail *Male*: 0% *African American*: 69%	*Level*: Group *Duration*: 16 two-hours sessions, twice weekly in prison; six booster sessions, monthly in community *Content*: HIV/AIDS risk behaviors, safe sex practices, self efficacy, problem solving, coping skills, social and support networks, injection related risks (delivered by women of similar ethnicity and substance use experience who received intensive 3-day training)	• No significant behavioral outcomes reportedRegardless of condition: • Increased coping skills (among those with less prior incarcerations) • Increased perception of emotional support (among those with greater prior incarcerations)

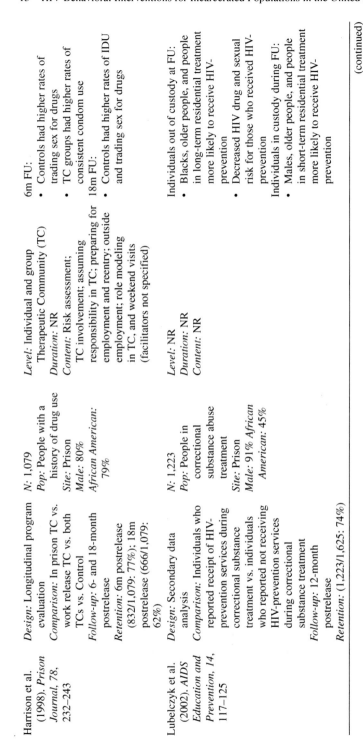

Harrison et al. (1998). *Prison Journal, 78,* 232–243	*Design:* Longitudinal program evaluation *Comparison:* In prison TC vs. work release TC vs. both TCs vs. Control *Follow-up:* 6- and 18-month postrelease *Retention:* 6m postrelease (832/1,079: 77%); 18m postrelease (666/1,079: 62%)	*N:* 1,079 *Pop:* People with a history of drug use *Site:* Prison *Male:* 80% *African American:* 79%	*Level:* Individual and group Therapeutic Community (TC) *Duration:* NR *Content:* Risk assessment; TC involvement; assuming responsibility in TC; preparing for employment and reentry; outside employment; role modeling in TC, and weekend visits (facilitators not specified)	6m FU: • Controls had higher rates of trading sex for drugs • TC groups had higher rates of consistent condom use 18m FU: • Controls had higher rates of IDU and trading sex for drugs
Lubelczyk et al. (2002). *AIDS Education and Prevention, 14,* 117–125	*Design:* Secondary data analysis *Comparison:* Individuals who reported receipt of HIV-prevention services during correctional substance treatment vs. individuals who reported not receiving HIV-prevention services during correctional substance treatment *Follow-up:* 12-month postrelease *Retention:* (1,223/1,625: 74%)	*N:* 1,223 *Pop:* People in correctional substance abuse treatment *Site:* Prison *Male:* 91% *African American:* 45%	*Level:* NR *Duration:* NR *Content:* NR	Individuals out of custody at FU: • Blacks, older people, and people in long-term residential treatment more likely to receive HIV-prevention • Decreased HIV drug and sexual risk for those who received HIV-prevention Individuals in custody during FU: • Males, older people, and people in short-term residential treatment more likely to receive HIV-prevention

(continued)

Table 15.1 (continued)

Study author and journal citation	Evaluation design	Sample description	Intervention description	Significant intervention effects (p ≤ 0.05)
Magura et al. (1995). *International Journal of the Addictions, 30*, 259–273	*Design:* Non-randomized design *Comparison:* Women who were released prior to intervention receipt *Follow-up:* 7-month post-release *Retention:* (101/134: 75%) (based on number of women contacted for FU)	*N:* 101 *Pop:* Drug users (analyses limited to first 53 intervention and first 48 control participants who completed FU) *Site:* Jail *Male:* 0% *African American:* 65%	*Level:* Group *Duration:* Four alternate-day 1-h sessions *Content:* Drug use, sexual behavior, and HIV/AIDS; guided by Problem-Solving Therapy approach, including role-play and rehearsal (delivered by White female counselor with a MA in psychology)	• No significant behavioral outcomes between groups • Women in drug dependency treatment at FU, regardless of condition, reported decreased heroin use, crack use, drug dealing, and criminal activity
Martin et al. (2003). *Journal of Psychoactive Drugs, 35*, 435–443	*Design:* Random assignment *Comparison:* ESI (enhanced NIDA standard intervention) vs. PFI (probation-focused intervention) *Follow-up:* 3- and 6-month postrelease *Retention:* Preliminary analysis before study complete, 6m postrelease (426/706: 60%)	*N:* 706 *Pop:* Drug-involved people on probation *Site:* Community *Male:* 72% *African American:* 70%	*Level:* Individual *Duration:* 3 sessions over 3-months (initial session, 2-week post-test results receipt and post-test counseling; brief 3-month booster) *Content:* ESI (HIV-testing; pre- and post-test counseling; information; demonstration and rehearsal of condom use, needle-cleaning; distribution of prevention materials) *Content:* PFI intervention added personal action plans and thought-mapping techniques to ESI (delivered by program staff)	At 6m FU: • Decreased heroin use, cocaine use, and IDU among both groups • Decreased multiple sex partners, unprotected sex acts, and pay in exchange for sex among both groups • Decreased sex in exchange for money among PFI group • Decreased % of women had unprotected sex in ESI group

Wexler et al. (1994). *The International Journal of the Addictions, 29,* 361–386	*Design:* Non-random assignment *Comparison:* ARRIVE intervention completers vs. eligible parolees who completed baseline but did not receive intervention *Follow-up:* 12-month postrelease *Retention:* (237/317: 75%)	*N:* 317 *Pop:* People on parole with a history of drug injection *Site:* Community *Male: 81% African American: 57%*	*Level:* Group *Duration:* Three 60–90 min sessions per week for 8 weeks *Content:* AIDS transmission, testing, and treatment information; AIDS risk reduction; depression and addiction; employment counseling; job interview role-play and resume preparation; relapse prevention; presentation skills (delivered by 2 clinical staff in recovery with criminal histories)	Intervention participants reported • Less steady IV drug use, recreational drug use, and association with injectors • More "always" condom use; greater condom acceptability • Less high risk sex partners • Less re-arrest and re-incarceration • More employment, educational training, and vocational training • More participation in drug treatment
Non-behavioral (n = 0) No identified studies *Descriptive (n = 0)* No identified studies Adults (N = 20) *Behavioral (n = 9)*				
Arriola et al (2007). *Journal of Health Care for the Poor and Underserved,* 18, 665–674 Also see Arriola et al. (2002)	*Design:* 1-group *Comparison:* NA *Follow-up:* 6-months post-release *Retention:* (226/647: 35%)	*N:* 647 *Pop:* Soon-to-be release HIV infected inmates *Site:* County Jail or Prison *Male: 100% African American: 18%*	*Level:* Individual and Group *Duration:* 1 visit per week for first month post release; 2 visits per month post release by fifth month *Content:* Post-release services include individual or group HIV prevention education, individual counseling, disease management education, and discharge planning (making appointments or referrals)	6m FU: • Increased likelihood of not engaging in sex exchange during subsequent 6 months • Increase likelihood of participating in drug or alcohol treatment

(continued)

Table 15.1 (continued)

Study author and journal citation	Evaluation design	Sample description	Intervention description	Significant intervention effects (p≤0.05)
Braithwaite et al. (2005). *Journal of Health Care for the Poor and Underserved, 16*, 130–139	*Design:* Random assignment *Comparison:* Of 4 modes of delivering videos on health promotion and disease prevention *Follow-up:* 3-month postrelease *Retention:* NR (Number of men recruited not reported)	*N:* 116 *Pop:* People who completed 3-month assessment *Site:* Prison *Male:* 100% African American: 69%	*Level:* Group *Duration:* 12 sessions over 6 weeks (length not specified) *Content:* All four intervention conditions had same content (health education, HIV/AIDS, substance abuse), but each group used a different mode of facilitation: − Passive facilitation − Didactic facilitation by health educator − Didactic facilitation by an HIV− peer − Didactic facilitation by an HIV+ peer	Didactic groups reported • Reduction in substance use • Reduction in risky sexual behavior • Reduction in marijuana use (health educator and HIV− peer groups only) • Increased condom self efficacy Passive facilitation group reported • Reduction in sexual self expectations (versus health educator and HIV+ peer groups only)
Grinstead et al. (1999). *Criminal Justice and Behavior, 26*, 468–480	*Design:* Non-biased block assignment *Comparison:* Access to HIV educational materials and informal consults with staff *Follow-up:* 2-week postrelease *Retention:* (176/414: 43%)	*N:* 414 *Pop:* General *Site:* Prison *Male:* 100% African American: 51%	*Level:* Individual *Duration:* One 30-min session *Content:* Risk assessment and risk reduction plan on acquiring or transmitting HIV, HIV knowledge, and risk behavior (delivered by an incarcerated peer educator)	Intervention participants reported • Increased condom use during oral, vaginal, or anal sex first time after release from prison
Grinstead et al. (2001). *AIDS Education and Prevention, 13*, 109–119 Also see Zack et al. (2004)	*Design:* Non-randomized design *Comparison:* Those who enrolled in the intervention but were unable to attend *Follow-up:* 8-month postrelease (average) *Retention:* (81/144: 56%)	*N:* 144 *Pop:* HIV+ *Site:* Prison *Male:* 100% African American: 55%	*Level:* Group *Duration:* Eight 2–2.5 h sessions in 1 week *Content:* HIV information and treatment, substance use, sexuality, inspirational speaker, nutrition, community service referrals (delivered by community service providers)	• No significant behavioral outcomes reported • Positive and negative intervention outcomes, primarily with small effect sizes

Citation	Methods	Sample	Intervention	Results
Harrison et al. (2001). *Culture, Health & Sexuality, 3*(1), 101–118	*Design:* 1-Group (pre/post) *Comparison:* NA *Follow-up:* 2 months post-release *Retention:* (163/246; 66%)	*N:* 246 *Pop:* General *Site:* Prison *Male:* 0% *African American:* 67%	*Level:* Group *Duration:* One 20 h course during confinement *Content:* Didactic health and HIV education course including information sharing, discussion, participant exercises, role playing, and hands on practice sessions on the female condom	• 0% of participants reported using the female condom prior to confinement • 62% reported using the female condom within 2 months post-release • Most used the female condom with their boyfriend/spouse Overall, 23% reported consistent female condom use and 27% consistent male condom use during all vaginal sex acts 2-months post-release
Lurigio et al. (1992). *AIDS Education and Prevention, 4,* 205–218	*Design:* Random assignment *Comparison:* Diet and exercise strategies *Follow-up:* 1-month postrelease *Retention:* (50/99; 51%)	*N:* 99 *Pop:* People on probation *Site:* Community *Male:* 90% *African American:* 86%	*Level:* Individual and Group *Duration:* One session (length not specified) *Content:* Condom use skills, needle cleaning skills, HIV CT information	Participants in two HIV education groups reported • Increased condom use • Increased HIV knowledge
Myers et al. (2005). *American Journal of Public Health, 95,* 1682–1684	*Design:* 1-Group *Comparison:* NA *Follow-up:* 2.5 months postrelease (immediate post; some still receiving PCM in community) *Retention:* (51/127: 40%)	*N:* 127 *Pop:* General *Site:* Prison *Male:* 55% *African American:* 48%	*Level:* Individual *Duration:* 2 months of PCM prior to release and up to 3 months in the community *Context:* Prevention case management, referrals to community resources, HIV risk reduction education and counseling (delivered by CBO case managers)	At FU: • Increased rates of abstinence or condom use • Reduced rates of drug use during sex

(continued)

Table 15.1 (continued)

Study author and journal citation	Evaluation design	Sample description	Intervention description	Significant intervention effects (p ≤ 0.05)
Needels et al. (2005). *Journal of Urban Health: Bulletin of the New York Academy of Medicine, 82,* 420–433	*Design:* Random assignment based on who was willing to meet conditions of enhanced intervention *Comparison:* Standard discharge planning services *Follow-up:* 15-month postrelease *Retention:* Adults (511/704: 73%) (Intervention: 60% had any postrelease contact, 51% retained at 6 months, 36% for full year)	*N:* 1,410 *Pop:* General (adult women = 704; adolescent males = 706) *Site:* Jail Adults: *Male:* 0% *African American:* NR	*Level:* Individual *Duration:* Adults averaged 6.5 h of contact during 1-year postrelease period *Content:* All participants received standard discharge planning (individual counseling + voluntary empowerment group meetings). Enhanced intervention also included community case management to help people successfully reintegrate and avoid problem behavior (in-jail services provided by jail caseworkers; community services provided by CBO case managers).	Adolescent males:See Adolescent Behavioral section above Adult women at FU: • Decreased arrest for serious charge during 1-year postrelease FU period • Higher percent participated in 1+ postrelease program or 1+ postrelease detox program • Increased # of acts of unprotected vaginal or anal sex • Lower mean # of times used drugs or alcohol during sex • Fewer times had sex for money or drugs Increased percent had sex with an HIV serostatus unknown partner
Wolitski et al. (2006). *American Journal of Public Health,* 96, 1854–1861	*Design:* Non-biased block assignment (intent-to-treat) *Comparison:* 1 session HIV risk reduction program *Follow-up:* 6-month postrelease *Retention:* (432/522: 83%)	*N:* 522 *Pop:* General *Site:* Prison *Male:* 100% *African American:* 52%	*Level:* Individual *Duration:* Two 60–90 min sessions prior to release and four 30–60 min sessions at 1, 3, 6, and 12 weeks post release *Content:* HIV risk reduction, skills training, referrals, community re-entry needs, problem solving (delivered by lay staff who attended 3-day intensive cross-site training)	At 6m FU: • Reduction in rates of unprotected vaginal or anal sex at last intercourse • Reduction in rates of unprotected vaginal or anal sex with main partner

Non-behavioral (n = 7)

Study	Design	Sample	Intervention	Outcomes
Bauserman et al. (2003). *AIDS Education and Prevention, 15*, 465–480	*Design:* 1-Group *Comparison:* NA *Follow-up:* Immediate post *Retention:* (745/2,610: 29%)	*N:* 2,610 *Pop:* General *Site:* Prison and jail *Male:* 50% *African American:* 64%	*Level:* Individual and group *Duration:* 4 required and 3 optional sessions (median: 11 h total) *Content:* Prevention case management, HIV education, skill building, case management, HIV risk reduction, condom use, substance abuse, transitioning back to the community, service referrals (delivered by health department case managers)	Immediate post: • Increased positive attitudes and self efficacy towards condoms • Increased self efficacy to reduce risk involving IDU and other substances • Increased safer sex intentions • Increased perceived future risk of having HIV/AIDS
Bryan et al. (2006). *Health Education and Behavior, 33*, 154–177	*Design:* 1-Group *Comparison:* NA *Follow-up:* Immediate post *Retention:* NR	*N:* 196 *Pop:* General *Site:* Prison *Male:* 90% *African American:* 40%	*Level:* Group *Duration:* One 90-min session per week for 6 weeks *Content:* HIV prevention, knowledge, fears, perceptions, peer educator training (trained and experienced male and female HIV prevention educators)	Immediate post: • Increased AIDS-related knowledge • Increased positive attitudes towards condoms, condom self efficacy, and condom intentions • Increased self efficacy for not sharing needles Increased peer education self efficacy, intentions, behaviors
Grinstead et al. (1997). *Journal of Health Education, 28*, 31–37	*Design:* Non-biased assignment *Comparison:* HIV presentation *Follow-up:* Immediate post *Retention:* NR	*N:* 2,295 *Pop:* General *Site:* Prison *Male:* 100% *African American:* 38%	*Level:* Group *Duration:* one 60–90 min session *Content:* HIV transmission routes, testing, substance use/abuse, correct condom use, needle cleaning (Group 1 led by professional HIV educator; Group 2 led by incarcerated HIV+ peer)	Intervention participants reported • Increased HIV knowledge • Increased condom use intentions • Increased HIV testing intentions

(continued)

Table 15.1 (continued)

Study author and journal citation	Evaluation design	Sample description	Intervention description	Significant intervention effects (p ≤ 0.05)
Pomeroy et al. (1999). *Research on Social Work Practice, 9,* 171–187	Quasi-experimental *Comparison:* Standard of care *Follow-up:* Immediate post *Retention:* (139/160: 87%)	*N:* 160 *Pop:* General *Site:* Jail *Male:* 0% *African American:* 55%	*Level:* Group *Duration:* Two 90-min sessions per week for 5 weeks *Content:* Overview of HIV/AIDS, opportunistic infections, medication issues, safer sex, nutritional needs, women and children with HIV, financial issues, future planning, trust, self esteem, depression, anxiety, unhealthy relationships, communication skills, parenting issues, coping skills, empowerment, goal setting (co-delivered by experienced MSW and second-year social work students)	Intervention participants reported • Reduction in depression, anxiety, and trauma symptomology • Increase in AIDS knowledge
Pomeroy et al. (2000). *Social Work Research, 24,* 156–166	*Design:* Quasi-experimental *Comparison:* Standard of care *Follow-up:* Immediate post *Retention:* (53/72: 74%)	*N:* 72 *Pop:* General *Site:* Jail *Male:* 100% African American: 46%	*Level:* Group *Duration:* Two 90-min sessions per week for 5 weeks *Content:* Same as Pomeroy (1999) above	Intervention participants reported • Reduction in depression, anxiety, and trauma symptomology • Increased AIDS knowledge
Ross et al. (2006). *AIDS Education and Prevention, 18,* 504–517/see Scott et al. (2004). *Journal of Correctional Health Care, 10,* 151–173	*Design:* 1-Group *Comparison:* NA *Follow-up:* 9-month post-baseline (peer educators); Immediate post (students) *Retention:* Peer educators (257/590: 44%)	*Ross et al:* *N:* 590 peer educators; 2,506 students *Pop:* General *Site:* Prison *Male:* 84% (educators) 86% (students) *African American:* 38% (educators) 38% (students)	*Level:* Group *Duration:* Six sessions lasting about 2 h each *Content:* HIV/AIDS education and risk reduction skills within cultural context (delivered by incarcerated women and men who received 40 h intensive peer educator training)	*Immediate post* • Increased HIV knowledge among students *At 9-m FU* • Increased HIV knowledge among peer educators • Increased proportion of peer educators had obtained an HIV test

St. Lawrence et al. (1997). *Journal of Consulting and Clinical Psychology, 65,* 504–509	*Design:* Random assignment *Comparison:* Demonstration project to compare an intervention based on social cognitive theory (SCT) against a comparison condition based on the theory of gender and power (GP) *Follow-up:* 6 months (Did not specify if Follow-up occurred pre- or post-release) *Retention:* NR	*N:* 90 *Pop:* General *Site:* Prison *Male:* 0% African American: 81%	*Level:* Group *Duration:* One 90-min session per week for 6 weeks *Content:* Skills training in correct condom use; partner negotiation, information provision skills; drug use and HIV risk, correct needle cleaning and drug refusal skills (delivered by experienced same-gender facilitators)	SCT intervention participants reported • Increased condom application skills (using model) Both groups reported • Increased self efficacy, self-esteem, attitudes towards prevention, AIDS knowledge, frequency of AIDS-related communication, and comfort with AIDS-related communication (no significant between-group differences)
Descriptive (n = 4) Boudin et al. (1999). *Journal of the Association of Nurses in Health Care, 10,* 90–98	*Design:* NA *Comparison:* NA *Follow-up:* NA *Retention:* NA	*N:* NR *Pop:* HIV+ *Site:* Prison *Male:* 0% African American: NR	*Level:* Individual and Group *Duration:* 3 h sessions daily for 3 weeks *Content:* Peer support program, adherence, HIV transmission, compassionate care standards, medical diaries, buddy system, skits and transitional issues (delivered by peers)	No formal evaluations reported

(continued)

Table 15.1 (continued)

Study author and journal citation	Evaluation design	Sample description	Intervention description	Significant intervention effects (p≤0.05)
Clark et al. (2006). *Maternal and Child Health Journal, 10,* 367–373	*Design:* NA *Comparison:* NA *Follow-up:* NA *Retention:* NA	*N:* 515 *Pop:* General *Site:* Jail *Male:* 0% *African American:* NR	*Level:* Not reported *Duration:* Not reported *Content:* Pregnancy and HIV testing, link to medical and supportive services, education about HIV/AIDS prevention, STDs, substance abuse, and domestic violence (delivered by outreach workers from local STD program)	Authors anecdotally reported that the intervention (no statistical analyses reported): • Increased prenatal care • Increased prenatal testing rates • Reduction in prenatal HIV transmission
El-Bassel et al. (1997). *Criminal Justice and Behavior, 24,* 205–223	*Design:* NA *Comparison:* NA *Follow-up:* NA *Retention:* NA	*N:* 30 (pilot); intervention trial currently being conducted with 400 women *Pop:* Women who used cocaine, heroin, or crack 3+ times/week prior to arrest *Site:* Prison *Male:* 0% *African American:* NR	*Level:* Group *Duration:* Eight 1.5 h weekly sessions, twice weekly in prison; eight community-based booster sessions within 2 months of release *Content:* Groups: HIV/AIDS risk behavior, knowledge, and perceived risk; safer sex and needle use practices; positive condom attitudes; social support and help-seeking skills; role-play and rehearsal. Boosters: Focus on transfer and application of skills to real-world situations (group sessions delivered by experienced social worker and a trained group leader; community booster sessions delivered by trained community counselors with a history of incarceration and who had work experience in substance abuse).	No formal evaluations reported

Citation	Design	Sample	Intervention	Outcomes
Loue et al. (2001). *Journal of Immigrant Health, 3*, 157–163	*Design:* 1-Group *Comparison:* NA *Follow-up:* NR *Retention:* NR	*N:* 50 *Pop:* General *Site:* INS detainment center *Male:* 50% *African American:* 0%	*Level:* Group *Duration:* One 1-h session *Content:* HIV knowledge, risk behaviors, condom use skills, self efficacy, video on HIV transmission, culturally appropriate for Mexicans and Puerto Ricans (delivered by P.I.)	No formal evaluations reported
System-wide (N = 1) **Descriptive (n = 1)** Klein et al. (2002a). *AIDS Education and Prevention, 14* (Suppl. B), 114–123Klein et al. (2002). *The Prison Journal, 82,* 69–83	*Design:* NA *Comparison:* NA *Follow-up:* NA *Retention:* NA	*N:* NR *Pop:* General *Site:* System-wide *Male:* NR *African American:* NR	*Level:* Systemic Intervention *Duration:* NR *Content:* Two articles report on a mandate to increase HIV prevention services within the New York State Correctional System *Article 1* describes the development of a collaborative network to provide prevention services throughout the state correctional system. *Article 2* reports on a survey HIV prevention services provided following initiation of the state plan	Following intervention initiation, compared to earlier surveys: • A broader range of HIV prevention interventions were available and accessible in state correctional facilities • Spanish-language services were more salient

FU follow-up; *NA* not applicable; *NR* not reported

Results

Behavioral Outcome Studies

We identified 24 published HIV prevention intervention articles that described 22 studies with behavioral outcome data. Of these, six were conducted with adolescents, seven with adult drug users, and nine with other adult populations.

Studies with Adolescents

Five of the adolescent studies utilized some form of a comparison trial that included a small-group intervention condition delivered prior to release, while one study compared two individual interventions. All six studies included a postrelease follow-up. The three most rigorous of the small group studies failed to demonstrate intervention effects. St. Lawrence, Crosby, Belcher, Yazdani, and Brasfield (1999) randomly assigned 361 predominantly African American (70%) juvenile males entering a state reformatory to either a 6-session sexual risk reduction skills training or an attention-controlled anger management cognitive-behavioral small-group intervention. At 6-month follow-up, there were no significant differences between groups for any outcome. However, it is noted that regardless of condition, participants at 6-month postrelease follow-up (89% retention) relative to baseline reported a smaller number of sexual partners and a lower frequency of oral sex, unprotected anal and vaginal sex, coercive or unwanted sexual activity, and exchange of drugs for sex. Both groups also reported less reliance on conflict in interpersonal interactions, and a lower frequency of alcohol and marijuana use, court appearances, and days in jail.

In another study, using a weekly block assignment, 282 heterosexually active youth (42% male, 46% African American) incarcerated in a juvenile detention center were enrolled into a comparison trial of three sexual risk reduction interventions: a 2-session group skills training curriculum with peer modeling and role-playing, a 27-min videotape presenting factual information and modeling vignettes, and a 16-page informational comic book (Gillmore et al., 1997). All three interventions provided factual information and emphasized skills development for communicating and negotiating condom use with partners. Intervention completion was high (81%) and about 60% were retained at 3- and 6-month follow-up. There were no differences between groups at either follow-up for number of sexual partners, condom use, or a range of non-behavioral outcomes. One exception was that group participants reported more comfort talking with sexual partners about condoms.

A study by Slonim-Nevo and Auslander (1996) enrolled 358 adolescents (56% male, 46% African American) who had been admitted to a residential center due to juvenile delinquency, child abuse, neglect, or mental health problems. Adolescents were assigned to a 9-session skills-building intervention, an attention-controlled HIV prevention intervention involving factual information and discussion only, or a no-intervention wait-list control (75% of group participants completed all nine sessions). There were no significant between-group differences for any of the sexual risk behavior outcomes at 9–12 month follow-up (81% retention).

The small group HIV prevention intervention that resulted in positive intervention outcomes involved a sample of predominantly African American (66%) and Latino (33%) adolescent male drug users who were incarcerated (Magura, Kang, & Shapiro, 1994). At 5-month postrelease follow-up, intervention participants compared to wait-list controls reported increased frequency of condom use for vaginal, oral, and anal sex and greater condom acceptability. However, the validity of these findings was limited by the decision to restrict follow-up to the first 58 intervention participants and the first 99 wait-list controls released prior to intervention receipt (38% of full baseline sample).

In a study that included both adolescent males (n=706) and adult women (n=704), individuals willing to meet program requirements were self-selected into a program of intensive discharge planning services combined with community-based case management services (Needles, James-Burdumy, & Burghardt, 2005). Other participants received a less intensive discharge planning service with no community-based follow-up. Both discharge planning programs included voluntary participation in a personal empowerment group supplemented with individual counseling. Among adolescent males, there were no significant differences between groups at 15-month postrelease follow-up (76% retention) for a range of HIV sexual risk, drug use, and recidivism outcomes. The efficacy of the intensive intervention may have been limited by a lack of postrelease contact. Only 29% maintained contact with their case manager for the full year and the average participant received less than 10 total hours of case management services.

The final study involved a randomized trial (N=114) to compare the effectiveness of a 2-session individualized Relaxation Training (RT) to a 2-session individualized Motivational Enhancement (ME) intervention (Rosengard et al., 2008). At 3-month post-release follow-up (97% retention), the strongest predictor of sexual risk was increased sexual risk prior to incarceration. However, among participants who reported lower levels of depression at baseline, those in the ME condition, compared to those in the RT condition, reported less condom non-use and less condom non-use in conjunction with the use of marijuana.

Studies with Adult Drug Users

There are seven studies that specifically targeted adult drug users. One study evaluated the impact of a therapeutic community (TC) in prison and after release on drug use and HIV risk behavior. Incarcerated people with a history of drug use who were eligible for parole or work release were assigned to primary drug treatment in prison (KEY), primary treatment in prison plus treatment in residential work-release (KEY-CREST), primary treatment in work-release alone (CREST), or an HIV-prevention education control condition (Harrison, Butzin, Inciardi, & Martin, 1998). In a longitudinal evaluation, the TCs (KEY; CREST; KEY-CREST) were compared to a control condition. Participants (n = 1,079; 80% male, 70% African American) were followed for 18 months (62% retention). No significant differences were found among the three TC conditions. However, control participants reported higher rates of injection drug use and trading sex for drugs and TC groups had higher rates of condom use.

Six interventions focused directly on HIV-risk reduction with drug users, rather than addressing HIV-risk reduction as a by-product of reductions in injection drug use. In one innovative study, an Enhanced Standard Intervention (ESI) developed for the NIDA Cooperative Agreement for AIDS Community-Based Research Initiative was compared to a Probationer-focused Intervention (PFI) (Martin, O'Connell, Inciardi, Beard, & Surratt, 2003). The ESI included community outreach, risk assessment, risk reduction counseling, optional HIV-testing, and crisis intervention if required; the PFI added personalized strategies for risk reduction and thought-mapping techniques to the ESI. In preliminary data analyses, with 426 of the projected 800 participants having completed the 3- and 6-month follow-up assessments, participants in both interventions showed marked reductions in drug use (cocaine and heroin), injection drug use, and sexual risk for HIV (multiple sex partners and unprotected sex acts). Only minor differences between groups were detected, notably a reduction in selling sex for PFI participants. Interestingly, the percentage who reported any unprotected sex decreased for all participants, except for women in the PFI, where the percentage remained unchanged at 77% from baseline assessment to 6-month follow-up.

ARRIVE, an AIDS education/relapse prevention model for recently released parolees with a history of IDU, was based on developing self-help and individual responsibility, adherence to therapeutic community principles, a social learning approach to prevention, and job readiness training (Wexler, Magura, Beardsley, & Josepher, 1994). The 24-session, 8-week structured group program was designed to train formerly incarcerated individuals to provide HIV-risk reduction services in the community. The training included information on AIDS transmission, testing, and treatment; AIDS risk reduction; the relationship between depression and addiction; employment counseling; job interview skills; relapse prevention and self-presentation skills. Three hundred and ninety-four individuals were recruited, 153 completed the baseline assessment but did not enroll in the training program (control group) and 164 completed the training program (intervention group). At 12-month follow-up for the 317 individuals in the intervention and control groups (81% male; 57% African-American), retention was 86% for individuals in the intervention group and 63% for individuals in the control group. Individuals in the intervention group were less likely to report steady injection drug use, using drugs as a recreational activity, associating with friends who injected drugs, or having sexual contact with high-risk persons. Program participants also were more likely to report always using a condom for vaginal, anal, and oral sex, greater condom acceptability, and fewer perceived barriers to HIV risk reduction behavior change; however, the study design leaves open the possibility that the effects were due to self-selection bias.

An RCT design was used to test two HIV prevention interventions for women who were incarcerated in jail and who used cocaine, crack, or heroin at least three times weekly prior to arrest (El-Bassel et al., 1995). In this study, 145 women (65% African American) were assigned to either a 3-session HIV/AIDS education small group intervention or a 16-session, multi-theory small group intervention consisting of HIV/AIDS education, skills building, and social support development. At 1-month postrelease (retention: 70%), there were no significant differences in HIV risk behavior between the two groups.

In a study involving people who were incarcerated in jail and who had injected drugs in the prior 6 months, participants were randomly assigned to an 8-h HIV/AIDS education program or a no-intervention control group (Baxter, 1991). Analysis of 3-month follow-up data from the first 200 participants showed minimal changes in HIV/AIDS knowledge, attitudes, or risk behavior. At 6-month follow-up, data collected from 134 participants (30% male, 11% African American) indicated that people in the experimental compared to the control condition reported fewer female sex partners who were IDUs, but increased sharing of needles, cookers/cleaners, and/or rinse water. There were no significant between-group differences in frequency of injection drug use, using new works, types of sexual behavior practiced, condom use, or number of sex partners.

In another jail-based AIDS education intervention for female IDUs, women (65% African American) who were expected to be incarcerated for at least 2 weeks were invited to participate in the 4-h small group intervention (Magura, Kang, Shapiro, & O'Day, 1995). A no-intervention control group was comprised of women who were expected to be incarcerated for less than 2 weeks and women who were released before participating in the intervention. Fifty-three women in the experimental condition and 48 in the control condition were interviewed about 7 months after release. No significant between-group differences were evident for any injection drug use or sexual behavior outcomes.

Secondary analyses were conducted on 12-month follow-up data (74% retention) collected from 1,223 incarcerated adults (91% male, 45% African American) who had been enrolled in one of nine correctional substance abuse treatment programs (Lubelczyk, Friedman, Lemon, Stein, & Gerstein, 2002). The analyses were stratified by custody status: individuals who were released from custody during the 12 month follow-up period (out of custody group) vs. individuals who remained in custody throughout the entire follow-up period (in custody group). Outcomes of interest were (a) the individual's report of receiving any in-custody HIV-prevention services during the follow-up period; and (b) HIV risk behavior during the follow-up period. There was no documentation of the content or nature of HIV-prevention services that people reported receiving. For individuals who were released from custody during the follow-up period, receipt of HIV-prevention services differed significantly by race/ethnicity, age, and the type of treatment program. For individuals who remained in custody for the entire follow-up period, receipt of HIV-prevention services differed significantly by gender, age, current alcohol treatment, and type of treatment program. However, report of lower HIV risk behavior during the follow-up period was associated with receipt of in-custody HIV-prevention services only for individuals who were released from custody during the follow-up period (out-of-custody group) and not for individuals who remained in custody through the follow-up period (in-custody group).

Studies with Other Adults

The nine studies that specifically targeted HIV risk behavior among adult correctional populations, but were not focused on HIV testing or limited to drug users, were provided either one-on-one or in small groups. Five programs were for men only, three were for both men and women, and one was for women only. In terms of evaluation designs, five studies were randomized control trials (RCTs) or used a non-biased block assignment, three studies used a 1-group design, and one study used a non-randomized design.

Among the five studies that used a RCT or non-biased block assignment, only one used an intent-to-treat design and had adequate retention at follow-up (Wolitski & the Project START Writing Group, for the Project START Study Group, 2006). In this intervention, 522 men (52% African American), ages 18–29, were systematically assigned to either a 1-session pre-release risk reduction intervention or a 6-session pre- and postrelease enhanced intervention. Both interventions addressed HIV, STI, and hepatitis risk behavior, including risk assessment, development of a risk-reduction plan, facilitated referrals for services, and postrelease condom provision. At the 24-week postrelease follow-up assessment (83% retention), men in the enhanced condition were significantly less likely to report unprotected vaginal or anal sex compared to men in the 1-session comparison condition. This finding was primarily due to reductions in sexual risk behavior with main partners. There were no differences between groups in sexual behavior with non-main partners or in patterns of substance use. Project START, the only HIV prevention intervention for incarcerated populations that meets the requirements for inclusion in the "Compendium of HIV Prevention Interventions with Evidence of Effectiveness" (http://www.cdc.gov/hiv/topics/research/prs/best-evidence-intervention.htm), is available for dissemination through CDC's DEBI (Diffusing Evidence-Based Interventions) program.

The four other studies that used a RCT or a non-biased block assignment had low retention rates or did not report retention, and three of them reported intervention efficacy with the sample that was retained. Lurigio, Petraitis, and Johnson (1992) evaluated the efficacy of an HIV education intervention for 99 people (90% male, 86% African American) on probation versus an attention-controlled heart disease education intervention. Both interventions were delivered in individual and group formats. People who received the HIV education intervention reported a significantly higher rate of condom use at 1-month post-intervention (51% retention) than those who received the control intervention. No between-group differences were observed for HIV testing behavior, communication about condom use or needle cleaning, or needle sharing behavior.

Grinstead, Zack, Faigeles, Grossman, and Blea (1999) evaluated the efficacy of a 30-min pre-release intervention delivered by an HIV-positive peer that included

HIV risk assessment and development of an HIV risk-reduction plan compared to a no-intervention control. Referrals for services were provided based on each individual participant's county of release. Data were collected from 414 men (51% African American) who had been assigned to one of the two conditions: interventions were offered on alternating weeks. At the 2-week postrelease follow-up (43% retention), a higher proportion of men in the intervention than in the control group reported condom use at first sex after release. The two groups did not differ significantly on their frequency of any drug use, injection drug use, or needle sharing.

Braithwaite, Stephens, Treadwell, Braithwaite, and Conerly (2005) randomized incarcerated men to one of four 12-session group interventions delivered prior to release: (1) a traditional, facility-based control that included a video on health promotion and disease prevention with limited facilitation, (2) an HIV and substance abuse curriculum with didactic presentations and video delivered by a facilitator, (3) an HIV and substance abuse curriculum with didactic presentations and video delivered by a HIV-negative peer educator; and (4) an HIV and substance abuse curriculum with didactic presentations and video delivered by an HIV-positive peer educator. All four interventions promoted HIV risk reduction behavior after release from prison. Based on data from 116 men (69% African American) who completed the 3-month postrelease follow-up, all four interventions showed reductions in overall substance use and sexual risk-taking, and increases in health and condom self-efficacy.

As described earlier, a study by Needels, James-Burdumy, and Burghardt (2005) for adult women (n = 704) willing to meet program requirements, provided a program of intensive discharge planning services combined with community-based case management services. Other participants received a less intensive program. Among the participants at 15-month postrelease follow-up (73% retention), women in the intensive case-management group reported more unprotected anal or vaginal sex, more sex while using drugs or alcohol, and more sex in exchange for sex or drugs. Women in the less intensive condition were more likely to report sex with partners whose HIV serostatus was unknown. No between-group differences were observed for the total number of sex partners or for the percent of participants who had multiple sex partners, exchanged sex for money or drugs, had sex with a partner whose HIV status was unknown, or injected drugs. It is noted that only 36% of women in the intensive condition maintained contact with their case manager for the full year.

The other four studies did not use a RCT or a non-biased block assignment. The study conducted by Arriola and her colleagues (Arriola, Braithwaite, Holmes, & Fortenberry, 2007; Arriola et al., 2002) evaluated a post-release intervention for soon-to-be released HIV positive inmates in county jails or prisons. The 1-group study provided services such as HIV prevention education, individual counseling, disease management, and discharge planning to 647 participants (100% male, 18% African American). The participants who completed the 6 month follow up (35%) reported a greater likelihood of not engaging in sex exchange as well as a greater likelihood of participating in drug or alcohol treatment. The second study reported on a 5-month prevention case management (PCM) program provided to 127 participants (55% male, 48% African American) who reported HIV risk behaviors (Myers et al., 2005). PCM activities were provided for 2 months before release and for 3 months after release from prison. Although a mean of 39 h per person of PCM was provided, only 51% completed the full program. Among those participants who received PCM services and who completed both the baseline and the 10-week postrelease assessments (40% retention), there was a significant increase in the percent of people who reported abstinence from sexual activity or 100% condom use during sex, and a decrease in the percent of people who reported drug use during sex. Although participants also reported fewer sex partners and less frequent use of alcohol during sex, these reductions were not significant.

Harrison, Bachman, Freeman, and Inciardi (2001) conducted a single group pre/post evaluation of a 20 h course for adult women during confinement that focused on HIV risks and the importance of using condoms post-release. The course was conducted in a small classroom within the correctional setting, and included generally ten or fewer women. The course included information sharing, discussion groups, participant exercises, role playing, and hands on practice sessions for the female condom. Data were collected from 246 women (67% African American). No participants reported prior use of the female condom at baseline. At the 2-month post-release follow-up (163/246, 66% retention), 62% of participants reported using the female condom, with most using the female condom with their boyfriend/spouse. Overall, 23% reported consistent female condom use, and 27% consistent male condom use during vaginal sex at 2-months post-release. One study evaluated an intervention which was aimed to assist HIV-positive participants (55% African American) to successfully access HIV-related services following release from custody (Grinstead, Zack, & Faigeles, 2001; Zack, Grinstead, & Faigeles, 2004). In this study (N = 144 eligible men), HIV education and referral services were provided to men who were within 6 months of their release. The intervention group consisted of 94 men who received the intervention, and the comparison group (n = 29) consisted of men who were unable to attend the intervention. An additional 21 men enrolled into the study and declined to participate in post-release follow-up assessments. A follow-up assessment conducted about 8 months after release (n = 81, 56% retention) revealed that men in the HIV-education intervention were less likely than the control group to have had sex since release and more likely to have used a condom the first time they had sex after release. They also were less likely to have used drugs or alcohol, injected drugs, or shared needles since release. The intervention group reported higher rates of first sex with a casual partner, marijuana and crack cocaine use than the comparison group. However, the findings were primarily associated with small effect sizes.

Non-behavioral Outcome Studies

We identified 15 HIV prevention interventions studies (16 published articles) that included non-behavioral outcome data (see Table 15.1 for summary details). Eight interventions were conducted with adolescents, seven interventions (eight articles) with adult populations, and none targeted drug users. Most of these intervention studies (n = 12) involved a small-group intervention ranging in duration from 3 to 40 h. Of the remaining three studies, two involved HIV prevention embedded within a therapeutic community approach and one evaluated the impact of low- versus high-fear messages.

Seven studies used comparison-group designs (two random assignments, three non-biased assignments, and two quasi-experimental), one study used a no-intervention control comparison, and eight studies used a single-group pre-post design. Follow-up in 13 studies was limited to a single immediate post-intervention assessment conducted prior to release, while two studies had follow-up times ranging from several weeks to 6 months post-intervention. Across studies, these interventions generally increased AIDS knowledge, self-efficacy for risk reduction and condom negotiation, favorable personal and normative beliefs about condoms, and self-esteem. Positive intervention effects were inconsistently observed for condom use intentions and AIDS risk perception. One study also found that a larger proportion of people who were trained to be HIV peer educators had been tested for HIV at 9-month follow-up compared to baseline (Ross, Harzke, Scott, McCann, & Kelley, 2006; Scott, Harzke, Mizwa, Pugh, & Ross, 2004). HIV testing rates within intervention prisons, compared to non-intervention facilities, were nearly twice has high at 12 and 18 months following intervention implementation.

Descriptive Studies

We identified eight published articles that described seven HIV prevention programs, but which did not provide any outcome data (see Table 15.1 for summary details). Of these studies, two were conducted with adolescents, four with adult populations, and one with correctional systems or staff. Although some of these programs were highly innovative, the lack of outcome data precludes evaluation of their efficacy.

One article described an empowerment model that actively integrated incarcerated adolescents into the intervention development process. Another adolescent program integrated HIV risk assessment and reduction activities with the provision of medical and substance abuse treatment services in a short-term detention center. Among adults, one article described a peer education program, two described small group interventions, and one described and compared three innovative methods for preventing perinatal HIV transmission in jails. The remaining two articles described a systemic approach to HIV prevention by increasing HIV prevention services within a state correctional system. This program is unique in that it attempts to alter the structure of prevention program availability and delivery within an entire correctional system.

Additionally, most correctional systems provide HIV education or prevention programming and all federal and state prison systems provide HIV testing (Maruschak, 2008). One in three prison systems provide HIV testing on entry, and most systems offer HIV testing upon request, when there are clinical indications suggesting HIV infection, when there has been possible exposure to HIV, or when a court order requires a test to be administered. Less HIV testing is provided in jails, primarily because of the greater numbers of people who are processed through the facilities and the shorter duration of their incarceration. Although the availability of the rapid HIV test makes it more feasible to conduct HIV testing in jails (MacGowan et al., 2007), and in 2007, the Centers for Disease Control and Prevention funded health departments to collaborate with jails to implement HIV testing (PS07-768).

Discussion

Research has documented elevated rates of HIV, STIs, and hepatitis among correctional populations. These infections were often associated with injection drug use, sexual risk behavior in the community, and infectious disease co-morbidity. These findings highlight an urgent public health need for comprehensive HIV risk reduction programs that address not only disease prevention but also the factors enabling disease transmission (Seal, 2005). Despite this urgent need, few rigorously designed and evaluated HIV prevention interventions for incarcerated populations have been reported in the literature to date, and we identified few non-U.S. studies in our literature search. Within the U.S., the most common HIV prevention programs were system-delivered standard-of-care HIV counseling and testing (CT) services or HIV educational programs. Unfortunately, there has been little rigorous evaluation of these programs and services to assess their efficacy in helping recipients reduce their HIV risk behavior during or after incarceration.

The vast majority of published evaluations of HIV prevention interventions with adolescents and non-injection drug using adults in correctional settings have reported on variations of educational or skills-based small group, individual risk reduction, or prevention case management intervention formats. HIV prevention interventions for IDUs in custody have centered on both drug treatment and sexual risk behavior. Regardless of format, most of the published studies had design limitations that affected the evaluation of efficacy for these interventions. These limitations included self-selection into programs, small sample size, lack of control or comparison groups, low retention rates, and no post-intervention behavioral outcome assessment.

Nonetheless, data from these studies suggests HIV prevention interventions can lead to short-term increases in HIV/AIDS knowledge, positive attitudes toward condom use, and self-efficacy for condom use communication and negotiation. Studies which reported behavioral outcomes further suggest that skills-based prevention programs at both the individual and small group level can help adults reduce HIV risk behavior following release from prison. This may be particularly true for interventions that prepare people for community reintegration or include a transitional intervention component. However, less positive effects were observed for adolescents. The only adolescent intervention study that resulted in behavioral risk reduction had a very low retention rate, undermining the validity of these findings.

Our review suggests that there are four major areas that represent significant missed opportunities for HIV-prevention interventions with correctional populations.

First, we identified only six intervention studies for adolescents that included behavioral outcomes. The three most rigorous of these interventions failed to have an effect. The strong co-occurrence of delinquency, substance use, and sexual risk behavior among adolescents has been well documented (Perrino, Gonzalez-Soldevilla, Pantin, & Szapocznik, 2000), and highlights an urgent need to develop risk reduction interventions for youth at highest risk for HIV infection (Donenberg, Emerson, Bryant, Wilson, & Weber-Shifrin, 2001; Ozechowski & Liddle, 2000). Such interventions may need to occur with at-risk adolescents prior to involvement with the legal system or with social systems that can underlie delinquent behavior (e.g., family dysfunction; Hanlon et al., 2005; Ozechowski & Liddle).

Second, despite significantly disproportionate rates of incarceration and HIV infection among African Americans and Latinos in the U.S., we did not identify a single U.S. study that specifically targeted or was specifically tailored for racial and ethnic minorities. Interventions targeted for specific racial or ethnic groups may be difficult in correctional settings due to the potential costs and complications of delivering targeted interventions and concerns about singling out particular groups for intervention. Nonetheless, incarceration is a societal phenomenon that is predominantly and disproportionately experienced by racial and ethnic minorities. Thus, any intervention with incarcerated people must include race and ethnicity as an underlying core context of a culturally sensitive and culturally competent intervention. Indeed, racially, ethnically, and culturally targeted interventions are possible and may enhance efficacy. The description by Peres et al. (2002) of their nationally-acclaimed intervention for incarcerated adolescents in Brazil illustrated ways that program participants can be empowered to tailor prevention messages and formats to their particular life circumstances. In this program, participants generated their own HIV prevention messages which were delivered through a range of modalities, including music, hip-hop arts, graffiti murals, and interactive workshops focused on issues relevant to their everyday lives (e.g., violence, drugs, paternity, sexuality, racism).

Disparities in access to and use of health care and other prevention services among racial and ethnic minorities exist in the U.S. Correctional settings can offer a unique opportunity to reduce these disparities by providing HIV prevention interventions to a substantial proportion of African Americans who have engaged in high-risk behaviors. Providing such interventions to African Americans before they are released is likely to offer protective benefits not only for them but also for their sexual partners upon return to the community.

Third, given high rates of recidivism (Glaze & Bonczar, 2009), HIV prevention activities focused on risk behavior in prison cannot be disassociated from risk behavior occurring in the community either prior to or after release from prison. As has been asserted elsewhere (Seal, 2005; Seal et al., 2007; Wolitski et al., 2006), there is an urgency to implement and evaluate HIV risk reduction interventions for incarcerated people focused on the period of community re-entry as people re-establish sexual or injection drug use relationships. Re-entry interventions to improve transitional health care, medication adherence, and behavioral risk reduction among HIV-positive individuals also are urgently needed.

Fourth, 70% of adults under U.S. correctional supervision are on probation or parole. However, we identified only three articles that specifically targeted people on probation or parole (excluding transitional interventions). People under community correctional supervision have greater opportunity to engage in HIV risk behavior than individuals who are incarcerated, and most incarcerated people who are HIV-positive were infected in the community. Thus, there is a critical need to develop HIV prevention interventions for people under community correctional supervision. Indeed, in two studies that we have conducted, we found that about one-fourth of 18- to 29-year old men were positive for hepatitis or another STI when tested 6 months after their release from prison (MacGowan et al., 2004; Sosman et al., 2005).

Finally, research and activism are needed to address structural factors impeding HIV prevention efforts for correctional populations. It is ironic that the punishment for illicit drug use in most countries is incarceration in a setting in which substance use is widespread and treatment and prevention opportunities are illegal or unavailable (Seal et al., 2004). The scarcity of substance use treatment and needle exchange programs (NEPs) for incarcerated people illuminates a systemic failure to address the very behavior underlying imprisonment, thus increasing the probability that individuals will become entrapped in a cycle of release, relapse to substance use, re-incarceration, and risk for HIV and other infectious diseases.

Nonetheless, evidence from evaluation of NEPs in European prisons suggests that such preventive efforts can be successfully and safely implemented (Jacob & Stöver, 2000; Menoyo, Zulaica, & Parras, 2000; Nelles, Bernasconi, Dobler-Mikola, & Kaufmann, 1997; Stark, Herrmann, Ehrhardt, & Bienzle, 2005). Despite evidence of continued in-prison injection drug use in these studies, the overall frequency of drug use did not increase, needle sharing was reduced or eliminated, the number of drug users in treatment increased, and no needle attacks or other adverse events were reported. Two of these studies further indicated that there were no new cases of HIV, hepatitis B, or hepatitis C during the evaluation period (Nelles et al.; Stark et al.).

Similarly, although methadone maintenance treatment (MMT) has been shown to reduce heroin use, HIV-risk behavior, and imprisonment, it is rarely available in correctional settings (see Dolan et al., 2005). One study conducted in an Australian prison found that MMT participants, compared to MMT non-participants, reported greater reductions in heroin injection, frequency of syringe sharing, and frequency of heroin injection (Dolan et al., 2003). Analysis of hair samples confirmed that heroin use was twice as prevalent in the control group (53%) as in the treatment group (27%). In another study, following an outbreak of eight cases of acute clinical hepatitis B and two cases of HIV-seroconversion among IDUs in a Scottish prison, a range of harm reduction measures were initiated, including the availability of hepatitis B vaccine, bleach tablets to clean injection equipment, a methadone detoxification program, increased training for prison officers, and improved access to drug and harm minimization counseling for people who were incarcerated (Goldberg et al., 1998). Follow-up investigations revealed no new HIV infections during the 12 months after these harm reduction measures were initiated.

Similar conclusions also were drawn in an evaluation of a free condom distribution program in another Australian prison (Dolan, Lowe, & Shearer, 2004). This study found that men reported substantial access and use of the condoms during incarceration. No adverse consequences related to condom distribution were reported by incarcerated men or correctional personnel. In the U.S., two state prison systems (Vermont and Mississippi) and five local jails (Los Angeles, New York, Philadelphia, San Francisco, and Washington DC) currently provide condoms to people who are incarcerated. Similar to the findings of Dolan et al., a survey of prison guards and people incarcerated in the Washington D.C. jail found that both groups generally supported the condom distribution program (May & Williams, 2002). No major infractions resulting from this program have been reported.

In sum, despite disproportionate rates of HIV, STIs, and hepatitis among correctional populations in the U.S., there is a dearth of effective prevention interventions specifically tailored for this population and for the ethnic and racial minorities who are disproportionately affected by both incarceration and HIV. Our review highlights the need to develop and rigorously evaluate HIV, STI, and hepatitis risk-reduction interventions for correctional populations. Risk-reduction programs for correctional populations should address both individual (e.g., substance abuse) and structural factors (e.g., substance abuse treatment, needle and condom distribution). Programs should also address risk behavior that occurs both within and outside the correctional facility. In accordance with World Health Organization (1992) recommendations for incarcerated populations, risk-reduction programs should focus on reducing HIV risks rather than punishment. The effectiveness of such programs may be enhanced through collaboration between agencies such as correctional departments, public health entities, researchers, and community-based organizations. Programs may be further enhanced through the use of trained peer educators within the correctional setting and through sustained support as people transition from prison to the community. The provision of HIV prevention programs to incarcerated populations will help to decrease the rates of HIV, STI, and hepatitis risk behavior and disease transmission among people who are incarcerated or under community correctional supervision.

References

Arriola, K. J., Braithwaite, R. L., Holmes, N. E., & Fortenberry, R. M. (2007). Post-release case management services and health seeking behavior among HIV infected ex-offenders. *Journal of Health Care for the Poor and Underserved, 18*, 665–674.

Arriola, K. J., Kennedy, S. S., Coltharp, J. C., Braithwaite, R. L., Hammett, T. M., & Tinsley, M. J. (2002). Development and implementation of the cross-site evaluation of the CDC/HRSA Corrections Demonstration Project. *AIDS Education and Prevention, 14*(Suppl. 3), 107–118.

Baillargeon, J., Black, S. A., Pulvino, J., & Dunn, K. (2000). The disease profile of Texas prison inmates. *Annals of Epidemiology, 10*, 74-B80.

Baxter, S. (1991). AIDS education in the jail setting. *Crime and Delinquency, 37*, 48–63.

Beck, A. J., & Harrison, P. M. (2006, July). *Sexual violence reported by correctional authorities, 2005.* Bureau of Justice Statistics, Office of Justice Programs, U.S. Department of Justice. Retrieved August 2006, from http://www.ojp.usdoj.gov/bjs/pub/pdf/svrca05.pdf.

Belenko, S., Langley, S., Crimmins, S., & Chaple, M. (2004). HIV risk behaviors, knowledge, and prevention education among offenders under community supervision: A hidden risk group. *AIDS Education and Prevention, 16,* 367–385.

Braithwaite, R., Stephens, T. T., Treadwell, H., Braithwaite, K., & Conerly, R. (2005). Short-term impact of an HIV risk reduction intervention for soon-to-be-released inmates in Georgia. *Journal of Health Care for the Poor and Underserved, 16,* 130–139.

Centers for Disease Control and Prevention. (2001). Hepatitis B outbreak in a state correctional facility, 2000. *Morbidity and Mortality Weekly Report, 50,* 529–532.

Clarke, J. G., Stein, M. D., Hanna, L., Sobota, M., & Rich, J. D. (2001). Active and former injection drug users report of HIV risk behaviors during periods of incarceration. *Substance Abuse, 22,* 209–216.

Dolan, K., Lowe, D., & Shearer, J. (2004). Evaluation of the condom distribution program in New South Wales prisons. *Australian Journal of Law, Medicine, & Ethics, 32,* 124–128.

Dolan, K. A., Shearer, J., MacDonald, M., Mattick, R. P., Hall, W., & Wodak, A. D. (2003). A randomized controlled trial of methadone maintenance treatment versus wait list control in an Australian prison system. *Drug and Alcohol Dependence, 72,* 59–65.

Dolan, K. A., Shearer, J., White, B., Zhou, J., Kaldor, J., & Wodak, A. D. (2005). Four-year follow-up of imprisoned male heroin users and methadone treatment: Mortality, reincarceration, and hepatitis C infection. *Addiction, 100,* 820–828.

Donenberg, G., Emerson, E., Bryant, F. B., Wilson, H., & Weber-Shifrin, E. (2001). Understanding AIDS-risk behavior among adolescents in psychiatric care: Links to psychopathology and peer relationships. *Journal of the American Academy of Child and Adolescent Psychiatry, 40,* 642–653.

El-Bassel, N., Ivanoff, A., Schilling, R. F., Gilbert, L., Borne, D., & Chen, D. R. (1995). Preventing HIV/AIDS in drug abusing incarcerated women through skills building and social support enhancement: Preliminary outcomes. *Social Work Research, 19,* 131–141.

Gillmore, M. R., Morrison, D. M., Richey, C. A., Balasonne, M. L., Gutierrez, L., & Farris, M. (1997). Effects of a skills-based intervention to encourage condom use among high risk heterosexually active adolescents. *AIDS Education and Prevention, 9*(Suppl. A), 22–43.

Glaze, L. E., & Bonczar, T. P. (2009, December). *Probation and parole in the United States.* Bureau of Justice Statistics, Office of Justice Programs, U.S. Department of Justice. Retrieved January 2010, from http://bjs.ojp.usdoj.gov/index.cfm?ty=pbdetail&iid=1764.

Goldberg, D., Taylor, A., McGregor, J., Davis, B., Wrench, J., & Gruer, L. (1998). A lasting public health response to an outbreak of HIV infection in a Scottish prison. *International Journal of STD and AIDS, 9,* 25–30.

Grinstead, O. A., Faigeles, B., Comfort, M., Seal, D., Sealey-Moore, J., Belcher, L., et al. (2005). HIV, STD, and hepatitis risk to primary female partners of men being released from prison. *Women and Health, 41,* 63–80.

Grinstead, O., Zack, B., & Faigeles, B. (2001). Reducing postrelease risk behavior among HIV seropositive prison inmates: The health promotion program. *AIDS Education and Prevention, 13,* 109–119.

Grinstead, O., Zack, B., Faigeles, B., Grossman, N., & Blea, L. (1999). Reducing postrelease HIV risk among male prison inmates: A peer-lead intervention. *Criminal Justice & Behavior, 26,* 468–480.

Hanlon, T. E., Blatchley, R. J., Bennett-Sears, T., O'Grady, K. E., Rose, M., & Callaman, J. M. (2005). Vulnerability of children of incarcerated addict mothers: Implications for preventive intervention. *Children and Youth Services Review, 27,* 67–84.

Harrison, L., Bachman, T., Freeman, C., & Inciardi, J. (2001). The Acceptability of the Female Condom among U.S. Women at High Risk for HIV. *Culture, Health and Sexuality, 3*(1), 101–118.

Harrison, L., Butzin, C., Inciardi, J., & Martin, S. (1998). Integrating HIV prevention strategies in a therapeutic community work-release program for criminal offenders. *Prison Journal, 78,* 232–243.

Hogben, M., St. Lawrence, J., & Eldridge, G. D. (2001). Sexual risk behavior, drug use, and STD rates among incarcerated women. *Women and Health, 34*, 63–78.

Jacob, J., & Stöver, H. (2000). The transfer of harm-reduction strategies into prisons: Needle exchange programmed in two German prisons. *International Journal of Drug Policy, 11*, 325–335.

Kelly, P. J., Bair, R. M., Baillargeon, J., & Gerrman, V. (2000). Risk behaviors and the prevalence of chlamydia in a juvenile detention facility. *Clinical Pediatrics, 39*, 521–527.

Lubelczyk, R. A. B., Friedman, P. E., Lemon, S. C., Stein, M. D., & Gerstein, D. R. (2002). HIV prevention services in correctional drug treatment programs: Do they change risk behaviors? *AIDS Education and Prevention, 14*, 117–125.

Lurigio, A. J., Petraitis, J., & Johnson, B. R. (1992). Joining the front line against HIV: An education program for adult probationers. *AIDS Education and Prevention, 4*, 205–218.

MacGowan, R. J., Margolis, A., Gaiter, J., Morrow, K., Zack, B., Askew, J., et al. (2003). Predictors of risky sex of young men after release from prison. *International Journal of STD and AIDS, 14*, 519–523.

MacGowan, R., Margolis, A., Richardson-Moore, A., Wang, T., LaLota, M., French, P., et al. (2007). Voluntary rapid HIV testing in Jails. *Journal of Sexually Transmitted Diseases, 34*, 11. DOI:10.1097/OLQ.0b013e318148b6b1.

MacGowan, R., Sosman, J., Eldridge, G., Moss, S., Margolis, A., Flanigan, T., et al. (2004). Sexually transmitted infections in men with a history of incarceration. Poster presented at the 2004 International AIDS Conference, Bangkok, Thailand.

Magura, S., Kang, S. Y., & Shapiro, J. L. (1994). Outcomes of an intensive AIDS education for male adolescent drug users in jail. *Journal of Adolescent Health, 15*, 457–463.

Magura, S., Kang, S. Y., Shapiro, J. L., & O'Day, J. (1995). Evaluation of an AIDS education model for women drug users in jail. *The International Journal of the Addictions, 30*, 259–273.

Margolis, A. D., MacGowan, R. J., Grinstead, O., Sosman, J., Iqbal, K., Flanigan, T. P., et al. (2006). Unprotected sex with multiple partners: Implications for HIV prevention among young men with a history of incarceration. *Sexually Transmitted Diseases, 33*, 175–180.

Martin, S. S., O'Connell, D. J., Inciardi, J. A., Beard, R. A., & Surratt, H. L. (2003). HIV/AIDS among probationers: An assessment of risk and results from brief interventions. *Journal of Psychoactive Drugs, 35*(4), 435–443.

Maruschak, L. M. (2008, April). *HIV in prisons, 2006*. Bureau of Justice Statistics Bulletin, Washington, DC: U.S. Department of Justice, Office of Justice Programs. Retrieved January 2010, from http://www.ojp.usdoj.gov/bjs/pub/pdf/hivp06.pdf.

May, J. P., & Williams, E. L. (2002). Acceptability of condom availability in a U.S. jail. *AIDS Education and Prevention, 14*(Suppl. B), 85–91.

Menoyo, C., Zulaica, D., & Parras, F. (2000). HIV/AIDS in prisons: Needle exchange programs in prisons in Spain. *Canadian HIV/AIDS Policy & Law Review, 5*, 20–21.

Mertz, K. J., Voigt, R. A., Hutchins, K., Levine, W. C., & the Jail STD Prevalence Monitoring Group. (2002). Findings from STD screening of adolescents and adults entering corrections facilities: Implications for STD control strategies. *Sexually Transmitted Diseases, 29*, 834–839.

Morris, R. E., Baker, C. J., Valentine, M., & Pennisi, A. J. (1998). Variations in HIV risk behaviors of incarcerated juveniles during a four-year period: 1989–1992. *Journal of Adolescent Health, 23*, 39–48.

Morris, R. E., Harrison, E. A., Knox, G. W., Tromanhauser, E., Marquis, D. K., & Watts, L. L. (1995). Health risk behavioral survey from 39 juvenile correctional facilities in the United States. *Journal of Adolescent Health, 17*, 334–344.

Morrow, K. M., Eldridge, G., Nealey-Moore, J., Grinstead, O., Belcher, L., & the Project START Study Group. (2007). HIV, STD, and hepatitis risk in the week following release from prison: An event level analysis. *Journal of Correctional Health Care, 13*(1), 27–38.

Moseley, K., & Tewksbury, R. (2006). Prevalence and predictors of HIV risk behaviors among male prison inmates. *Journal of Correctional Health Care, 12*, 132–144.

Myers, J., Zack, B., Kramer, K., Gardner, M., Rucobo, G., & Costa-Taylor, S. (2005). Get connected: An HIV prevention case management program for men and women leaving California prisons. *American Journal of Public Health, 95*, 1682–1684.

Needels, K., James-Burdumy, S., & Burghardt, J. (2005). Community case-management for former jail inmates: Its impact on re-arrest, drug use, and HIV risk. *Journal of Urban Health:
Bulletin of the New York Academy of Medicine, 82*, 420–433.

Nelles, J., Bernasconi, S., Dobler-Mikola, A., & Kaufmann, B. (1997). Provision of syringes and
prescription of heroin in prison: The Swiss experience in the prisons of Hindelbank and
Obershöngrün. *The International Journal of Drug Policy, 8*, 40–52.

Oh, M. K., Smith, K. R., O'Cain, M., Kilmer, D., Johnson, J., & Hook, E. W. (1998). Urine-based
screening of adolescents in detention to guide the treatment for gonococcal and chlamydial infections: Translating research into intervention. *Archives of Pediatric Adolescent Medicine, 152*,
52–56.

Ozechowski, T. J., & Liddle, H. A. (2000). Family-based therapy for adolescent drug abuse:
Knowns and unknowns. *Clinical Child and Family Psychology Review, 3*, 269–298.

Peres, C. A., Peres, R. A., da Silveira, F., Paiva, V., Hudes, E. S., & Hearst, N. (2002). Developing
an AIDS prevention intervention for incarcerated male adolescents in Brazil. *AIDS Education
and Prevention, 14*(Suppl. B), 36–44.

Perrino, T., Gonzalez-Soldevilla, A., Pantin, H., & Szapocznik, J. (2000). The role of families in
adolescent HIV prevention: A review. *Clinical Child and family Psychology Review, 3*,
81–96.

Rosengard, C., Stein, L. A. R., Barnett, N. P., Monti, P. M., Golembeske, C., Lebeau-Craven, R., et al.
(2008). Randomized clinical trial of motivational enhancement of substance use treatment among
incarcerated adolescents. *Journal of HIV/AIDS Prevention in Children and Youth, 8*, 45–64.

Ross, M. W., Harzke, A. J., Scott, D. P., McCann, K., & Kelley, M. (2006). Outcomes of Project
Wall Talk: An HIV/AIDS peer education program implemented within the Texas state prison
system. *AIDS Education and Prevention, 18*, 504–517.

Scott, D., Harzke, A., Mizwa, M., Pugh, M., & Ross, M. (2004). Evaluations of an HIV peer
education program in Texas. *Journal of Correctional Health Care, 10*, 151–173.

Seal, D. W. (2005). HIV-related issues and concerns for imprisoned persons throughout the world.
Current Opinion in Psychiatry, 18, 530–535.

Seal, D. W., Belcher, L., Morrow, K., Eldridge, G., Binson, D., Kacanek, D., et al. (2004). A qualitative study of substance use and sexual behavior among 18- to 29-year-old men while incarcerated in the United States. *Health Education and Behavior, 31*, 775–789.

Seal, D. W., Eldridge, G. D., Kacanek, D., Binson, D., MacGowan, R. J., & the Project START
Study Group. (2007). A longitudinal, qualitative analysis of the context of substance use and
sexual behavior among 18- to 29-year-old men following their release from prison. *Social
Science and Medicine, 11*, 2394–2406.

Seal, D. W., Margolis, A. D., Morrow, K. M., Belcher, L., Sosman, J., Askew, J., et al. (2008).
Substance use and sexual behavior during incarceration among 18- to 29-year old men:
Prevalence and correlates. *AIDS and Behavior, 12*, 27–40.

Slonim-Nevo, V., & Auslander, W. F. (1996). The long-term impact of AIDS-preventive interventions for delinquent and abused adolescents. *Adolescence, 31*, 409–421.

Sosman, J. M., MacGowan, R. J., Margolis, A. D., Eldridge, G., Flanigan, T., Vardaman, J., et al.
(2005). The feasibility of STD and hepatitis screening among 18–29 year old men recently
released from prison. *International Journal of STDS and AIDS, 16*, 117–122.

St. Lawrence, J. S., Crosby, R. A., Belcher, L., Yazdani, N., & Brasfield, T. L. (1999). Sexual risk
reduction and anger management interventions for incarcerated male adolescents: A randomized controlled trial of two interventions. *Journal of Sex Education and Therapy, 24*, 9–17.

Stark, K., Herrmann, U., Ehrhardt, S., & Bienzle, U. (2005). A syringe exchange programme in
prison as prevention strategy against HIV infection and hepatitis B and C in Berlin, Germany.
Epidemiology & Infection, 134, 814–819.

Struckman-Johnson, C., & Struckman-Johnson, D. (2006). A comparison of coercion experiences
reported by men and women in prison. *Journal of Interpersonal Violence, 21*, 1591–1615.

Taussig, J., Shouse, R. L., LaMarre, M., Fitzpatrick, L., McElroy, P., Borkowf, C. B., et al. (2006).
HIV transmission among male inmates in a state prison system – Georgia, 1992–2005.
Morbidity and Mortality Weekly Report, 55, 421–426.

Teplin, L. A., Mericle, A. A., McClelland, G. M., & Abram, K. M. (2003). HIV and AIDS risk behaviors in juvenile detainees: Implications for public health policy. *American Journal of Public Health, 93*, 906–912.

West, H. C., & Sabol, W. J. (2009, March). *Prison inmates at midyear 2008 – Statistical tables.* Bureau of Justice Statistics, Office of Justice Programs, U.S. Department of Justice. Retrieved January 2010, from http://bjs.ojp.usdoj.gov/index.cfm?ty=pbdetail&iid=839.

Wexler, H. K., Magura, S., Beardsley, M. M., & Josepher, H. (1994). ARRIVE: An AIDS education/relapse prevention model for high-risk parolees. *The International Journal of the Addictions, 29*, 361–386.

Wolfe, M. I., Fujie, X., Patel, P., O'Cain, M., Schillinger, J. A., St. Louis, M. E., et al. (2001). An outbreak of syphilis in Alabama prisons: Correctional health policy and communicable disease control. *American Journal of Public Health, 91*, 1220–1225.

Wolitski, R. J., & the Project START Writing Group, for the Project START Study Group. (2006). Relative efficacy of a multisession sexual risk-reduction intervention for young men released from prisons in 4 states. *American Journal of Public Health, 96*, 1854–1861.

World Health Organization. (1992). *Drug users in prison: Managing their health problems.* Copenhagen: WHO Regional Publications. European Series, No. 27.

Zack, B., Grinstead, O., & Faigeles, B. (2004). Health promotion intervention for prison inmates with HIV. In B. P. Bowser, S. I. Mishra, et al. (Eds.), *Preventing AIDS: Community-science collaborations* (pp. 97–114). New York: Haworth Press.

Chapter 16
The HIV/AIDS Epidemic in the African American Community: Where Do We Go from Here?*

Ann O'Leary, Kenneth Terrill Jones, and Donna Hubbard McCree

Introduction

The chapters in this book review several contextual factors affecting the HIV/AIDS epidemic in the African American community. These chapters also present reviews of interventions designed to reduce behavioral risk among subpopulations most at risk for HIV acquisition and transmission. With some notable exceptions (male-to-female transgender persons, American Indians, and monolingual Asians), behavioral interventions for the most at-risk groups are available through the Diffusion of Effective Behavioral Interventions (DEBI) (Lyles, Crepaz, Herbst, & Kay, 2006). Further, a process for adapting these interventions for different populations has also been developed (McKleroy et al., 2006). Among structural interventions (see Chap. 14), only the distribution of sterile injection equipment to reduce HIV transmission among intravenous drug users has come into widespread use (see Chap. 13). While many of the contextual chapters describe important social determinants of health (SDH), the available literature shows that there is a paucity of interventions to address them. In the absence of appropriate data, it is impossible to estimate the relative effectiveness of a particular structural intervention targeting a SDH against that of an HIV-specific behavioral intervention. However, it is likely that some structural interventions – microenterprise, for example (Stratford, Mizuno, Williams, Courtenay-Quirk, & O'Leary, 2008) – may be considerably more efficacious than interventions targeting individual behaviors (Adimora & Schoenback, 2005; Aral, Adimora, & Fenton, 2008; Hallfors, Iritani, Miller, & Bauer, 2007; Hogben & Leichliter, 2008).

---

*The contents of this article are solely the responsibility of the authors and do not necessarily represent the views of the Centers for Disease Control and Prevention

A. O'Leary (✉)
Prevention Research Branch Division of HIV/AIDS Prevention, National Center for HIV/AIDS, Viral Hepatitis, STD and TB Prevention, Centers for Disease Control and Prevention, 1600 Clifton Road, MS E-37, Atlanta, GA 30333, USA
e-mail: aoleary@cdc.gov

D.H. McCree et al. (eds.), *African Americans and HIV/AIDS*,
DOI 10.1007/978-0-387-78321-5_16,

311

Specifically, these interventions might further reduce the risk of multiple health outcomes and disparities by reducing stress, sex exchange, and poor lifestyle habits and increasing access to health promotion and care.

In October 2007, the CDC convened a research consultation to explore new, un- or under-utilized, research issues and innovative intervention strategies for HIV/AIDS prevention among African Americans. Articles authored by several consultation participants were published in a theme issue of the *American Journal of Public Health* (June, 2009), and several were published in a later issue including a commentary highlighting key recommendations from the meeting (Purcell & McCree, 2009). We now use this forum to give additional voice to the consultation participants, as well as to provide our own views.

Summary of the Consultation

Some criticism was made of the CDC and other funding agencies and researchers' use of the "scientific method," to develop HIV/AIDS prevention strategies for African Americans. It was suggested that this method does not address the historical oppression of black people. Participants voiced that this historical oppression was associated with how HIV/AIDS and other health disparities within the African American community are understood and subsequently addressed.

Additionally, some participants felt it important that the field identify novel study designs for testing the efficacy of intervention strategies. Criticism was specifically directed toward the use of randomized controlled trials (RCT) for community-level interventions because of the difficulty in identifying well-matched communities for these trials, the enormous costs, and the difficulty in assessing relative effectiveness.

Also voiced was the opinion that the scientific criteria used to classify (i.e., as best and promising evidence) and determine the efficacy of behavioral interventions (i.e., criteria used to make decisions about which interventions should be disseminated) were not developed with input from affected communities. Further, some consultants mentioned that scientists of color who possessed expertise and training in behavioral interventions and were also members of affected communities were not included in discussions about the criteria cutoffs used to determine strength of efficacy. Additionally, a specific concern was that most of the interventions identified as efficacious were individual level with outcomes focused on increasing condom use and decreasing numbers of sex partners. Additionally, the behavioral risk group (BRG) framework (i.e., categorizing individuals based on their sexual behavior, e.g., men who have sex with men or heterosexually active men), while useful and understandable, was thought to be limiting. Some consultants felt that continuing research focused on behavior alone is not sufficient to end the epidemic because this type of research excludes social determinants of health (as discussed in this volume) that often influence and may be more important than behavior.

Barriers to prevention science and translation were also discussed. Some participants expressed concerns that proposals submitted to federal funders and papers submitted to peer-reviewed journals describing interventions that attempt to address contextual factors such as oppression, power, racism, and the media are unsuccessful in the review process, in obtaining sufficient funding or dissemination as originally intended. Further, there were also concerns that community-based organizations (CBOs) charged with delivering evidence-based interventions (EBIs), are grossly underfunded and lack capacity for these activities. The suggestion was made to provide research funding directly to CBOs as opposed to research-based agencies that often partner with these organizations. Additionally, participants pointed out that scientific collaboration with CBOs can be made difficult by power imbalances in the research process and negative feelings against funders sometimes held by CBO staff. It was further stated that potential participants may distrust research and some researchers, given historical factors like the Tuskegee Syphilis study.

Regarding decisions about identifying and funding efficacious interventions for African American communities, the participants noted that CDC is perceived by some in the community as engaging in top-down decision-making rather than involving affected communities from the beginning. Factors influencing behaviors like condom use are complex and may involve the "drive toward extinction." Interventions would be more effective if they succeeded in "lifting them up." In other words, building on strengths rather than reducing deficits may be precluded by current intervention efforts.

Issues raised in break-out groups (ironically, organized by BRG, i.e., heterosexual transmission, MSM and men who have sex with men and women, and youth) pointed out further inadequacies in existing intervention approaches. One issue discussed was sexuality and a lack of understanding of HIV transmission and acquisition among some groups in the African American community, particularly MSM (see Chap. 10). There remains a paucity of research on black sexuality generally. Black male sexuality has often been considered to be artificially dichotomized into "homosexual" and "heterosexual". As such, participants echoed the need for a baseline study of black sexuality in the US and prospective and sexual network studies.

Ethical concern was also expressed about the biomedical interventions circumcision and pre-exposure prophylaxis (PrEP – providing antiviral medications to individuals who are at risk for HIV). Regarding the former, some participants offered that African American men are sensitive about their genitalia for political, cultural and historical reasons. Regarding the latter, participants offered that many HIV-positive individuals do not receive antiretroviral medication; therefore it seems inappropriate to provide medication for uninfected individuals. The participants also noted that it will be important to bring the community to the table for discussions before mounting such efforts. Moreover, participants were concerned about the relative allocation of funds for biomedical versus behavioral interventions.

Finally, participants noted, importantly, that in order for structural interventions to be mounted, collaboration between federal and other agencies including the Departments of Justice, Labor, and Education, will be necessary. Beyond this, participants offered that it may be important to change policies and procedures of institutions themselves (e.g., reorganizing HHS so that it does not consist of disease-specific silos).

Our Views

Eliminating scientific rigor from decisions regarding which interventions work may not be appropriate. While it is true that many of the EBIs were designed to favor internal validity over external validity (although note that it is possible to maximize both, Warner et al., 2008), and involving the community is certainly desirable, needed and quite appropriate, scientists should take a lead on scientific decisions with appropriate community input. Further, participatory methods that engage affected communities in these scientific decisions must be considered. The fact that science alone has not cured all social ills implies that activism and political activity will be necessary to reduce the SDH without which the HIV epidemic and many related ones – drug addiction, poverty, violence, and so on – will not be eliminated. But we need not pit individual behavior change interventions against political activism. The interventions that are being disseminated have worked in studies. Effectiveness research will be necessary to determine if they continue to work when delivered in the field and by CBO staff.

With respect to individual interventions and their characteristics, some of the issues raised during the consultation are amenable to empirical study. These include aspects of the male-female relationship, acceptability, uptake, and adherence to circumcision and PrEP, and whether strength-models produce more behavior change than deficit models.

We do agree wholeheartedly that further progress against the epidemic will not be possible until structural interventions targeting social determinants of health are mounted. Poverty, racism, homophobia, drug distribution systems, and policies producing disproportionate rates of incarceration of African Americans, especially men, all exert substantial effects on the spread of HIV among African Americans. The great irony is that health disparities and injustices are greatest for the same people across health outcomes. Most health problems are located geographically in the same places: inner cities and the rural south. Moreover, the sorts of structural interventions that could address HIV could also reduce other health disparities. Public health efforts are hampered severely from being used this way by "siloiza-tion," or the fragmentation of funding along disease lines. This prevents "bundling" of preventive and health care services and militates strongly against collaborative efforts such as microenterprise or mass media interventions. These collaborations, if feasible, might be a very cost-effective method for influencing multiple facets of health. Even beyond collaboration among health service entities, we agree with the consultation participants that collaborations with the Departments of Housing and Urban Development, Labor Justice, and Education are necessary.

At present, however, those of us whose responsibility it is to produce solutions for a single health issue – in our case, HIV/AIDS – but knowing that addressing structural issues such as poverty is likely to be the most potent public health response possible, are in a nearly untenable position. We are often in a position neither to fund nor to administer structural interventions and other poverty-reduction programs without the collaborations of other entities, which are very difficult to forge. A single federal agency could foster and support such interventions only through extensive collaborations with other federal agencies.

As we face the likely future of "combination prevention" (Coates, Richter, & Caceres, 2008; Merson et al., 2008), deploying an array of behavioral and biomedical approaches to reduce the HIV epidemic in this country, a number of questions will need to be answered. Allocation of resources to different strategies will indeed be complex and difficult, and will need to be based on cost-effectiveness models for which necessary data will be incomplete for some time. For example, most of the PrEP trials are occurring overseas, leaving unanswered the levels of adherence that will be seen in the U.S.

Among the other issues that will need to be addressed is how dual- messages, especially inconsistent ones, will be understood. For example, efforts to persuade individuals to adhere to PrEP and also to use condoms are likely to be confusing: if one works, why is the other being recommended? Indeed, in a recent randomized trial of diaphragm and gel in which both groups were encouraged to use male condoms, null effects were obtained (Padian et al., 2008). However, participants in the control group not using diaphragms reported more condom use than those in the intervention group, rendering interpretation of the findings impossible. Identifying the optimal mix of intervention strategies for individuals with particular characteristics will be very difficult: some are able to change behavior after a single, brief risk reduction intervention; some will be unable to adhere to antiretroviral medication, etc.

It is now 30 years since we in the U.S. first learned of AIDS. We have watched it uncannily affect the most discriminated-against and stigmatized groups: illegal drug users, men who have sex with men, the poor, and increasingly, African Americans in all transmission risk groups, including heterosexually active people. Unfortunately, efforts to direct public health attention to blacks have the potential to further stigmatize the population. To avoid this, it will be important to contextualize epidemiologic or clinical information we are providing to the public. African Americans do not engage in more risk behavior than whites (Espinoza, Hall, Hardnett, Seik, Ling, & Lee, 2007; Hallfors et al., 2007; Millett, Peterson, Wolitski, & Stall, 2006; Tillerson, 2008) – rather, delayed prevention efforts combined with assortative mating (the tendency to have sex with members of one's own racial/ethnic group) plus higher HIV/STI morbidity prevalence are responsible – and this is part of the context within which racial disparities in sexual health should be reported.

Unfortunately, HIV/AIDS is but one of a myriad of health conditions disproportionately impacting African Americans. As is true with HIV, these health disparities (e.g., cancer, cardiovascular diseases) are driven largely by the contextual and structural factors presented in this volume and less by individual risk behavior. Hence, the need, as previously stated, to focus efforts on contextual and structural factors for a positive solution to the disparities. Tackling these factors will require a coordinated, focused, sustained, collaborative effort from federal, state, local and community-based agencies; academicians; advocates and providers and dedicated sources of funding. Time is of the essence given the toll of health disparities, specifically HIV/AIDS, on our society. And yes, we believe that the problem lies not with affected communities alone, but rather with society as a whole. We offer that the time to begin this focus is now.

References

Adimora, A. A., & Schoenbach, J. V. (2005). Social context, sexual networks, and racial disparities in rates of sexually transmitted infections. *The Journal of Infectious Diseases, 191*, S115–S122.

Aral, S. O., Adimora, A. A., & Fenton, K. A. (2008). Understanding and responding to disparities in HIV and other sexually transmitted infections in American Americans. *Lancet, 372*, 337–340.

Clark-Tasker, V. A., Wutoh, A. K., & Mohammed, T. (2005). HIV risk behaviors in African American males. *The ABNF Journal, 16*(3), 56–59.

Coates, T. J., Richter, L., & Caceres, C. (2008). Behavioral strategies to reduce HIV transmission: How to make them work better. *Lancet, 372*, 669–684.

Espinoza, L., Hall, H. I., Hardnett, F., Selik, R. M., Ling, Q., & Lee, L. M. (2007). Characteristics of persons with heterosexually acquired HIV infection, United States, 1999–2004. *American Journal of Public Health, 97*, 144–149.

Hallfors, D. D., Miller, I. B. J., & WC, B. D. (2007). Sexual and drug behavior patterns and HIV and STD racial disparities: The need for new directions. *American Journal of Public Health, 97*(1), 125–132.

Hogben, M., & Leichliter, J. S. (2008). Social determinants and sexually transmitted disease disparities. *Sexually Transmitted Diseases, 35*(12 Suppl), S13–S18.

Lyles, C. M., Crepaz, N., Herbst, J. H., Kay, L. S., & HIV/AIDS Prevention Research Team. (2006). Evidence-based HIV behavioral prevention from the perspective of the CDC's HIV/ AIDS prevention research synthesis team. *AIDS Education and Prevention, 18*(A), 21–31.

McKleroy, V. S., Galbraith, J. S., Cummings, B., Jones, P., Harshbarger, C., Collins, C., et al. (2006). Adapting evidence-based behavioral interventions for new settings and target populations. *AIDS Education and Prevention, 18*(A), 59–73.

Merson, M., Padian, N., Coates, T. J., Gupta, G. R., Bertozzi, S. M., Piot, P., et al. (2008). Combination HIV prevention. *Lancet, 372*, 1805–1806.

Millett, G. A., Peterson, J. L., Wolitski, R. J., & Stall, R. (2006). Greater risk for HIV infection of black men who have sex with men: A critical literature review. *American Journal of Public Health, 96*(6), 1007–1019.

Padian, N. S., van der Straten, A., Ramjee, G., Chipato, T., de Btuyn, G., Blanchard, K., et al. (2008). Diaphragm and lubricant gel for prevention of HIV acquisition in southern African women: A randomized controlled trial. *Lancet, 370*, 251–261.

Purcell, D. W., & McCree, D. H. (2009). Recommendations from a research consultation to address intervention strategies for HIV/AIDS prevention focused on African Americans. *American Journal of Public Health, 99*(11), 1937–1940.

Stratford, D., Mizuno, Y., Williams, K., Courtenay-Quirk, C., & O'Leary, A. (2008). Addressing poverty as risk for disease: Recommendations from CDC's consultation on microenterprise as HIV prevention. *Public Health Reports, 123*, 9–20.

Tillerson, K. (2008). Explaining racial disparities in HIV/AIDS incidence among women in the US: A systematic review. *Statistics in Medicine, 27*(2), 4132–4143.

Warner, L., Klausner, J. D., Rietmeijer, C. A., Malotte, C. K., O'Donnell, L., Margolis, A. D., et al. (2008). Effect of a brief video intervention on incident infection among patients attending sexually transmitted disease clinics. *PLoS Medicine, 5*(6), e135.

Index

Breinigsville, PA USA
01 October 2010
246477BV00004B/7/P